Manual of Sperm Function Testing in Human Assisted Reproduction

Cambridge Laboratory Manuals in Assisted Reproductive Technology

Titles in the series:

Manual of Oocyte Retrieval and Preparation in Human Assisted Reproduction, Rachel Cutting & Mostafa Metwally

Manual of Sperm Retrieval and Preparation in Human Assisted Reproduction, Ashok Agarwal, Ahmad Majzoub & Sandro C. Esteves

Manual of Intracytoplasmic Sperm Injection in Human Assisted Reproduction: With Other Advanced Micromanipulation Techniques to Edit the Genetic and Cytoplasmic Content of the Oocyte, Gianpiero D. Palermo & Peter Nagy

Manual of Embryo Selection in Human Assisted Reproduction, Catherine Racowsky, Jacques Cohen & Nick Macklon

Manual of Embryo Culture in Human Assisted Reproduction, Kersti Lundin & Aisling Ahlström

Manual of Cryopreservation in Human Assisted Reproduction, Sally Catt, Kiri Beilby & Denny Sakkas

Manual of Sperm Function Testing in Human Assisted Reproduction

Edited by

Ashok Agarwal
The Cleveland Clinic Foundation, Cleveland, OH, USA

Ralf Henkel
University of the Western Cape, Bellville, South Africa, Imperial College London, London, UK, and
LogixX Pharma Ltd., Theale, Reading, UK

Ahmad Majzoub
Hamad Medical Corporation, Weill Cornell Medicine – Qatar, Doha, Qatar

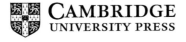

CAMBRIDGE
UNIVERSITY PRESS

University Printing House, Cambridge CB2 8BS, United Kingdom

One Liberty Plaza, 20th Floor, New York, NY 10006, USA

477 Williamstown Road, Port Melbourne, VIC 3207, Australia

314–321, 3rd Floor, Plot 3, Splendor Forum, Jasola District Centre, New Delhi – 110025, India

79 Anson Road, #06–04/06, Singapore 079906

Cambridge University Press is part of the University of Cambridge.

It furthers the University's mission by disseminating knowledge in the pursuit of
education, learning, and research at the highest international levels of excellence.

www.cambridge.org
Information on this title: www.cambridge.org/9781108793537
DOI: 10.1017/9781108878715

First published 2021

Printed in the United Kingdom by TJ Books Limited, Padstow Cornwall

A catalogue record for this publication is available from the British Library.

Library of Congress Cataloging-in-Publication Data
Names: Agarwal, Ashok, editor. | Henkel, Ralf (Ralf R.), editor. | Majzoub, Ahmad, editor.
Title: Manual of sperm function testing in human assisted reproduction / edited by Ashok Agarwal, Ralf Henkel,
    Ahmad Majzoub.
Description: Cambridge, United Kingdom ; New York, NY : Cambridge University Press, 2020. | Includes
    bibliographical references and index.
Identifiers: LCCN 2020041955 (print) | LCCN 2020041956 (ebook) | ISBN 9781108793537 (paperback) |
    ISBN 9781108878715 (epub)
Subjects: MESH: Spermatozoa–pathology | Infertility, Male–etiology | Semen Analysis–methods | Molecular
    Diagnostic Techniques–methods | Reproductive Techniques, Assisted
Classification: LCC QP255 (print) | LCC QP255 (ebook) | NLM WJ 834 | DDC 571.8/451–dc23
LC record available at https://lccn.loc.gov/2020041955
LC ebook record available at https://lccn.loc.gov/2020041956

ISBN 978-1-108-79353-7 Paperback

....

To my father Professor RC Agarwal (late) for instilling the virtues of honesty, dedication, and hard work. To my wonderful wife, Meenu, sons, Rishi and Neil-Yogi, for their unconditional love and support. To Prof. Kevin Loughlin (Harvard Medical School), Prof. Anthony Thomas (late) (Cleveland Clinic), and Prof. Edmund Sabanegh (Cleveland Clinic) for their friendship, guidance, and support and for making an indelible positive impression on my life. To my associates at work, large number of researchers and students, and most importantly the patients who placed their trust in our work.

–**Ashok Agarwal**

To my late parents Waldemar and Helga Henkel for instilling the values of hard work, perseverance, and dedication. To my academic teachers, Professor Christoph Kirchner (Philipps University, Marburg, Germany) and Professor Wolf-Bernhard Schill (Justus Liebig University, Giessen, Germany) for guiding me in my academic career and continuous support. To my wife, Adv. Sharon Henkel for her unconditional love and support, without which I would not be able to do this work.

–**Ralf Henkel**

I would like to dedicate this book to my wife, Zeinab, and our two lovely daughters, Sarah and Tala, for their love and support; to my mentors, Dr. Edmund Sabanegh and Prof. Ashok Agarwal (Cleveland Clinic), for their guidance and support and for all the opportunities they made possible.

–**Ahmad Majzoub**

Contents

Contributors

Ashok Agarwal, Ph.D.
Professor of Urology at Case Western Reserve
University; Director of Andrology Center; Director,
American Center for Reproductive Medicine,
Cleveland Clinic Foundation, Cleveland, Ohio, USA

R. John Aitken FRSE, FRSN, FAHMS, FAA
Distinguished Laureate Professor of Biological
Sciences, Priority Research Centre for Reproductive
Science, University of Newcastle, Callaghan NSW
2308, Australia

Elisabetta Baldi, Ph.D.
Associate Professor of Clinical Pathology,
Department of Clinical and Experimental Medicine,
University of Florence, Viale Pieraccini 6, 50139
Florence, Italy

Saradha Baskaran, Ph.D.
American Center for Reproductive Medicine,
Cleveland Clinic, Cleveland, OH, USA

Francesca Benini
Senior Embryologist, Centro Procreazione Assistita
Demetra (Florence, Italy)

Lars Björndahl, M.D. Ph.D.
Licensed Swedish Physician, Specialist in Clinical
Chemistry, Senior Consultant Physician, Andrology
Laboratory Director, ANOVA – Karolinska
University Hospital.

Elizabeth G. Bromfield, B Biotech (Hons), Ph.D.
Priority Research Centre for Reproductive Science,
School of Environmental and Life Sciences, The
University of Newcastle, Callaghan, NSW 2308,
Australia, and Hunter Medical Research Institute,
Pregnancy and Reproduction Program, New
Lambton Heights, NSW 2305, Australia

Shenae L. Cafe, B Biotech (Hons)
Priority Research Centre for Reproductive Science,
School of Environmental and Life Sciences,
The University of Newcastle, Callaghan, NSW 2308,
Australia, and Hunter Medical Research Institute,
Pregnancy and Reproduction Program,
New Lambton Heights, NSW 2305, Australia.

Douglas T. Carrell
Department of Surgery (Urology), University of Utah
School of Medicine, Salt Lake City, UT, USA, and
Department of Human Genetics, University of Utah
School of Medicine, Salt Lake City, UT, USA

Rima Dada, M.D., Ph.D.
Laboratory for Molecular Reproduction and Genetics,
Department of Anatomy, AIIMS, N Delhi

Christopher Douglas, BS.
American Center for Reproductive Medicine,
Cleveland Clinic, Cleveland, OH, USA, and Texas
College of Osteopathic Medicine, Fort Worth,
TX, USA

Matthew D. Dun, B Biotech (Hons), Ph.D.
Hunter Medical Research Institute, Pregnancy and
Reproduction Program, New Lambton Heights, NSW
2305, Australia; Cancer Signaling Research Group,
School of Biomedical Sciences and Pharmacy, Faculty
of Health and Medicine, University of Newcastle,
Callaghan, NSW 2308, Australia; and Priority
Research Centre for Cancer Research Innovation and
Translation, Hunter Medical Research Institute,
Lambton, NSW 2305, Australia.

Benjamin R. Emery
Department of Surgery (Urology), University
of Utah School of Medicine, Salt Lake City,
UT, USA

Donald P Evenson, Ph.D., HCLD
President and Director, SCSA Diagnostics, Inc., Brookings, SD; Emeritus Distinguished Professor, South Dakota State University, Brookings, SD; Adjunct Professor, Sanford Medical School, Dept OB/GYN, University of South Dakota, Sioux Falls, SD; former faculty, Sloan Kettering Research Institute, NY, USA

José Luís Fernández
Unidad de Genética, Instituto de Investigación Biomédica de A Coruña (INIBIC), Complexo Hospitalario Universitario de A Coruña (CHUAC), Sergas, Universidade de A Coruña (UDC), Spain, and Laboratorio de Genética, Centro Oncológico de Galicia, A Coruña, Spain.

Renata Finelli
American Centre for Reproductive Medicine, Cleveland Clinic, Cleveland, Ohio, USA

Daniel R Franken, Ph.D.
Emeritus Professor, Department of Obstetrics and Gynecology, Tygerberg Hospital, Stellenbosch University, Tygerberg, South Africa; Emeritus Professor, Department of Obstetrics and Gynecology, University of the Free State, Bloemfontein, South Africa; Former Adjunct Professor, Eastern Virginia Medical School, Norfolk, VA; and Consultant, SARhealth Line Chennai, India

Nicolas GERMAIN, M.D.
University of Lille, CNRS, Inserm, CHU Lille, UMR9020-U1277 - CANTHER - Cancer Heterogeneity Plasticity and Resistance to Therapies, F-59000 Lille, France

Jaime Gosálvez
Unidad de Genética, Facultad de Biología, Universidad Autónoma de Madrid, Madrid, Spain.

Sezgin GunesOndokuz Mayis
University Medical Faculty Department of Medical Biology, 55139 Atakum, Samsun, Turkey

Ralf Henkel
American Center for Reproductive Medicine, Cleveland Clinic, Department of Urology, Cleveland, Ohio, USA; Department of Medical Bioscience, University of the Western Cape, Bellville, South Africa; and Department of Metabolism, Digestion and Reproduction, Imperial College London, London, UK

Kathleen Hwang, M.D.
Associate Professor of Urology, Department of Urology, University of Pittsburgh Medical Center, Pittsburgh, Pennsylvania

Nathalie JOUY, Ph.D.
University of Lille, CNRS, Inserm, CHU Lille, Institut Pasteur de Lille, US 41 - UMS 2014 - PLBS, F-59000 Lille, France

De Yi Liu, Ph.D.
Chengdu Xinan Gynecology Hospital, Chengdu, China and Department of Obstetrics & Gynecology, University of Melbourne, Australia

Concetta Iovine
American Center for Reproductive Medicine, Cleveland Clinic, Cleveland, OH, USA

Geoffry N. De Iuliis, BSc (Hons), Ph.D.
Priority Research Centre for Reproductive Science, School of Environmental and Life Sciences, The University of Newcastle, Callaghan, NSW 2308, Australia, and Hunter Medical Research Institute, Pregnancy and Reproduction Program, New Lambton Heights, NSW 2305, Australia.

Jesse JP, M.D.
Laboratory for Molecular Reproduction and Genetics, Department of Anatomy, AIIMS, N Delhi

Rajasingam S. Jeyendran, B.V.Sc., M.S., Ph.D., HCLD, ALD
Androlab Inc., Chicago, IL 60611, USA

Ahmad Majzoub
Department of Urology, Hamad Medical Corporation Doha, Qatar, and Weill Cornell Medicine – Qatar, Doha, Qatar

Carole MARCHETTI, M.D., Ph.D.
Cerballiance 44 avenue Max Dormoy, F-59000 Lille, France

Philippe MARCHETTI, M.D., Ph.D.
University of Lille, CNRS, Inserm, CHU Lille, UMR9020-U1277 - CANTHER - Cancer Heterogeneity Plasticity and Resistance to Therapies, F-59000 Lille, France

Sara Marchiani, Ph.D.
Scholarship at Sodc di Medicina della Sessualità e Andrologia afferente al DAI Materno Infantile, Azienda Ospedaliero Universitaria Careggi, Florence, Italy

Liana Maree Ph.D.
Department of Medical Biosciences, University of the Western Cape, Bellville, South Africa

Roelof Menkveld, Ph.D.
Department of Obstetrics and Gynaecology, Faculty of Medicine and Health Sciences, Stellenbosch University, Tygerberg 7505, South Africa

Mohammad Hossein Nasr-Esfahani, Ph.D
Department of Animal Biotechnology, Reproductive Biomedicine Research Center, Royan Institute for Biotechnology, ACECR, Isfahan, Iran and Isfahan Fertility and Infertility Center, Isfahan, Iran

Brett Nixon, BSc (Hons), Ph.D.
Priority Research Centre for Reproductive Science, School of Environmental and Life Sciences, The University of Newcastle, Callaghan, NSW 2308, Australia, and Hunter Medical Research Institute, Pregnancy and Reproduction Program, New Lambton Heights, NSW 2305, Australia.

Kathy A. Robert
American Center for Reproductive Medicine, Cleveland Clinic, Cleveland, Ohio, USA

Alexandre Rouen, M.D., Ph.D.
Medical Genetics Department, Trousseau Hospital, Paris, France

Shubhadeep Roychoudhury, Ph.D.
Assistant Professor, Department of Life Science and Bioinformatics, Assam University, Silchar, India, and Visiting Professor, Department of Morphology, Physiology and Animal Genetics, Mendel University in Brno, Czech Republic.

Raúl Sánchez, M.D.
Center of Excellence in Translational Medicine-Scientific and Technological Bioresource Nucleus (CEMT – BIOREN), Department of Preclinical Sciences, Faculty of Medicine, University of La Frontera, Temuco, Chile.

Manesh Kumar Panner Selvam, Ph.D.
American Center for Reproductive Medicine, Cleveland Clinic, Cleveland, OH, USA

Sandra Pellegrini, M.D.
gynecologist, Centro Procreazione Assistita Demetra (Florence, Italy)

Anup A. Shah, M.D.
Department of Urology, University of Pittsburgh Medical Center, Pittsburgh, Pennsylvania

Rakesh Sharma
American Center for Reproductive Medicine, Cleveland Clinic, Cleveland, USA

Luke Simon
Department of Surgery (Urology), University of Utah School of Medicine, Salt Lake City, UT, USA

Tamburrino Lara, Ph.D.
Research Fellowship at Department of Clinical and Experimental Medicine, University of Florence, Viale Pieraccini 6, 50139 Florence, Italy

Marziyeh Tavalaee, Ph.D
Department of Animal Biotechnology, Reproductive Biomedicine Research Center, Royan Institute for Biotechnology, ACECR, Isfahan, Iran.

Pamela Uribe, Ph.D.
Center of Excellence in Translational Medicine-Scientific and Technological Bioresource Nucleus (CEMT – BIOREN), Department of Internal Medicine, Faculty of Medicine, Universidad de La Frontera, Temuco, Chile

Vidhu Dhawan, M.D.
Laboratory for Molecular Reproduction and Genetics, Department of Anatomy, AIIMS, N Delhi

Zi-Na Wen, M.Sc.
Chengdu Xinan Gynecology Hospital, Chengdu, China

Fabiola Zambrano, Ph.D.
Center of Excellence in Translational Medicine-Scientific and Technological Bioresource Nucleus (CEMT – BIOREN), Department of Preclinical Sciences, Faculty of Medicine, University of La Frontera, Temuco, Chile.

Ying Zhong, M.D.
Chengdu Xinan Gynecology Hospital, Chengdu, China

Short Biography

Dr. Ashok Agarwal is the Head of Andrology Center and Director of Research at the American Center for Reproductive Medicine. He holds these positions at The Cleveland Clinic Foundation, where he is Professor of Surgery (Urology) at the Lerner College of Medicine of Case Western Reserve University. Ashok was trained in Male Infertility and Andrology at the Brigham and Women's Hospital and Harvard Medical School and has over 28 years of experience in directing busy male infertility diagnostic and fertility preservation services. He is an editor of over 40 medical text books on male infertility, assisted reproductive technology (ART), fertility preservation, DNA damage, and antioxidants.

Ralf Henkel, B.Ed., Ph.D., Habil., studied Biology and Chemistry at the University of Marburg, Germany, and obtained his Ph.D. in 1990. Ralf continued his post-doctoral training and obtained his Habilitation at the University of Giessen, School of Medicine in 1998. From 1998 to 2004, he was an Assistant, Associate and Extraordinary Professor, at the Justus-Liebig University of Giessen, Germany, before he accepted a Full Professorship at the Department of Urology at the University of Jena, Germany. From 2005 to 2020, he was Professor and Head of Department at the Department of Medical Bioscience at the University of the Western Cape, Bellville, South Africa. Currently, he is Chief Scientific Advisor at LogixX Pharma, Reading, UK, and holds a Visiting Reader Position in the Department of Metabolism, Digestion and Reproduction at Imperial College London, London, UK. He is also Honorary Professor at the Universidad Peruana Cayetano Heredia, Lima, Peru, and Editor-in-Chief of Andrologia. Ralf has published more than 165 original and review articles as well as 46 book chapters and supervised more than 70 Hons/M.Sc./M.D./Ph.D. postgraduate students' theses. For his research, Ralf received 16 awards. Ralf has received 26 research grants for numerous research projects to investigate the impact of oxidative stress on sperm functions, DNA fragmentation and fertilization, as well as the effects of Herbal Medicine on male reproductive functions including prostate cancer and benign prostatic hyperplasia.

Dr. Ahmad Majzoub is a Consultant at the department of Urology and the program director of the andrology and male infertility fellowship at Hamad Medical Corporation, Doha, Qatar. He is an Arab Board Certified Urologist and has undergone Clinical and Research Fellowship in Andrology at the world-famous Glickman Urological and Kidney Institute and the American Center for Reproductive Medicine at Cleveland Clinic Foundation, Cleveland, United States. He is actively involved in the field of Medical Research with over 150 research publications at peer reviewed journals and several book chapters mainly focusing on Andrology and men's health. He also co-edited several books and special issues on various aspects of male infertility.

Foreword

Infertility is ranked as the fifth highest serious global disability (among populations under the age of 60) by the World Health Organization. Human Assisted Reproduction Treatments have enabled many infertile couples to discard the tag of infertility. Nowhere has the impact of Assisted Reproduction been more apparent than in the treatment of male infertility. Male infertility is known to solely affect one third of all infertile couples and in another 10–20 percent of the couples seeking medical assistance it is paired with a female factor resulting in the fact that male factor infertility is found as a reason of infertility in about half of all infertile couples.

Sadly, sperm biology has taken a back seat in Assisted Reproduction and unfortunately, the male is somewhat overlooked as a major clinical contributor to a couple's chances of achieving a live birth. Much of this arose because of the advent of intra-cytoplasmic sperm injection (ICSI) in the early 1990s. This also led to a loss of interest in developing sperm function tests. Although ICSI has proven a savior for many men, it is now becoming evident that there is more than meets the eye about sperm. It is now clear that paternal factors may be responsible for miscarriages and repeated failures after Assisted Reproduction. It is also clear that the sperm epigenome can impact present and future pregnancies and offspring. Finally, the knowledge that sperm quality declines with age has refocused our attention on the male. The tide has therefore swung and researchers are now looking to develop new classes of sperm function tests and improve older ones.

In this excellent publication, many of the stalwarts of sperm research and other up and coming researchers have provided their impactful insights into the intricacies of preparation and analysis of semen. The book, entitled a *Manual of Sperm Function Testing in Human Assisted Reproduction*, outlines the experiences of many leaders in the field. It provides chapters on semen analysis, different assay techniques and finally the clinical utility of the old and new sperm function tests. The book finishes with a look into the future of sperm diagnostics using techniques adapted from genomics, transcriptomics, proteomics and metabolomics. The editors, Professor Ashok Agarwal, Professor Ralf Henkel and Dr Ahmad Majzoub, are all highly respected members in the field and bring together their foresight into how sperm function tests should and will be used in the future.

It is my hope that this book will be a resource not only to clinicians and scientists already practicing in the field of Assisted Reproduction, but will encourage young researchers and clinicians to embrace research in the area of sperm function so that future patients can benefit from their discoveries.

Denny Sakkas Ph.D.
Chief Scientific Officer, Boston IVF
Associate Professor
Department of OBGYN
Yale University of Medicine

Preface

Infertility is a global health concern as it affects over 190 million couples at reproductive age of which half is due to a male factor. According to the literature, about 50 percent of the global incidence of male infertility is due to known causes, while the causes for the remaining percent are unknown. Since male infertility seriously affects not only the physical well-being of individual patients, but also the psychological health of couples desiring their own children, it is the responsibility of clinicians and scientists to identify the causes of male infertility and possible treatment options. This includes an assessment of the functionality of the male germ cells in order to predict the chances of a man to father a child. The primary aim of a standard semen analysis according to the WHO guidelines is to evaluate the basic semen parameters, which over the years have been found to be insufficient in predicting the male fertilizing potential. The increased knowledge about the sperm functional parameters such as capacitation, acrosome reaction, zona binding or chromatin condensation has increased our understanding of the physiology and pathology of fertilization, and possible treatment options. This has also resulted in the development of several advanced diagnostic methods and treatments for male infertility in cases of impaired sperm function.

Our book provides a detailed description of the currently known sperm function properties including their physiological and pathological background. Renowned experts from 14 countries have generously contributed 26 state-of-the-art chapters for this book. We have provided detailed information on the role of functional sperm parameters in physiology and pathology with essential up-to-date diagnostic and clinical information to improve andrological diagnosis and treatment. The most common diagnostic tests to determine sperm function are described in a clinically relevant manner.

The combination of basic and clinical information makes our book one of its kind and highly suited for fertility practitioners, andrologists, urologists, medical doctors, reproductive professionals and research students. We are grateful to our contributors, who are distinguished leaders in the field with extensive experience from around the world.

This book would not have been possible without the excellent support of Cambridge University Press. We are thankful to Nick Dunton, Senior Acquisition Editor and Camille Lee-Own, Editorial Project Manager for excellent management of this project. The editors are grateful to their families for their love and support. We genuinely hope that this volume will support and enrich your clinical practice in clinical andrology.

Cleveland, OH, USA	*Ashok Agarwal, Ph.D., HCLD (ABB), EMB (ACE)*
Bellville, South Africa and London, UK	*Ralf Henkel, BEd, Ph.D., Habil.*
Doha, Qatar	*Ahmad Majzoub, M.D.*

Introduction
Sperm Function Testing: Historical Perspectives and Future Horizons

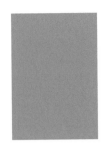

R. John Aitken

In this impressive volume, the editors have pulled together an international cast of distinguished authors, who present a detailed account of sperm function testing in terms of rationale, methodologies and clinical significance. In this introduction, my intention is to give a historical perspective on the evolution of these techniques and a view of where this field will head in the future. For what it is worth, I should also mention that these reflections are presented from the standpoint of someone who has spent the best part of half-a-century considering how we can reliably and effectively monitor the functional quality of human spermatozoa.

0.1 In the Beginning …

When a male patient comes into a clinic asking for an assessment of his fertility, the first instrument we reach for is the conventional semen profile. The assumption that underpins such traditional diagnostic assessments is that fertility is only possible if a patient possesses more than a certain critical number of motile, morphologically normal spermatozoa in his ejaculate. It is, ultimately, a descriptive approach to infertility diagnosis designed to indicate whether the various parameters of semen quality are within the normal range. The World Health Organization has played a major role in both the standardization of the laboratory techniques used to create a conventional semen profile and the thresholds of normality that can be used for calibration purposes, via the publication of its laboratory manual [1]. This manual is now in its fifth edition, available online, and is a credit to the hard work and dedication displayed by a small group of andrologists over many years, to bring this project to fruition. Its publication has helped build a significant level of consensus around the laboratory techniques that we should use to analyse human semen and has provided the field with a careful,

detailed analysis of what "normal" looks like [2]. Notwithstanding the amount of effort that has gone into refining the conventional semen analyses, there are still areas where disagreement abounds.

The first, and most fundamental, is whether the diagnosis of infertility can be approached on the basis of "thresholds of normality", no matter how carefully the latter are established. I am sure that most will agree that the binary classification of males as "fertile" or "infertile" is a gross oversimplification of the truth. In reality, fertility is a continuous variable; it cannot be depicted in terms of black and white but should acknowledge the existence of multiple shades of grey. This may mean that we have to educate patients not to expect a diagnosis of "fertile" or "infertile" but a "percentage probability of spontaneous conception as a function of time". In practice, we shall only be able to create the data bases needed to establish such prognoses if we contemplate establishing pre-conception cohort studies, which involve the collection of semen quality data and the long-term follow-up of couples to determine their reproductive fate.

Even if we did go to the expense and considerable effort of establishing such databases, what would we learn? Those limited prospective studies that have been conducted suggest that the conventional semen profile is of little diagnostic value outside of extreme oligo- or azoo- spermia [3, 4]. It is for this reason that we see a high (~30 percent) incidence of unexplained infertility in the general patient population, where the semen profile is normal and yet functional deficiencies exist [5]. Such poor prognostic value is a reflection of the obvious limitations of the semen profile since all it can provide is an assessment of "normality" relative to a spontaneously fertile population. It may generate an indication of the relative quality of the underlying spermatogenic process but the descriptive criteria at its core cannot supply accurate information on the fertilizing capacity of the ejaculate.

1

0.2 The Birth of Functional Assays

Realization that descriptive criteria were of little value in determining the fertilizing potential of human spermatozoa sparked interest in developing a more functional approach to male infertility diagnoses. One of the first aspects of sperm function to be considered during this phase in the evolution of diagnostic laboratory andrology was sperm motility. A quantum leap in the quality of sperm motility data was achieved with the development of Computer Aided Sperm Analysis (CASA) systems that permitted accurate quantification of the movement characteristics of human spermatozoa and research into which aspects of sperm movement are significant in defining the fertilizing potential of these cells.

One of the first areas to be addressed using this newly developed technology was the quality of sperm movement needed to achieve penetration of cervical mucus since failure to penetrate this barrier was, at the time, a well-established cause of infertility [6]. In these studies, the amplitude of the flagellar wave was shown to be critical for mucus penetration, as reflected in the amplitude of lateral sperm head displacement [7, 8]. Interestingly, this research revealed patients in whom inadequacies in the flagellar waveform was the only detectable defect in their ejaculate [8]. For those laboratories not possessing CASA systems, the identification of such patients was achieved using simple penetration tests based on human or bovine cervical mucus or artificial polymers possessing similar physico-chemical characteristics [9, 10].

Failure to penetrate the zona pellucida was another recognized cause of infertility related to the movement characteristics of the spermatozoa defined by CASA technology. In this case, the key attribute of sperm motility needed to effect zona penetration was their ability to establish a state of hyperactivation, characterized by large amplitude, high frequency, asymmetrical flagellar waves capable of generating significant propulsive force. Accordingly, CASA criteria were developed to enable the accurate classification of such cells [11]. Such measurements were shown to be helpful in positively identifying sperm populations capable of fertilizing human oocytes *in vitro*. However, they were much less effective in identifying cases of fertilization failure [12]. Clearly, not all aspects of sperm function are reflected in the capacity of these cells for movement.

0.3 Fertilization Bioassays

In order to address this deficiency, the field searched for an *in vitro* fertilization bioassay that could be used to address other aspects of sperm function aside from their motility including their ability to capacitate, acrosome react and achieve fusion with the oocyte. Of course, human oocytes could not be used for such diagnostic purposes for ethical reasons. However, an alternative was identified by one of the greatest gamete biologists the world has ever seen, Ryuzo Yanagimachi (Yana). Yana made the unexpected discovery that the vitelline membrane of hamster oocytes was able to fuse with human spermatozoa providing these cells had capacitated, acrosome reacted and generated a fusogenic equatorial segment, just as they must *in vivo* [13]. The ultrastructural details of sperm-oocyte fusion in this heterologous model exactly reflected the homologous situation, inviting speculation that this *in vitro* fertilization model might be used to generate diagnostic information of clinical significance. In the event, this test was found to be a very good diagnostic criterion for sperm function, accurately predicting the fertility of male patients in prospective studies, under circumstances where the conventional semen profile was shown to be of limited diagnostic value [3, 14–16]. When the results of this assay were combined with data describing sperm movement and the conventional semen profile, multivariate discriminant equations could be written that predicted the fertility of cryostored semen samples in a donor insemination program with more than 80 percent accuracy [17]. While the biochemical basis for this bioassay has recently been resolved (the hamster egg receptor, Juno, apparently binding to the human sperm ligand, Izumo1 [18]), the test is clearly not a key part of our current diagnostic armamentarium. Why is this?

The fundamental problem with the hamster oocyte penetration test is that it is a bioassay. It is complex, extremely labour intensive, involves the use of animals and is difficult, if not impossible, to standardize. The World Health Organization did everything it could to generate a standard method for performing the assay [19]. However, a survey of the relevant literature reveals a wide range of protocols used to conduct this assay and a correspondingly wide variation in the conclusions drawn as to its diagnostic validity. In truth, this assay was never intended to be a routine diagnostic test but rather a unique model that might help us understand the biochemical basis of defective sperm function. Achievement of this goal would provide a logical basis for the development of standardize-able biochemical assays with which to generate the same diagnostic information as provided by the bioassay.

Exactly the same argument could be made for bioassays looking at sperm-zona interaction. In the right hands, assessments of sperm-zona interaction using, for example, the hemi-zona assay, are highly predictive of fertility [20]. However, the logistical complexities of running and standardizing the assay has meant that it has not been widely adopted as a front-line diagnostic procedure. As our understanding of the fundamental biochemical processes underpinning sperm-zona interaction improves [21] so we can anticipate opportunities arising to replace this bioassay with biochemical tests that will generate the same information at a fraction of the cost and time required to run the bioassay.

0.4 Oxidative Stress

One of the key findings secured with the hamster egg penetration assay was that in infertile males, levels of sperm-oocyte fusion were reduced even if a calcium signal was artificially generated in the cell using the ionophore, A23187 [22]. These data suggested that a common defect in human spermatozoa is an inability to complete membrane fusion events, such as the acrosome reaction and oocyte fusion, in response to a calcium stimulus. In looking for a membrane defect that might impair the responsiveness of the sperm plasma membrane to calcium, we established the importance of reactive oxygen species (ROS) generation and lipid peroxidation [23–25] in the pathophysiology of defective sperm function. Insertion of the terms "oxidative stress" and "male infertility" into PubMed currently generates 1465 hits. Several chapters of this book are devoted to this particular topic so I shall not elaborate here. Suffice it to say that exposure to ROS emanating from infiltrating leukocytes or the spermatozoa themselves and/or exposure to an environment low in extracellular antioxidant protection leads to a state of oxidative stress in these cells. A major consequence of this stress is to initiate lipid peroxidation cascades that culminate in the generation of toxic electrophilic aldehydes such as 4-hydroxynonenal and acrolein [26]. These aldehydes bind to the vulnerable

nucleophilic centres of proteins in the immediate vicinity (cysteine, histidine and lysine residues in particular) stimulating increased levels of ROS generation by the mitochondria, the suppression of sperm motility and the impairment of sperm-egg recognition [27–29]. In addition, oxidative stress attacks the DNA in the sperm nucleus leading to oxidative DNA damage and strand breakage [30]. There are chapters in this book by internationally recognized pioneers in the field such as Don Evenson, who was among the first to understand that DNA damage to the male germ line is a determinant not just of fertility but also, potentially, the mutational load carried by the offspring [31].

0.5 The Future of Sperm Function Testing

We have moved a long way since the conventional semen profile was established as the foundation stone of male infertility assessments. It is now clear that defective sperm function can exist under conditions where the conventional semen profile is normal, due to biochemical lesions in the spermatozoa that impair both their fertilizing potential and their ability to establish a normal pregnancy. Unfortunately, research in this important area suffered a setback from the introduction of ICSI as a method of oocyte insemination. ICSI is very forgiving of defects in the functional competence and genetic integrity of spermatozoa and, as a result, the clinical demand for sperm function testing waned. Hopefully, we have now reached a point in the evolution of this field where the importance of assessing sperm quality is becoming more apparent. Such assessments may help us develop rational approaches towards the assignment of patients to IVF or ICSI, or even avoid assisted conception altogether. Furthermore, measurements of DNA damage may help us to understand potential paternal impacts on the health and wellbeing of offspring and open the door to therapies that will reduce levels of DNA damage prior to the initiation of assisted reproductive technology (ART).

It has been a long journey but the time for more extensive sperm function testing may have finally arrived. For anyone engaging with this complex field, this book will provide the reader with an authoritative snapshot of all that is current in assessing the functional qualities of these infinitely complex, fascinating cells.

References

1. World Health Organization. (2010). *WHO Laboratory Manual for the Examination and Processing of Human Semen*, 5th ed. Geneva: The WHO Press. www.who.int/reproductivehealth/publications/infertility/9789241547789/en/

2. Cooper TG, Noonan E, von Eckardstein S, Auger J, Baker HW, Behre HM, Haugen TB, Kruger T, Wang C, Mbizvo MT, Vogelsong KM. World Health Organization reference values for human semen characteristics. *Hum Reprod Update* 2010; **16**: 231–45.

3. Aitken RJ, Irvine DS, Wu FC. Prospective analysis of sperm-oocyte fusion and reactive oxygen species generation as criteria for the diagnosis of infertility. *Am J Obstet Gynecol* 1991; **164**: 542–51.

4. Aitken RJ, Best FS, Warner P, Templeton A. A prospective study of the relationship between semen quality and fertility in cases of unexplained infertility. *J Androl* 1984; **5**: 297–303.

5. Templeton A, Aitken J, Mortimer D, Best F. Sperm function in patients with unexplained infertility. *Br J Obstet Gynaecol* 1982; **89**: 550–4.

6. Kremer J, Jager S. The sperm-cervical mucus contact test: a preliminary report. *Fertil Steril* 1976; **27**: 335–40.

7. Aitken RJ, Sutton M, Warner P, Richardson DW. Relationship between the movement characteristics of human spermatozoa and their ability to penetrate cervical mucus and zona-free hamster oocytes. *J Reprod Fertil* 1985; **73**: 441–9.

8. Feneux D, Serres C, Jouannet P. Sliding spermatozoa: a dyskinesia responsible for human infertility? *Fertil Steril* 1985; **44**: 508–11.

9. Mortimer D, Mortimer ST, Shu MA, Swart R. A simplified approach to sperm-cervical mucus interaction testing using a hyaluronate migration test. *Hum Reprod* 1990; **5**: 835–41.

10. Aitken RJ, Bowie H, Buckingham D, Harkiss D, Richardson DW, West KM. Sperm penetration into a hyaluronic acid polymer as a means of monitoring functional competence. *J Androl* 1992; **13**: 44–54.

11. Sukcharoen N, Keith J, Irvine DS, Aitken RJ. Definition of the optimal criteria for identifying hyperactivated human spermatozoa at 25 Hz using in-vitro fertilization as a functional end-point. *Hum Reprod* 1995; **10**: 2928–37.

12. De Geyter C, De Geyter M, Koppers B, Nieschlag E. Diagnostic accuracy of computer-assisted sperm motion analysis. *Hum Reprod* 1998; **13**: 2512–20.

13. Yanagimachi R, Yanagimachi H, Rogers BJ. The use of zona-free animal ova as a test-system for the assessment of the fertilizing capacity of human spermatozoa. *Biol Reprod* 1976; **15**: 471–6.

14. Aitken RJ. Diagnostic value of the zona-free hamster oocyte penetration test and sperm movement characteristics in oligozoospermia. *Int J Androl* 1985; **8**: 348–56.

15. Gwatkin RB, Collins JA, Jarrell JF, Kohut J, Milner RA. The value of semen analysis and sperm function assays in predicting pregnancy among infertile couples. *Fertil Steril* 1990; **53**: 693–9.

16. Margalioth EJ, Feinmesser M, Navot D, Mordel N, Bronson RA. The long-term predictive value of the zona-free hamster ova sperm penetration assay. *Fertil Steril* 1989; **52**: 490–4.

17. Irvine DS, Aitken RJ. Predictive value of in-vitro sperm function tests in the context of an AID service. *Hum Reprod* 1986; **1**: 539–45.

18. Bianchi E, Wright GJ. Cross-species fertilization: the hamster egg receptor, Juno, binds the human sperm ligand, Izumo1. *Philos Trans R Soc Lond B Biol Sci* 2015; **370**: 20140101.

19. Aitken RJ. (ed.) The zona-free hamster oocyte penetration test and the diagnosis of male fertility. World Health Organisation Symposium. *Int J Androl* 1986; Supplement 6.

20. Oehninger S, Morshedi M, Franken D. The hemizona assay for assessment of sperm function. *Methods Mol Biol* 2013; **927**: 91–102.

21. Redgrove KA, Nixon B, Baker MA, Hetherington L, Baker G, Liu DY, Aitken RJ. The molecular chaperone HSPA2 plays a key role in regulating the expression of sperm surface receptors that mediate sperm-egg recognition. *PLoS One* 2012; **7**: e50851.

22. Aitken RJ, Buckingham DW, Fang HG. Analysis of the responses of human spermatozoa to A23187 employing a novel technique for assessing the acrosome reaction. *J Androl* 1993; **14**: 132–41.

23. Aitken RJ, Clarkson JS. Cellular basis of defective sperm function and its association with the genesis of reactive oxygen species by human spermatozoa. *J Reprod Fertil* 1987; **81**: 459–69.

24. Aitken RJ, Clarkson JS, Fishel S. Generation of reactive oxygen species, lipid peroxidation, and human sperm function. *Biol Reprod* 1989; **41**: 183–97.

25. Aitken RJ, Clarkson JS, Hargreave TB, Irvine DS, Wu FC. Analysis of the relationship between defective sperm function and the generation of reactive oxygen species in cases of oligozoospermia. *J Androl* 1989; **10**: 214–20.

26. Moazamian R, Polhemus A, Connaughton H, Fraser B, Whiting S, Gharagozloo P, Aitken RJ. Oxidative stress and human spermatozoa: diagnostic and functional significance of aldehydes generated as a result of lipid peroxidation. *Mol Hum Reprod* 2015; **21**: 502–15.

27. Aitken RJ, Whiting S, De Iuliis GN, McClymont S, Mitchell LA, Baker MA. Electrophilic aldehydes generated by sperm metabolism activate mitochondrial reactive oxygen species generation and apoptosis by targeting succinate

dehydrogenase. *J Biol Chem* 2012; **287**: 33048–60.

28. Baker MA, Weinberg A, Hetherington L, Villaverde AI, Velkov T, Baell J, Gordon CP. Defining the mechanisms by which the reactive oxygen species by-product, 4-hydroxynonenal, affects human sperm cell function. *Biol Reprod* 2015; **92**: 108.

29. Bromfield EG, Aitken RJ, Anderson AL, McLaughlin EA, Nixon B. The impact of oxidative stress on chaperone-mediated human sperm-egg interaction. *Hum Reprod* 2015; **30**: 2597–613.

30. Drevet JR, Aitken RJ. Oxidation of sperm nucleus in mammals: a physiological necessity to some extent with adverse impacts on oocyte and offspring. *Antioxidants* 2020; **9**(2): 95–109.

31. Wyrobek AJ, Eskenazi B, Young S, Arnheim N, Tiemann-Boege I, Jabs EW, Glaser RL, Pearson FS, Evenson D. Advancing age has differential effects on DNA damage, chromatin integrity, gene mutations, and aneuploidies in sperm. *Proc Natl Acad Sci U S A* 2006; **103**: 9601–6.

Standard Semen Examination: Manual Semen Analysis

Lars Björndahl

1.1 Introduction

The aim of this chapter is not to provide all practical details necessary for proper semen examination. There already exist other sources for that type of information [1, 2]. The purpose of this chapter is therefore to focus on biological and physiological aspects that are relevant to the examination of human ejaculates. It is aimed to give the clinician a proper background to set requirements for a qualitative laboratory service needed to diagnose and treat men with disorders in the male reproductive organs contributing to couple infertility.

The investigation of the human ejaculate includes observations (e.g. color, odor, viscosity and liquefaction) as well as measurements and assessments (volume, concentration, motility, vitality and morphology). It is therefore adequate to refer to semen examination that is considered to be a concept that is wider than analysis, also including observations and not only measurements.

The examination of the ejaculate is an essential cornerstone in the evaluation of the reproductive functions of the human male. The ejaculate is different from all other body fluids possible to analyze in a modern medical laboratory, and many delusions still exist concerning what the ejaculate is and what it can tell about the man and his fertility. Since the rise of Assisted Reproductive Technologies (ART) with the introduction and the development of *In Vitro* Fertilization (IVF) and Intra Cytoplasmic Sperm Injection (ICSI), the main focus in studies of ejaculate examination has been on its usefulness to predict the probability for spontaneous and assisted conceptions, pregnancies and live births of children. However, since many factors affecting a couple's fertility are independent from semen examination results, most isolated male or female factors cannot be expected to solely be a major determinant of a couple's probability for a successful pregnancy. Still, if simplistic

testing of isolated ejaculate parameters is abandoned in favor of multifactorial ejaculate evaluations, useful predictive information regarding spontaneous and assisted pregnancies can be achieved [3, 4]. Thus, although not completely without interest, this predominant focus on ejaculate examination as a pregnancy predictor has drawn the attention from the information that can be gained about the functions of the male reproductive organs. In the light of a possible decrease in general human male reproductive function [5] it is essential that ejaculate examination for the evaluation of the function of the male reproductive organs is in focus.

Another aspect that is essential to the understanding of semen examination is that the "semen sample" only exists in the laboratory. Semen does not even exist in the body: the ejaculate is formed instantly during the process of ejaculation: spermatozoa are transported from the cauda epididymides to the urethra where they are suspended in prostatic fluid concomitantly emptied from the small prostatic gland acini and expelled in the first ejaculate fractions. The seminal vesicles empty into the urethra after the bulk of spermatozoa has been ejaculated [6]. In general, the seminal vesicular fluid appears to be hostile to sperm function (motility), survival and DNA protection [7]. There is no evidence that the seminal vesicular fluid is in any way beneficial for sperm function *in vivo* and there is no evidence that exposure of spermatozoa to seminal vesicular fluid ever occurs *in vivo* [6, 8]. In contrast, examination of ejaculates *in vitro* is based on collection of all parts of the ejaculate in one device, where the entire ejaculate is included in the gel-like substance originating from the seminal vesicles. This structure is then subsequently decomposed by enzymes of prostatic origin. The effect of this process – called liquefaction – is not only that the ejaculate becomes more watery in appearance, but the process also means that the osmolality of ejaculates increase *in vitro* [9, 10].

1.2 Pre-Examination Aspects

The composition and quantity of each ejaculate depends on several factors, among them the rate of sperm production but not limited to that. The procurement of an ejaculate for examination is highly dependent on the man himself. Frequency of ejaculation – and not only time of sexual abstinence before collection of the examination sample – will have influence on characteristics like sperm number, motility and morphology. Also the duration and quality of sexual arousal during sample collection is important [11]. In addition, truthful information on the completeness of sample collection is required for correct interpretation of ejaculate examination results.

Due to the continuous changes (osmolality, pH) occurring in the ejaculate *in vitro* leading to deterioration of sperm motility and changes in morphological appearance, standardized temperature and time to initiation of assessments is required.

1.3 Examination Aspects

1.3.1 Ejaculate Volume

The ejaculate volume is important to achieve reliable data on total sperm number as well as measures of secretory contributions from the epididymides, prostate and seminal vesicles.

There is a highly variable and significant volume loss when using pipettes for measuring ejaculate volume or transferring to reliable measuring devices [12]. Practically, a reliable and more correct volume is best obtained by weighing the collection device before and after sample collection. The specific weight (density) of human semen has been assessed to be 1.03–1.04 g/mL [13], indicating that the error in volume, based on ejaculate weight, would be less than 4 percent even when assuming a specific weight of 1.0 g/mL. A 4 percent error is much less than can be expected from measurements where the ejaculate must be removed from the collection device and an unknown volume is left in the collection device.

1.3.2 Sperm Concentration

The accuracy of sperm concentration assessment depends on several factors. The most basic is that the examined aliquots are representative of the entire ejaculate. Macroscopically well mixed ejaculates quite often still show considerable variation between different fields of vision in the microscope (10 μL aliquot). Based on this typical finding the recommendation is that aliquots of at least 50 μL should be used to reduce the risk for poor representation of the entire ejaculate. Furthermore, comparison of two separate aliquots should be examined and compared, to further reduce the risk for poor representation and other errors that may occur in the process of establishing the correct number of spermatozoa.

Another essential aspect is the use of dilutions. One important reason is that it is much easier to assess non-moving objects than live motile spermatozoa. Another equally important reason is that with adequate dilutions counting is easier when spermatozoa are evenly spread within and between the microscopic fields; densely packed spermatozoa or too diluted makes counting more difficult, time consuming, exhausting and less reliable.

A third important aspect is to reduce the influence of random factors that cause a spermatozoon to occur or not occur in the area of observation. If only a few spermatozoa are observed, the influence of random factors can influence the final result considerably. Therefore, the number of observations is crucial. As can be seen in Figure 1.1, the uncertainty of a cell counting result varies with the number of observations. The recommendation of assessing at least 400 spermatozoa is based on the fact that statistically a total of 400 observations reduces the random variability to ±10 percent of the observed value [2].

Further sources of possible causes of significant errors and variability lie in the accuracy of the volume assessed in the counting chamber. While the area examined can be very precisely determined, the depth can vary. A shallow chamber (10 μm) would cause a 10 percent volume error if the cover is only 1 μm wrong. However, in a 100-μm deep hemocytometer, the same absolute error would only cause a 1 percent error in the volume.

1.3.3 Sperm Motility

The only practical way of assessing sperm motility "manually" in the microscope means using wet preparations with a depth of approximately 10–20 μm, meaning that a 10 μL aliquot under a 22 mm × 22 mm cover slip is appropriate. It is necessary also for the representativity of the aliquots to examine at least two aliquots and compare results to minimize random error.

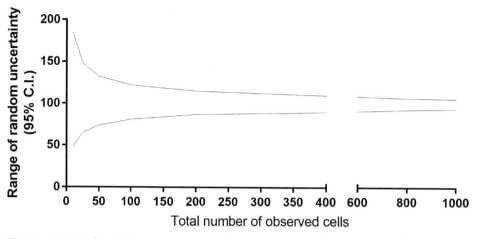

Figure 1.1 Range of uncertainty of sperm concentration results based on different numbers of observations (100 represents calculated value; lines show range of 95 percent Confidence Interval for the different numbers of observations).

Sperm velocity is very dependent on the temperature. While "room temperature" is not well defined and can vary significantly in most laboratories, the recommendation is to standardize microscope stage temperature to 37°C and preferably to use pre-warmed slides.

The same statistical consideration as for sperm concentration assessment is relevant for the motility assessment. Thus, at least 400 spermatozoa should be included in the assessment of each sample to reduce the random error to ±10 percent of the observed value.

1.3.4 Sperm Vitality

Vitality assessment is only important when many spermatozoa are immotile. The investigation is essential to identify samples with many live but immotile spermatozoa to distinguish from disorders where reduced sperm motility is due to poor sperm survival.

Since the assessment of sperm vitality by eosin-nigrosine staining [14, 15] does not appear to be sensitive to aliquot representativity (compared to sperm concentration and sperm motility assessment), replicate assessment and comparison is not considered necessary for the purpose of distinguishing between samples with immotile dead spermatozoa and samples with immotile live spermatozoa [16]. It is more important to use adequate equipment (bright field, high magnification (x1000), high resolution microscopy) and count at least 200 spermatozoa in each ejaculate.

1.3.5 Sperm Morphology

The assessment of human sperm morphology may be the most controversial part of basic semen examination. The usefulness of the examination has mainly been assessed in relation to ART. There are, however, many reasons why this is a too simplistic argumentation. One important point is that investigations of spermatozoa that have been able to reach the site of fertilization are much more uniform in appearance than spermatozoa in the ejaculate [17, 18]. The definition of sperm morphology based on observations of spermatozoa passing through cervical mucus and binding to the zona pellucida (Tygerberg Strict Criteria) is the basis for the current World Health Organization recommendations [1]. One argument raised against the use of the Tygerberg Strict Criteria is that very few spermatozoa in the ejaculate have a morphology that fulfil the criteria. However, the number of spermatozoa that can reach the site of fertilization is very low, in the magnitude of 100–1000 spermatozoa from a normal ejaculate [19]. From a statistical point of view, sufficient numbers of spermatozoa with "normal" morphology are very likely to exist, although not possible to detect when 200 or 400 spermatozoa from the ejaculate are randomly chosen and assessed. The distribution of morphological abnormalities still gives information about the function of the spermatogenesis. Therefore, a very important use of sperm morphology is to understand the function of the testicles, rather than only predict the outcome of spontaneous or assisted fertilization. Together with data on sperm number and motility, morphology data provides information on qualitative and quantitative aspects of testicular function.

The general assessment of the morphology of each spermatozoon should include at least four aspects: head, neck/midpiece, tail and presence of cytoplasmic residues. Only recording head abnormalities excludes essential information. Presence of more than one type of abnormality appears to indicate more severe problems, often testicular problems [18, 20]. A specific assessment that is useful when evaluating fertilization failure is the acrosome index, measuring the presence of normal acrosomes [21].

To obtain useful data, the choice of staining is essential. Without staining, phase contrast is necessary to see spermatozoa, but the level of details possible to discern will be too low. Among the different staining procedures available, the sperm adapted Papanicolaou stain is considered the best overall staining of all parts of the spermatozoon [1]. Replicate assessments with comparisons appear to be less critical than correct equipment, as well as proper training to obtain reliable and consistent results [16].

1.4 Post-Examination Aspects

For the proper interpretation of data, it is essential that the laboratory not only presents the basic examination result. Critical information like time between ejaculate collection and initiation of assessments should always be included, as well as the abstinence time (days). Any aberrant macroscopic property (color, liquefaction, odor, viscosity) should also be reported. The total number of spermatozoa is more important than concentration, since the latter is largely dependent on the rate of secretion from the seminal vesicles and the prostate. For motility not only the proportion of motile spermatozoa is of interest, rather the proportion of progressively motile spermatozoa is important. In contrast to the 2010 edition of the World Health Organization recommendations [1], the proportion of rapidly progressive spermatozoa provides essential information: lack of rapid progressive spermatozoa is the strongest negative predictor of common IVF success [16, 22].

1.5 Conclusions

Examination of the human ejaculate is basic to the evaluation of the man in an infertile couple. Results primarily provide information about the functions of the male reproductive organs and can thereby give clues to essential investigations and treatments of the man. Ejaculate examination can also contribute to the choice of proper modalities for assisted fertilization for the couple.

As the case with all laboratory investigations, basic semen examination must be performed with insights of possible causes for errors and how systematic and random errors can be minimized. With proper training, and internal and external quality control, reliable results can be obtained, but also patients must be involved to provide essential information on abstinence time and sample collection.

References

1. World Health Organization. (2010) *WHO Laboratory Manual for the Examination and Processing of Human Semen*, 5th ed. Cooper TG, Aitken J, Auger J, Baker HWG, Barratt CLR, Behre HM, et al., eds. Geneva: The WHO Press, p. 286.

2. Björndahl L, Mortimer D, Barratt CLR, Castilla JA, Menkveld R, Kvist U, et al. (2010) *A Practical Guide to Basic Laboratory Andrology*. Cambridge and New York: Cambridge University Press, pp. xii, 336.

3. Jedrzejczak P, Taszarek-Hauke G, Hauke J, Pawelczyk L, Duleba AJ. Prediction of spontaneous conception based on semen parameters. *Int J Androl* 2008; **31**(5): 499–507.

4. Guzick DS, Overstreet JW, Factor-Litvak P, Brazil CK, Nakajima ST, Coutifaris C, et al. Sperm morphology, motility, and concentration in fertile and infertile men. *N Engl J Med* 2001; **345**(19): 1388–93.

5. Levine H, Mohri H, Ekbom A, Ramos L, Parker G, Roldan E, et al. Male reproductive health statement. XIIIth International Symposium on Spermatology, May 9–12, 2018, Stockholm, Sweden. *Basic Clin Androl* 2018; **28**: 13.

6. Björndahl L, Kvist U. Sequence of ejaculation affects the spermatozoon as a carrier and its message. *Reprod Biomed Online* 2003; **7**(4): 440–8.

7. Björndahl L, Kvist U. Human sperm chromatin stabilization: a proposed model including zinc bridges. *MHR* 2010; **16**(1): 23–9.

8. MacLeod J, Gold RZ. The male factor in fertility and infertility. III. An analysis of motile activity in the spermatozoa of 1000 fertile

men and 1000 men in infertile marriage. *Fertil Steril* 1951; **2**(3): 187–204.

9. Holmes E, Björndahl L, Kvist U. Post-ejaculatory increase in human semen osmolality in vitro. *Andrologia* 2019: e13311.

10. Holmes E, Bjorndahl L, Kvist U. Possible factors influencing post-ejaculatory changes of the osmolality of human semen in vitro. *Andrologia* 2019: e13443.

11. Pound N, Javed MH, Ruberto C, Shaikh MA, Del Valle AP. Duration of sexual arousal predicts semen parameters for masturbatory ejaculates. *Physiol Behav* 2002; **76**(4–5): 685–9.

12. Cooper TG, Brazil C, Swan SH, Overstreet JW. Ejaculate volume is seriously underestimated when semen is pipetted or decanted into cylinders from the collection vessel. *J Androl* 2007; **28**(1): 1–4.

13. Woodward B, Gossen N, Meadows J, Tomlinson M. Uncertainty associated with assessing semen volume: are volumetric and gravimetric methods that different? *Hum Fertil* 2016; **19**(4): 249–53.

14. Björndahl L, Soderlund I, Johansson S, Mohammadieh M, Pourian MR, Kvist U. Why the WHO recommendations for eosin-nigrosin staining techniques for human sperm vitality assessment must change. *J Androl* 2004; **25**(5): 671–8.

15. Björndahl L, Soderlund I, Kvist U. Evaluation of the one-step eosin-nigrosin staining technique for human sperm vitality assessment. *Hum Reprod* 2003; **18**(4): 813–16.

16. Barratt CL, Björndahl L, Menkveld R, Mortimer D. ESHRE special interest group for andrology basic semen analysis course: a continued focus on accuracy, quality, efficiency and clinical relevance. *Hum Reprod* 2011; **26**(12): 3207–12.

17. Menkveld R, Stander FS, Kotze TJ, Kruger TF, van Zyl JA. The evaluation of morphological characteristics of human spermatozoa according to stricter criteria. *Hum Reprod* 1990; **5**(5): 586–92.

18. Mortimer D, Menkveld R. Sperm morphology assessment: historical perspectives and current opinions. *J Androl* 2001; **22**(2): 192–205.

19. Ahlgren M. Sperm transport to and survival in the human fallopian tube. *Gynecol Invest* 1975; **6**(3–4): 206–14.

20. Jouannet P, Ducot B, Feneux D, Spira A. Male factors and the likelihood of pregnancy in infertile couples. I. Study of sperm characteristics. *Int J Androl* 1988; **11**(5): 379–94.

21. Menkveld R, Rhemrev JP, Franken DR, Vermeiden JP, Kruger TF. Acrosomal morphology as a novel criterion for male fertility diagnosis: relation with acrosin activity, morphology (strict criteria), and fertilization in vitro. *Fertil Steril* 1996; **65**(3): 637–44.

22. Björndahl L. The usefulness and significance of assessing rapidly progressive spermatozoa. *Asian J Androl* 2010; **12**(1): 33–5.

Standard Semen Analysis: Computer-Assisted Semen Analysis

Liana Maree

2.1 Introduction

Computer-assisted semen analysis (CASA) is an automated and objective method to evaluate several sperm parameters, either in conjunction with or instead of routine manual semen analysis. CASA systems have undergone a complete metamorphosis since the initial systems were developed to track sperm motion four decades ago [see 1, 2 for detailed history]. Various innovations in bioengineering, software algorithms and computational power have led to more than 14 CASA systems (Figure 2.1) currently available across the globe for commercial use in evaluating both human and animal spermatozoa [3, 4, 5]. Although CASA was initially introduced as a research tool and not commonly used for semen analysis in the clinical setting [1], more and more fertility clinics are investing in and switching to automated systems.

The major difference between CASA and manual semen analysis is inherent in the subjectivity of evaluations. In routine manual analysis, both inter-

individual and -laboratory variation have been reported, mainly due to subjective scoring of sperm characteristics by laboratory staff and lack of quality assurance (e.g. methodology standardization and adherence to international guidelines) [2, 6]. Modern CASA systems have been designed to objectively and quantitatively measure several aspects of sperm structure and function, aiming to provide high levels of intra- and inter-laboratory consistency [7]. However, CASA systems are not ready-to-use devices and its usefulness in semen analysis rely on numerous factors discussed below [4, 8]. Despite these differences, it is important to note that both manual and automated semen analysis for humans are based on the same "gold standard", namely the World Health Organization's (WHO) laboratory manual [9, 10], as guideline for semen assessment. Several studies have compared values scored or generated for sperm concentration, motility and morphology between manual and CASA analysis, with contradictory results being

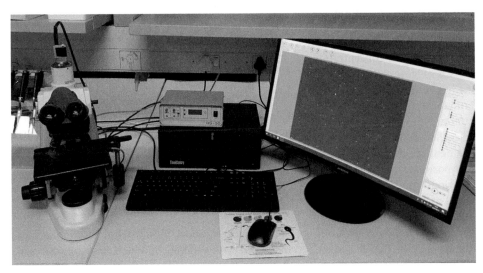

Figure 2.1 Example of a typical modern CASA system.

reported [8, 11–14]. Vendors should provide proof that their CASA systems have been validated [2] and internal quality control should be performed by each laboratory [15].

Any semen analysis typically includes evaluation of sperm concentration, motility and morphology and these three parameters will thus be addressed in this chapter. Since sperm morphology is the focus of Chapter 5, CASA of this parameter is only briefly touched on in the sections below. One of the limitations of a standard semen analysis is that it can only determine basic semen quality and cannot predict or be used to diagnose unexplained (idiopathic) infertility as is the case in around 30 percent of males affected by infertility [6]. The CASA measurement of these sperm parameters includes a much more detailed assessment of individual spermatozoon's attributes and thus results in more comprehensive biological information that might be directly correlated to sperm quality and fertility potential. In addition, high-end CASA systems now include modules that allow for less routinely evaluated parameters such as vitality (membrane integrity), DNA fragmentation and acrosome integrity, which could elucidate possible reasons for sperm dysfunction [4, 6].

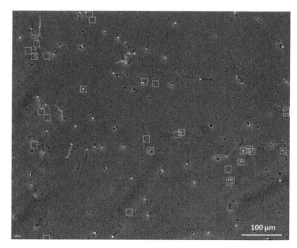

Figure 2.2 Sperm motility analysis at 50 frames per second illustrating correct identification and tracking of individual spermatozoa. Red tracks = rapid-progressive swimming sperm, green tracks = rapid-swimming sperm, blue tracks = medium-progressive swimming sperm, yellow circles = static sperm, turquoise blocks = hyperactivated sperm. The detailed kinematics measured for each spermatozoon are indicated in Figure 2.3.

2.2 Principle of Computer-Assisted Semen Analysis

2.2.1 Sperm Concentration and Motility

Most CASA systems use phase contrast optics to establish a centroid for each spermatozoon by registering the location of its head in two dimensions (x- and y-coordinates). Once the sperm heads have successfully been detected, both sperm concentration and motility can be assessed (Figure 2.2). Although sperm motility is essentially a result of flagellar bending that propels the spermatozoon forward, using the sperm head to measure motility is currently accepted as a representation of flagellar motion [16]. Sperm head trajectory and movement are therefore assessed by tracking the sequential position of the head using serial digital imaging. Various sperm motility percentages (Table 2.1) as well as kinematic parameters (Figure 2.3A) are subsequently calculated. It should be noted that alternative technologies used for motility analysis are employed by certain CASA systems [2]. The possibility of including high-throughput real-time flagellar capture and three-dimensional sperm

motion tracking into CASA motility analysis in future would open up new avenues for clinical semen analysis [17].

2.2.2 Sperm Morphology

Both wet preparations and dry preparations of stained spermatozoa can be accommodated by CASA systems to assess sperm morphology. Automated sperm morphology analysis (ASMA) generally uses algorithms to detect similar sperm component abnormalities as recommended by the WHO [10] for manual analysis [18]. Whereas the latter method depends on a trained set of human eyes to decide whether a sperm component is normal or abnormal, CASA employs several quantitative sperm morphometry parameters (Table 2.1) in order to qualify sperm morphology (Figure 2.3B) [3]. In addition, certain CASA systems automatically determine indices of multiple sperm defects, such as the multiple anomalies index (MAI), the teratozoospermia index (TZI) and the sperm deformity index (SDI) [10].

2.3 Equipment and Methods

Sperm concentration, motility and morphology are measured with different modules in the CASA software. A digital or video camera is mounted on a microscope, fitted with a temperature-controlled

Table 2.1 Typical Sperm Motility and Morphology Parameters Assessed by Computer-Assisted Semen Analysis

Motility	Morphology
Percentages	**Morphology**
Total motility	Normal (%)
Progressive motility	Abnormal (%)
Fast progressive [Type A*]	Head defects (%)
Slow progressive [Type B*]	Midpiece defects (%)
Non-progressive [Type C*]	Tail defects (%)
Immotile [Type D*]	Cytoplasmic droplets (%)
Rapid#	Acrosome coverage (%)
Medium#	Tetrazoospermia index
Slow#	Defortmity index
Sperm mucous penetration	Multiple anomalies index
Hyperactivation	
Kinematics	**Morphometry**
VCL (µm/s)	Head length (µm)
VAP (µm/s)	Head width (µm)
VSL (µm/s)	Head area (µm^2)
LIN (%)	Head perimeter (µm)
STR (%)	Head elipticity
WOB (%)	Head elongation
ALH (µm)	Head roughness
BCF (Hz)	Head regularity
	Midpiece width (µm)
	Midpiece area (µm^2)
	Midpiece insertion angle

* According to 4th ed. of WHO manual [10]
# Sperm swimming speed classes defined according to CASA sort function [3]
VCL = curvilinear velocity, VAP = average path velocity, VSL = straight-line velocity, LIN = linearity, STR = straightness, WOB = wobble, ALH = amplitude of lateral head displacement, BCF = beat cross frequency.

stage and phase contrast as well as bright field objectives (Figure 2.1). Semen or a sperm preparation is loaded into disposable, chambered slides (concentration and motility) or stained sperm smears are mounted (morphology) prior to analysis. Specific analysis properties are pre-set as recommended for standardized human sperm analysis [3].

2.4 Reference Values and How to Calculate Cut-Off Values

Central to accurate automated semen/sperm analysis is the employment of standardized protocols and analysis properties. Any deviations from recommended guidelines [10, 15] will result in unreliable data generated (see Section 2.6 below). In turn, incorrect data will be compared to reference values for sperm parameters (Table 2.2) and might influence the clinical interpretation of the analysis results (see Section 2.7 below). Apart from employing the WHO manual's reference values for sperm concentration, total number of sperm in the ejaculate, percentage total and progressive motility as well as normal sperm morphology [10], several other sperm parameter reference values can be incorporated in CASA systems (Table 2.2).

Cut-off values for specific sperm kinematic parameters are used to assess features of sperm motility which are virtually impossible with manual analysis. For instance, evaluation of sperm subpopulations portraying rapid-, medium- and slow-swimming speed, mucous penetration and hyperactivation characteristics are already incorporated in some systems or can be manually added by the technician using cut-offs incorporated into a "sort" function [6, Figure 2.2]. CASA sperm morphology assessments are traditionally based on minimum and maximum cut-off values for sperm head, midpiece and tail morphometry parameters as well as percentage acrosome coverage [3]. In certain CASA systems additional sperm motility or morphology features of interest can be assessed (e.g. subfertile population) by establishing cut-off values by using visual pattern recognition and receiver operating characteristic (ROC) curve analysis [1, 19] or 90–95 percent confidence intervals [3, 19].

2.5 Advantages and Disadvantages of Computer-Assisted Semen Analysis

2.5.1 Advantages of Computer-Assisted Semen Analysis Systems

Since the development of the earliest CASA systems it was reported that automated analysis is (or has the potential to be) more accurate, consistent (precise) and repeatable than manual and subjective semen analysis [4, 8]. Due to the use of algorithms to measure

13

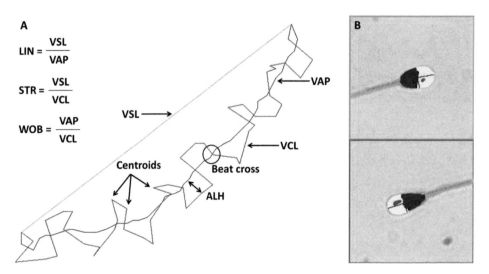

Figure 2.3 Motility and morphology analysis of individual spermatozoa. A) Centroid-based tracking of the sperm head results in eight kinematic parameters directly measured or calculated as a fraction. VCL = curvilinear velocity, VAP = average path velocity, VSL = straight-line velocity, LIN = linearity, STR = straightness, WOB = wobble, ALH = amplitude of lateral head displacement, BCF = beat cross frequency. B) Sperm morphology is assessed by incorporating various sperm morphometry parameters. Top sperm = normal morphology, bottom = abnormal morphology, yellow = acrosome, blue = head, red = vacuole, green = midpiece.

sperm parameters with CASA, there is reduced potential for human error and less analytical variance, although operator subjectivity is not completely eliminated [14]. CASA also provides a lower turnaround time per individual analysis and provides rapid results [8, 14] that can immediately be made available in a report to the doctor or patient (Figure 2.4). This also implies that when the same sample (e.g. morphology slide) is used for CASA analysis on similar systems in different laboratories, there should be no significant differences in the generated results [20]. These advantages of CASA can, however, only be achieved by employing well-trained technicians and optimized CASA settings (see disadvantages below) [8].

Modern CASA systems are much more user-friendly and allow for input and adjustments to be made by the technician. Not only can one change the configuration settings for different hardware (e.g. microscope and camera) and consumables (e.g. slides and staining method) available, in many systems, the initial analysis can be viewed again for verification of accuracy. For example, for motility analysis the "playback" option of the software can be used to identify and remove incorrect sperm tracks or add uncaptured spermatozoa. It is of particular importance that the analysis of curvilinear velocity (VCL) and average path velocity (VAP) are correctly assessed, since these

two parameters are used to calculate most other kinematic parameters.

A further indisputable advantage of CASA is the vast amount of data that is generated which can both be used for conventional clinical interpretations and be incorporated into multivariate statistical analyses to predict fertility potential. Apart from the array of motility and morphology/morphometry parameters CASA generates (Table 2.1), the detailed analysis of individually measured spermatozoa can also be accessed (Figure 2.3) and extracted for further analysis [4]. By evaluating additional and more detailed sperm parameters, CASA allows for the detection of subtle changes in sperm motion and morphometry that cannot be identified by conventional, manual sperm motility analysis.

The most recent advancement in human CASA is the fully automated systems where minimum input and no interaction during the analysis are required by the technician. Two examples of such systems are the LensHooke Semen Quality Analyzer (Bonraybio Co., Ltd, Taichung City, Taiwan) and the SCA SCOPE (Microptic S.L., Barcelona, Spain). The LensHooke system only requires loading of the sample in a disposable counting chamber to measure pH, sperm concentration, morphology and motility (percentage total, progressive and non-progressive motility). The

Concentration					
8.14 M/mL		20.35 M/Sample		Volume (mL): 2.50	
(≥46M/mL)		(≥16%)		Dilution 1:0	

WHO 5		Total	%	M/mL	M/Sample
Progressive (PR)	(≥34%)	261	60.70	4.94	12.35
Non-progressive (NP)		54	12.58	1.02	2.58
Immotile (IM)		115	26.74	2.18	5.44

		Total	%	M/mL	M/Sample
Motile	(≥42%)	315	73.26	5.98	14.91

Velocity	Total	%	M/mL	M/Sample
Rapid	237	55.12	4.49	11.22
Medium	49	11.40	0.93	2.32
Slow	29	6.74	0.55	1.37
Immotile (IM)	115	26.74	2.18	5.44

WHO 4	Total	%	M/mL	M/Sample
Rapid progressive (type A)	146	33.95	2.76	6.91
Medium progressive (type B)	115	26.74	2.18	5.44
Non progressive (type C)	54	12.56	1.02	2.56
Immotile (type D)	115	26.74	2.18	5.44

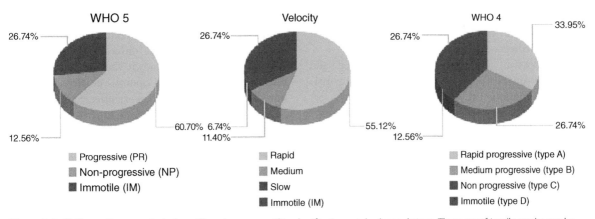

Figure 2.4 CASA motility report including different sperm motility classifications and subpopulations. These user-friendly results can be presented in various formats and can be extracted for alternative use. Semen parameters with measured values less the lower reference limits recommended by WHO [10] are highlighted in red in the report (sperm concentration in this example).

SCA SCOPE provides a more comprehensive device that includes all analysis modules available for the Sperm Class Analyzer (SCA) CASA system (motility and concentration, morphology, vitality, DNA fragmentation and leukocytes) and assesses more than 100 parameters. The development and use of such automated systems will possibly eliminate variations in CASA results inflicted by the user.

2.5.2 Disadvantages

2.5.2.1 Biological Factors Affecting Computer-Assisted Semen Analysis

A historic drawback in the use of CASA in the clinical setting, compared to the veterinary and wildlife fields, is that the inherent nature of human semen samples can limit CASA's ability to accurately assess sperm concentration and motility. Freshly ejaculated human semen can vary greatly in terms of its viscosity, presence of non-sperm cells and debris, sperm heterogeneity (e.g. pleomorphic heads), sperm aggregations and sperm count [1, 18]. These semen attributes as well as sperm motility will be modified if the sample is diluted (dependent on media used), washed or frozen-thawed and will require standardized CASA settings for each of these conditions [3, 4].

Several improvements in modern CASA systems produce more robust detection of spermatozoa and thus more accurate measurements by checking for the presence of the sperm tail [17] or using intelligent filters (advanced black and white mode) to eliminate particles in the seminal plasma being detected as spermatozoa [1]. If non-sperm cells or debris are included in the automated analysis, there will be an overestimation of sperm count/concentration and an underestimation of percentage total sperm motility.

2.5.2.2 Equipment, Software and User Factors Affecting Computer-Assisted Semen Analysis

An in-depth discussion of non-biological factors that may influence CASA measurements of sperm concentration, motility and morphology is beyond the scope of this publication and have been reviewed elsewhere [2, 4, 16]. Below is a brief introduction to some of these factors and settings that should be standardized to avoid incorrect set-ups and analysis.

In terms of equipment, the microscope and camera set-up as well as the slides used may contribute to variations in CASA results. CASA users should standardize the settings for the microscope stage (e.g. temperature control and automation), illumination (e.g. Köhler and power of light source) and objective selected (e.g. magnification and phase contrast vs. bright field). It is highly recommended that the digital or video camera and software used should have accreditation (e.g. ISO 9001 and EN 62304) as medical devices to assure quality and accuracy of the generated output.

Various reusable, drop-displacement counting chambers (e.g. Makler and Neubauer) and disposable, capillary-loaded counting chambers (e.g. Leja and CellVision) are commercially available for sperm concentration and motility analysis. Each of these chambers or slides has its own disadvantages in terms of distribution of sperm in the chamber, subjectivity to Segre-Silberberg effect and specimen "drifting" [2, 16]. Since spermatozoa swim in a helical pattern and need

enough space to develop this type of motility, particular attention should be paid to chamber depth. Most studies are in agreement that a chamber depth of 20 μm is adequate for human sperm motility analysis in different physiological and capacitation media [15, 16]. For this reason, it is also important to use a high-quality, certified chamber and to correctly set the chamber depth in the software [2].

As is the case with all software systems, incorrect input will result in incorrect output. All fertility clinics or reproductive specialists should eliminate or reduce incorrect results by adopting standardized protocols and software set-ups. Since configuration settings for accurate analysis of semen parameters are different for each CASA system, settings cannot be specified, but will include options for calibration, frame rate, number of images to capture, type of slide used, chamber depth, range of sperm head area, subpopulation settings, connectivity, stain used (for morphology) and criteria for analysis (e.g. WHO, Strict Criteria, David's Classification for morphology). Examples for the influence of different settings of frame rate and staining method on results generated are given below.

Centroid-based CASA motility analysis is tracking the sperm head for the specified number of frames per second (fps) (e.g. 50 fps for a digital camera and 60 fps for a video camera). While changes in frame rate will not influence the different sperm motility percentages, it is well-known that increased frame rates result in increased sperm velocity. However, not all kinematic parameters are affected to the same degree, with the most sensitive parameter being VCL and the straight-line velocity (VSL) basically staying constant (no change in first and last centroid detected) [16]. Thus, if the configuration setting for frame rate is halved (e.g. 25 fps instead of 50 fps], a large proportion of information on sperm head movement is not "tracked" due to the lower number of frames measured in the second that data is captured for (Figure 2.5). It should also be noted that the cut-off values selected for assessing sperm subpopulations are based upon kinematic values measured at a certain frame rate and will not give a true reflection of sperm classifications for the specific semen sample or sperm preparation.

For sperm motility analysis it is important to specify the staining method used, since the various commercially available fixatives and stains contain different chemicals that can influence sperm head

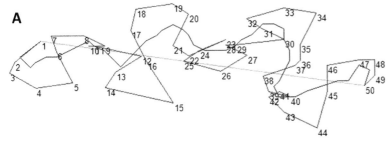

50 fps	Single sperm	Whole field
VCL (μm/s)	136.5	99.5
VAP (μm/s)	55.5	50.1
VSL (μm/s)	33.2	34.5
LIN (%)	24.4	36.9
STR (%)	59.8	67.4
WOB (%)	40.7	52.4
ALH (μm)	3.9	3.1
BCF (Hz)	19.0	18.6

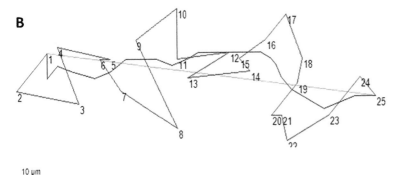

25 fps	Single sperm	Whole field
VCL (μm/s)	100.9	81.2
VAP (μm/s)	39.5	45.7
VSL (μm/s)	34.2	37.1
LIN (%)	33.9	47.0
STR (%)	86.6	78.8
WOB (%)	39.1	57.4
ALH (μm)	5.2	3.7
BCF (Hz)	9.0	11.5

10 μm

Figure 2.5 Sperm motility analysis at different frame rates. A) A sperm track captured at 50 fps for one second. B) The same sperm track reanalyzed at 25 fps for one second. Initial data was captured at 50 fps and an analyzed field was imported into VirtualDub 1.10.4 for re-analyses using every second frame and creating tracks of 25 fps. In both the individual and whole field sperm kinematic data it is clear that with half the number of centroid points tracked, less information is taken into consideration when calculating the sperm motion characteristics. Red line = VCL, blue line = VAP, turquoise line = VSL.

morphometry [20] and therefore potentially also the measurement of percentage sperm normality. Modern CASA systems can accommodate and assess sperm morphology with various staining methods, but the correct option should be selected in the configuration settings. Due to the fact that different cut-off values are used for different stains in terms of their range for normal sperm head, midpiece and tail morphometry, the same spermatozoon can be classified as "normal" in one morphology analysis set-up and "abnormal" in a different set-up (Figure 2.6). This could technically result in a male's semen morphology being classified as normal with one type of stain selected (e.g. 5 percent with SpermBlue) and abnormal with another (incorrect) stain selected (e.g. 2.5 percent with Papanicoulaou).

An important source of variation in measurements by CASA is related to the expertise of the CASA user [4]. Most of the above mentioned non-biological disadvantages can be avoided by technicians that receive proper training in standardizing the preparation of the sample before and during

analysis; selecting the correct analysis set-up; and accurate interpretation of the data generated [6, 18].

2.6 Laboratory and Clinical Interpretation of Computer-Assisted Semen Analysis Results

In a clinical unit, streamlining the information flow between the laboratory and the clinician would be a great advantage prior to communication of test results to the patient. Most CASA systems provide the technician or clinician with a summary report with analysed fields that can be extracted in different formats and is available immediately after a male's semen analysis has been completed (Figure 2.4). Moreover, modern systems also allow the technician to store all the patient's information and analysis results for various semen parameters on a CASA database that can easily be accessed during follow-up visits (Figure 2.7).

As CASA systems used for human semen analysis have incorporated the fifth WHO lower reference

17

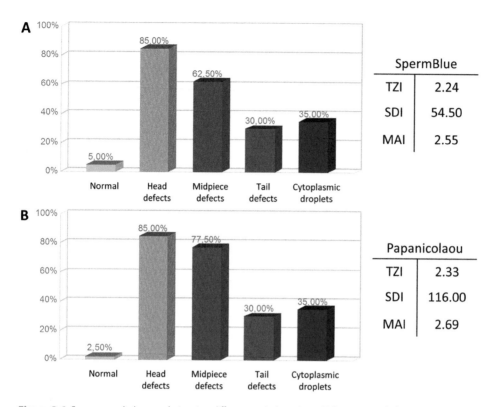

Figure 2.6 Sperm morphology analysis using different analysis settings. A) Sperm morphology assessed with SpermBlue stain. B) The same semen sample assessed but using Papanicolaou stain (incorrect setting). The latter setting influenced the percentage midpiece defects as well as the abnormal morphology indices. TZI = teratozoospermia index; SDI = sperm deformity index; MAI = multiple anomalies index.

limits for various semen parameters [10] into the software, it is possible for the software to make a diagnosis of infertility based upon a single semen parameter (e.g. motility or morphology) or a combination of all the parameters evaluated by CASA and additional manual inputs (e.g. semen volume and pH). Typically, classifications of a patient's sample are based upon semen nomenclature, for instance normozoospermia, asthenozoospermia, oligozoospermia and teratozoospermia (or a combination of the abnormalities). These classifications can then be used by the clinician to recommend a specific type of assisted reproductive technologies (ART) treatment for the infertile couple.

2.7 Clinical Significance of Computer-Assisted Semen Analysis Parameters

While any standard semen analysis (CASA or manual) can assist to define the quality of a semen sample, it is essential to highlight that such an assessment cannot predict fertility per se [6]. Furthermore, when either neat semen or semen diluted with an appropriate medium is evaluated in vitro, spermatozoa are not exposed to the fluids of the female reproductive tract as in vivo after ejaculation. Thus, no laboratory assessment of sperm motility reflects exactly its capabilities in the female's variable micro-environments up until the oocyte is reached [2]. However, CASA provides additional information (e.g. kinematics and subpopulations) on sperm motility and morphology that can be used in making deductions of a patient's fertility potential or decisions regarding a treatment protocol.

Investigations between motility parameters measured with earlier CASA systems and fertilization and pregnancy (both natural and assisted) have been controversial, but generally have indicated significant relationships with various sperm velocities (VCL and VAP) and progressiveness [5, 18]. In terms of sperm morphology analysis, little evidence exists that there is any relationship between percentage of

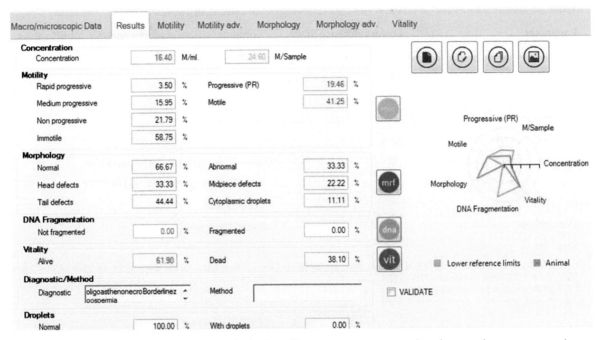

Figure 2.7 Example of a semen analysis using a CASA database. All semen parameters assessed are shown on the same screen and any parameters with values less than the reference limits or borderline cases are indicated in red.

normal forms and pregnancy after in vitro fertilization (IVF) or intracytoplasmic sperm injection (ICSI). This lack in prognostic value of normal sperm morphology is rather related to the description of what is deemed "normal", whether manual or CASA have been used [18]. Combining CASA results on sperm concentration, motility and morphology with other sperm parameters into multiple regression models will have a stronger predictive value for male fertility [5].

Evaluation of sperm subpopulations using CASA is highly recommended and will assist the andrologist to determine whether an ejaculate contains enough functional spermatozoa to potentially reach and fertilize the oocyte [1]. For instance, measurement of percentage of sperm mucous penetration and hyperactivation (Table 2.2) can form part of an integrated assessment of sperm functional potential and more robust determination of the level of ART an infertile couple might require [1, 18]. Furthermore, human ejaculates are known to contain several sperm subpopulations (Figure 2.8) and it is recommended that such subpopulations are evaluated rather than relying on mean values for the entire ejaculate [3]. In many ART applications, only the most motile sperm population are selected for assisted conception treatment

and might reveal a different sperm quality profile than the standard semen analysis.

2.8 When to Order the Test

Routine semen evaluations can be done by using either manual or CASA semen analysis. Conversely, subtle changes in sperm motility or morphology of a patient exposed to environmental factors (e.g. pesticides, heavy metals, tobacco and alcohol) or prescribed drugs [21, 22] will be impossible to detect with manual semen analysis. Thus, if the andrologist suspects that such exposures could have influenced a male's fertility, but his manual semen analysis reveals normozoospermia, it is recommended to order a CASA semen evaluation to possibly reveal elusive abnormalities.

2.9 Clinical Case Scenario where Computer-Assisted Semen Analysis May Be Needed and Helpful

2.9.1 Effect of Abstinence on Semen Parameters

A married couple is booked for a follow-up visit to your fertility clinic. After struggling to fall pregnant

Table 2.2 References Values and Cut-Off Values Typically Incorporated by Computer-Assisted Semen Analysis

Parameter	Lower reference limit	Computer-assisted semen analysis cut-off values
Sperm concentration (10^6/mL)	15	
Total sperm count (10^6/mL)	39	
Normal morphology (%)	4	
Total motility (%)	40	
Progressive motility (%)	32	
Sperm mucous penetration (%)	5	VAP>25 μm/s, STR>80%, ALH>2.5(5)*
Hyperactivation (%)	20	VCL>150 μm/s, LIN<50%, ALH>3.5(7)*
Rapid[#] (%)		VCL>89 μm/s
Medium[#] (%)		89<VCL>60 μm/s
Slow[#] (%)		60<VCL>23 μm/s

* Cut-off values as recommended in [6], ALH values given are for Sperm Class Analyzer and values in brackets are for other CASA systems using the full VCL wave to calculate ALH.
[#] Cut-off values as recommended in [3].

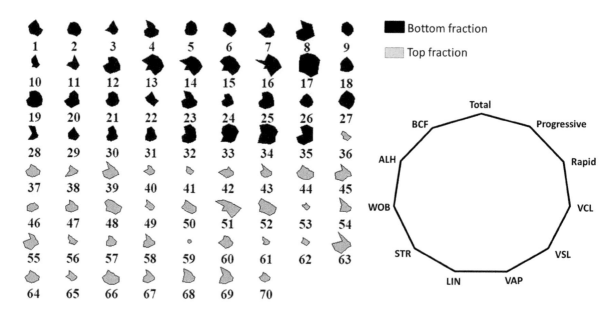

Figure 2.8 Sunray plots for 35 ejaculates to distinguish cases that have similar values for 11 input variables (see key on the right). Bottom and top fractions represent different subpoulations of spermatozoa in human semen and were extracted after density gradient centrifugation. The bottom fraction contains the most motile spermatozoa and clearly had higher percentages of motility as well as superior kinematic parameters compared to the top fraction. Total = total motility, Progressive = progressive motility, Rapid = rapid-swimming spermatozoa, VCL = curvilinear velocity, VAP = average path velocity, VSL = straight-line velocity, LIN = linearity, STR = straightness, WOB = wobble, ALH = amplitude of lateral head displacement, BCF = beat cross frequency. (Figure provided by Shannen Keyser.)

for more than three years, the couple's medical history and reproductive health have been assessed by the clinic's fertility specialist. Due to the fact that the couple presents with unexplained infertility, an intrauterine insemination (IUI) was recommended as ART treatment.

For IUI it is essential that the most motile spermatozoa should be selected for the insemination

Table 2.3 Hypothetical Data* for a Patient's Semen Analysis Using Computer-Assisted Semen Analysis after Long (Five Days) and Short (Three Hours) Abstinence Periods

	Sample 1 (Five days)	Sample 2 (Three hours)
Semen volume (mL)	3.1	2.0
Sperm concentration (10^6/mL)	54.4	43.2
Total sperm count (10^6/mL)	168.6	86.4
Total motile sperm count (10^6/mL)	119.4	65.8
Normal morphology (%)	16.3	16.1
Total motility (%)	70.8	76.2
Progressive motility (%)	53.1	57.8
Rapid-swimming sperm (%)	50.2	55.3
VCL (μm/s)	77.3	83.5
VAP (μm/s)	48.3	52.1
VSL (μm/s)	32.4	35.6
LIN (%)	38.5	41.5
STR (%)	61.0	62.6
WOB (%)	64.8	65.1
ALH (μm)	1.9	2.0
BCF (Hz)	13.1	14.5

* Data generated using average values reported [23, 24]. VCL = curvilinear velocity, VAP = average path velocity, VSL = straight-line velocity, LIN = linearity, STR = straightness, WOB = wobble, ALH = amplitude of lateral head displacement, BCF = beat cross frequency.

process. The husband was asked to produce two semen samples for comparison of sperm number and motility parameters, namely the first sample after two to seven days of abstinence [10] and the second after two to four hours of abstinence [23, 24]. You are using a CASA system to evaluate his standard semen characteristics and obtain the hypothetical results indicated in Table 2.3. The semen sample produced after just three hours abstinence has both a lower volume and lower sperm counts, but the sperm motility percentages and sperm velocities in this sample are superior to the five days abstinence. For this reason, you select the second sample for insemination, which, despite its lower total motile sperm count, will still produce enough motile spermatozoa (five to six million) for IUI purposes after the semen has been washed.

Several recent studies have shown that semen quality improves after short abstinence periods and these results challenge the generally accepted guidelines of prolonged abstinence periods [10, 23, 24]. Many of the differences reported in these studies for sperm motility are related to sperm subpopulations, including progressive motility, sperm velocity and hyperactivation. With the aid of CASA it is thus possible to objectively and accurately quantify the differences between subsequent semen samples.

2.10 Conclusion

During the past two decades several advancements in CASA technologies have ascertained this automated method of semen analysis both as an essential tool for research and routine clinical assessments. Modern CASA systems are more sophisticated than in the past and, if standardized protocols are adhered to, it reduces variability in data, while increasing the repeatability and precision of the measurements. As it is envisaged that additional applications of sperm functional testing will be incorporated into CASA in future, this assessment approach should be embraced by andrologists and reproductive medicine specialists alike.

References

1. Mortimer ST, van der Horst G, Mortimer D. The future of computer-aided sperm analysis. *Asian J Androl* 2015; **17**: 545–53.

2. Amann RP, Waberski D. Computer-assisted sperm analysis (CASA): capabilities and potential developments. *Theriogenology* 2014; **81**: 5–17.

3. van der Horst G, Maree L, du Plessis SS. Current perspectives of CASA applications in diverse mammalian sperm. *Reprod Fertil Dev* 2018; **30**: 875–88.

4. Yeste M, Bonet S, Rodríguez-Gil JE, Rivera Del Álamo MM. Evaluation of sperm motility with CASA-Mot: which factors may influence our measurements? *Reprod Fertil Dev* 2018; **30**: 789–98.

5. Ýaniz JL, Silvestre MA, Santolaria P, Soler C. CASA-Mot in mammals: an update. *Reprod Fertil Dev* 2018; **30**: 799–809.

6. van der Horst G, du Plessis SS. Not just the marriage of Figaro: but the marriage of WHO/ESHRE semen analysis criteria with sperm functionality. *Adv Androl Online* 2017; **4**: 6–21.

7. Tomlinson MJ, Pooley K, Simpson T, Newton T, Hopkisson J, Jayaprakasan K, Jayaprakasan R, Naeem A, Pridmore A. Validation of a novel computer-assisted sperm analysis (CASA) system using multitarget-tracking algorithms. *Fertil Steril* 2010; **93**: 1911–20.

8. Dearing CG, Kilkburn S, Lindsay KS. Validation of the sperm class analyser CASA system for sperm counting in a busy diagnostic semen analysis laboratory. *Human Fertil* 2014; **17**: 37–44.

9. World Health Organization. (1999) *Laboratory Manual for the Examination of Human Semen and Sperm-Cervical Mucus Interaction*, 4th ed. Cambridge: Cambridge University Press.

10. World Health Organization. (2010) *WHO Laboratory Manual for the Examination and Processing of Human Semen*, 5th ed. Geneva: The WHO Press.

11. Talarczyk-Desole J, Berger A, Taszarek-Hauke G, Hauke J, Pawelczyk L, Jedrzejczak P. Manual vs. computer-assisted sperm analysis: can CASA replace manual assessment of human semen in clinical practice? *Ginekol Pol* 2017; **88**: 56–60.

12. Dearing C, Jayasena C, Lindsay K. Can the Sperm Class Analyser (SCA) CASA-Mot system for human sperm motility analysis reduce imprecision and operator subjectivity and improve semen analysis? *Human Fertil* 2019; **6**: 11.

13. Kochman D, Marchlewska K, Walczak-Jedrzejowska R, Słowikowska-Hilczer J, Kula K, du Plessis S, Blignaut R, van der Horst G. Comparison of manual and computer aided sperm morphology analysis. *Adv Androl Online* 2016; **3**: 75.

14. Lammers J, Splingart C, Barrière Jean M, Fréour T. Double-blind prospective study comparing two automated sperm analyzers versus manual semen assessment. *J Assist Reprod Genet* 2014; **31**: 35–43.

15. European Society for Human Reproduction and Embryology (ESHRE). Guidelines on the application of CASA technology in the analysis of spermatozoa. *Hum Reprod* 1998; **13**: 142–5.

16. Bompart D, García-Molina A, Valverde A, Caldeira C, Yániz J, Núñez de Murga M, Soler C. CASA-Mot technology: how results are affected by the frame rate and counting chamber. *Reprod Fertil Dev* 2018; **30**: 810–19.

17. Gallagher MT, Smith DJ, Kirkman-Brown JC. CASA: tracking the past and plotting the future. *Reprod Fertil Dev* 2018; **30**: 867–74.

18. Tomlinson MJ, Naeem A. CASA in the medical laboratory: CASA in diagnostic andrology and assisted conception. *Reprod Fertil Dev* 2018; **30**: 850–9.

19. Menkveld R, Wong WY, Lombard CJ, Wetzels AMM, Thomas CMG, Merkus HMWM, Steegers-Theunissen RPM. Semen parameters, including WHO and strict criteria morphology, in a fertile and subfertile population: an effort towards standardization of in-vivo thresholds. *Hum Reprod* 2001; **16**: 1165–71.

20. Maree L, Menkveld R, du Plessis SS, van der Horst G. Morphometric dimensions of the human sperm head depend on the staining method used. *Hum Reprod* 2010; **25**: 1369–82.

21. Mukhopadhyay D, Varghese AC, Nandi P, Banerjee SK, Bhattacharyya AK. CASA-based sperm kinematics of environmental risk factor-exposed human semen samples designated as normozoospermic in conventional analysis. *Andrologia* 2010; **42**: 242–6.

22. Semet M, Paci M, Saïas-Magnan J, Metzler-Guillemain C, Boissier R, Lejeune H, Perrin J. The impact of drugs on male fertility: a review. *Andrology* 2017; **5**: 640–63.

23. Ayad BM, van der Horst G, du Plessis SS. Short abstinence: a potential strategy for the improvement of sperm quality. *Middle East Fertil Soc J* 2018; **23**: 37–43.

24. Alipour H, van der Horst G, Christiansen OB, Dardmeh F, Jørgensen N, Nielsen HI, Hnida C. Improved sperm kinematics in semen samples collected after 2 h versus 4–7 days of ejaculation abstinence. *Hum Reprod* 2017; **32**: 1364–72.

Chapter 3

Standard Semen Analysis: Home Sperm Testing

Manesh Kumar Panner Selvam, Christopher Douglas, Ashok Agarwal

3.1 Background

The definition of infertility is often described as the inability of a couple to conceive after one year of regular, unprotected sexual intercourse. Male factor infertility is present in approximately 50 percent of the cases and is the primary cause of the infertility in 30 percent of the cases [1]. Male factor infertility can be due to a variety of causes such as trauma, disease, anatomical or genetic abnormalities and many more. However, idiopathic male infertility comprises 30–40 percent of all cases [1].

Standard semen analysis (SA) is considered a fundamental diagnostic tool in the workup of the male fertility status. This essential test evaluates multiple semen parameters such as concentration, motility, morphology, volume and pH [2]. The results of the SA are then compared with reference ranges dictated by the World Health Organization's (WHO) Laboratory Manual for the examination and processing of human semen [2, 3]. If the results of a SA find parameters to be below the WHO 95th percentile reference range, the likelihood of pregnancy by intercourse becomes less probable [2, 3].

Although the SA is a cornerstone of the male infertility workup, many limitations inherent to the process exist, which facilitate the introduction of random errors into the test and thus cause significant variability in the results [4]. Observer subjectivity, insufficiencies in technician training and an absence of uniform laboratory protocol standardization are just a few of the ways in which the results of SA may be inaccurate and unreproducible [4]. An important additional limitation of laboratory-based SA is the reluctance of some men to make an office visit due the social stigma and embarrassment of infertility-related issues [5]. In light of this, men tend to be less likely than women to seek the care of a medical provider, while men that do seek medical attention are often better educated with higher paying occupations [6].

Since its inception in 1677 with Antonie van Leeuwenhoek's construction of a self-made microscope, SA has undergone many technological advancements [7]. The advent and application of more sophisticated microscopy has later been met by the rise of the digital age and the advent of computer-assisted sperm analysis (CASA) [8]. More recently, home SA devices have entered the market, with each device having its own unique operational platform designed to measure different semen parameters. The platforms by which these novel diagnostic tools function range from the use of immunochromatography and microfluidics to the utilization of centrifugal technology and smartphone-based applications [5, 9–12].

The increased use of point-of-care monitoring devices over the past two decades has made a dramatic impact on the way medical care is carried out. Sleep apnea diagnosis [13], fall risk [14] and blood glucose [15] monitoring are examples of ways patients now have increased control and knowledge over their health status in the privacy of their homes. However, the social stigma surrounding male infertility often prevents patients from getting the care they need and thus prolonging a couple's infertile status and chances of a successful pregnancy [5]. As a result, at-home testing devices has allowed men to check their semen quality in the comfort of their home and afterwards contact a fertility specialist if the results are abnormal [16].

3.2 Home Sperm Testing Devices

Several types of home sperm testing devices are available on the market. We have classified them based on the technology and working principle (Table 3.1).

3.2.1 Smartphone-Based Devices

The use of cellphones around the world has steadily expanded, reaching a global subscription in 2015 of

Table 3.1 Comparison of Commercially Available Home Sperm Testing Devices

Testing devices	Technology/working principle	Semen parameters measured
Smartphone Based (YO home sperm test)	YO clip mini-microscope, user's phone light source and camera	MSC, sperm concentration and motility
Microscope Based (Micra Sperm Test)	Manual microscope evaluation of semen parameters	Sperm concentration, motility and volume
Microfluidic Based	Analysis of motile sperm as they progress through differing chambers via channels or pores	Varies per device
Centrifugation Based (Trak®)	CentriFluidic™ technology which initiates centrifugal force on sperm and analyzes the condensed pellet	Sperm concentration
Immunodiagnostic Based (SpermCheck®)	Chemical labeling of spermatids and sperm-specific proteins to provide an indirect sperm concentration measurement.	Sperm concentration
Immunodiagnostic Based (SwimCount™)	SwimCount also utilizes 'swim up' method to separate and count progressively motile sperm.	TPMSC, morphology and DNA fragmentation

MSC: motile sperm concentration, TPMSC: total progressively motile sperm concentration

96.8 percent [17]. Smartphones, in particular, have a unique application in medicine because they are portable, have considerable processing power, contain high resolution cameras and can connect to the Internet [5]. Although each smartphone-based at-home sperm testing kit is unique, in general terms, most of these devices contain an attachable microscope, multiple sample loading chambers, and operate based on pre-programed software in "app" format, which is compatible with the majority of smartphone operating systems [10, 16].

3.2.2 Microfluidic-Based Devices

The utilization of microfluidic technology to measure semen parameters is found in a variety of home-based SA devices, such as the smartphone based YO Home Sperm Kit and the centrifugal-based Trak Male Fertility Testing System [10, 11]. Based on the principle of counting motile spermatozoa as they swim from one chamber to another (through a pore or channel), microfluidics can provide measures such as a sample's sperm concentration, motility and the motile sperm concentration (MSC) [10, 16].

3.2.3 Centrifugation-Based Devices

Centrifugation-based devices such as the "Trak Male Fertility Testing System" operate based on the principle of centrifugal force. Trak utilizes the induced movement of sperm cells from an initial loading inlet chamber (containing a pre-loaded density medium), through a progressively narrowing collection channel and into a column where the cells are condensed for evaluation [11].

3.2.4 Manually Operated Microscope Devices

Home SA devices based solely on the manual use of a microscope are currently available to the public. Priced at $85, the FDA-approved Micra Sperm Test includes a microscope, slides and a counting grid for the user to manually determine their own sperm count, motility and volume. However, studies have shown that the correct use of Micra requires an experienced operator as it is highly susceptible to user error by the layperson [10].

3.2.5 Immunodiagnostic-Based Devices

Immunodiagnostic home sperm tests operate based on unique principles designed for each individual device. Generally, these devices provide an indirect measure of sperm concentration via a lateral flow immunochromatographic test, which uses monoclonal antibodies designed for sperm specific antigens [12]. The signal generated when these antibodies bind to or "label" their respective antigens has a direct relation to sperm count and thus facilitates the enzyme-linked immunosorbent assay (ELISA)-based visualization of a semen sample's concentration [12].

3.3 Performance of Food and Drug Administration-Approved Home Sperm Testing Devices

3.3.1 YO Home Sperm Test

Developed in 2017, the YO Home Sperm Test (Medical Electronics Systems, Ltd., Caesarea Industrial Park, Israel) utilizes the video function built into most smartphones and operates based upon the software programed in its app [16]. The YO Home Sperm Test operates by mixing a liquefaction powder into a semen sample, transferring 20 μL of that sample onto a YO slide via the fixed transfer pipette and inserting it into the YO device [16]. Next, the YO device's microscope, in conjunction with the phone's camera and light source, record a 30-second video of the sperm; the built-in software then analyzes the sample (Figure 3.1) [16].

The YO Home Sperm Test measures a semen sample's motile sperm concentration (MSC), a composite value of the sample's concentration and motility. MSC is a unique measurement that provides greater insight into a patient's fertility outlook as opposed to simply reporting a patient's semen parameters [16]. Recent data has shown that, when compared to the laboratory-based automated sperm quality analyzer (SQA-Vision), the YO Home Sperm

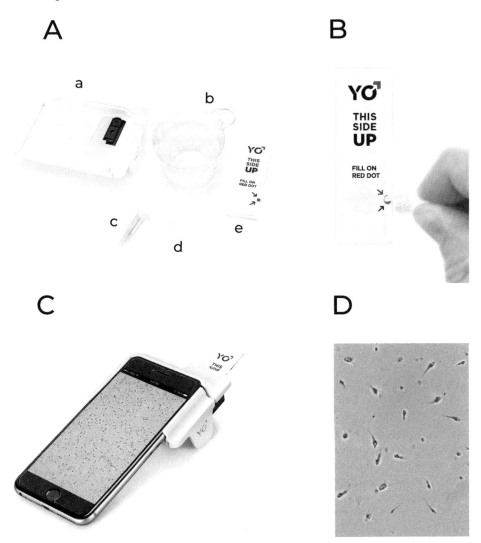

Figure 3.1 Components of the YO Home Sperm Test. (A) Photo of the YO kit contents, including (a) YO testing clip, (b) collection cup, (c) vial of liquefaction powder, (d) fixed volume transfer pipettes, and (e) fixed coverslip slide. (B) Sample loading into the filling chamber (highlighted in pink). (C) The assembled YO clip with inserted testing slide. (D) Screenshot of the captured sample as seen on the phone screen.

Test's MSC results present a moderate to good correlation with SQA-Vision. For example, the Pearson and Concordance correlations for sperm concentration utilizing the YO iPhone 7 was observed to be 0.96 and 0.96, respectively [16]. However, the correlations were 0.97 and 0.92, respectively, when utilizing the YO Galaxy S7.

An advantage of the YO Home Sperm Test includes the software's compatibility with both PC and Mac products, with the user interface being simple and easy to operate for both operating systems. Additionally, running of multiple tests is made easy by the YO Refill Kit which is readily available for purchase. The ability to measure MSC and generate an easy to interpret "YO Score" of low, moderate or high is based upon a cut-off value of 6×10^6/mL MSC. The advantage is that this integrated parameter consisting of the concentration and the motility provides valuable information regarding the patient's fertility status [16].

Disadvantages of this device include the price of the YO products, which range from $45.95 to $89.95 (yospermtest.com/shop/). Similarly, the number of semen parameters evaluated by the YO Home Sperm Test is lacking when compared to other such devices. Although there are many benefits inherent to smartphone-based tests, the simple fact that the YO Home Sperm Test requires a smartphone will prevent some underserved patients from being able to use the device.

3.3.2 SpermCheck Fertility

Developed in 1999, SpermCheck Fertility (similar to Fertilmarq) is an immunodiagnostic at-home SA device, which operates based upon the principle of lateral flow immunochromatography [12]. Utilizing monoclonal antibodies, which bind or "label" only spermatids and the sperm specific acrosome-protein SP-10, SpermCheck provides an indirect measure of the sperm concentration in approximately seven minutes [12].

SpermCheck is operated by collecting 100 µL of liquefied semen via a calibrated pipette and thoroughly mixing the sample with a detergent buffer used to solubilize the SP-10 protein. Next, the test cassette is loaded by adding four drops of sample into each of the two sample wells (Denoted "S") found below the two test strips. Initially, "control lines" denoted "C" will appear to indicate the test is functioning properly (Figure 3.2). After approximately seven minutes, the

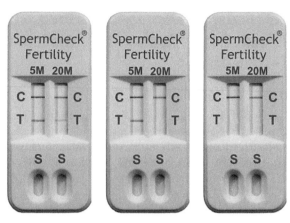

Figure 3.2 Presentation of differing sperm concentration results detected using SpermCheck® Fertility.

test lines denoted "T" should appear on both strips (the strip labeled "20M" and the strip labeled "5M"), if the sperm concentration is $>20 \times 10^6$ sperm/mL [12]. However, if the sperm concentration is $<20 \times 10^6$ sperm/mL but $>5 \times 10^6$ sperm/mL, the test line will appear only in the "5M" strip on the left. Similarly, if the concentration is $<5 \times 10^6$ sperm/mL, no test lines will appear (Figure 3.2) [12].

The accuracy of this device was evaluated in a study involving 225 semen samples, and compared sperm concentration results between SpermCheck and a hemocytometer as the reference. Coppola et al. reported that SpermCheck was able to accurately categorize patients into the proper sperm concentration category (normozoospermic, oligozoospermic, or severely oligozoospermic), 96 percent of the time [12]. Although this agreement shows SpermCheck's high level of reliability and apparent accuracy, the fact that this test only assesses one semen parameter is a significant limitation to its ability to fully assess semen quality. In an additional study involving postvasectomy men (n=144), SpermCheck's ability to accurately measure sperm concentration above or below the threshold value of 250,000/mL was (as determined by hemocytometer) 96 percent. The positive predictive value (PPV) and negative predictive value (NPV) were 93 percent and 97 percent, respectively [18].

3.3.3 SwimCount

The SwimCount™ device has been commonly used since 2015 to evaluate the male patient's reproductive status. Based on the use of antibody-mediated dyeing techniques, as well as the "swim up" principle, which is commonly used to increase the percentage of recovered motile sperm [10, 19], SwimCount™ is comprised of two macro-chambers separated by a filter composed of 10 µm pores. This "filtering" process enables the device to dye, capture and analyze only spermatozoa that are progressively motile, of normal form [9] and have low DNA fragmentation [20]. As the motile sperm reach the final "separation chamber", sperm density is quantified by an analysis of the darkness of the stain appearing in the "results window" [10]. The darker the stain in the results window, the higher the sperm density, as noted on the color-coded labels (Figure 3.3).

An advantage of this novel device is the number of semen parameters it measures in addition to the qualitative measure of the samples total progressively motile sperm concentration (TPMSC). TPMSC has been shown to be an important parameter when evaluating for male infertility [21, 22]. In light of this information, users of SwimCount™ could be men who are interested to learn more than just their semen quality, but are interested in their fertility status [9, 23]. SwimCount™ does have its share of limitations

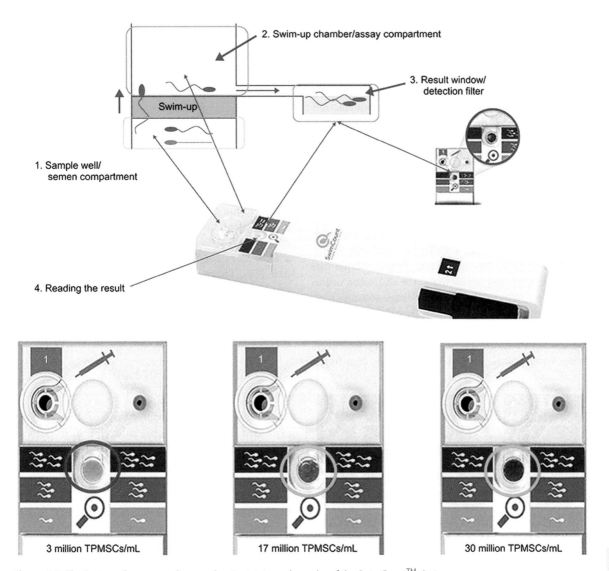

Figure 3.3 The "swim up" process and sperm density staining color-codes of the SwimCount™ device.

such as the device is disposable and multiple usages are not allowed. Furthermore, this device does not check and account for infection, pH or vitality and thus the results have the potential to be incorrect [9].

3.3.4 Trak

The Trak Male Fertility home-based semen test utilizes both microfluidic technology combined with the process of centrifugation. Producing results based on sperm concentration, Trak distributes the findings into three categories low ($\leq 15 \times 10^6$ sperm/mL), moderate ($15–55 \times 10^6$ sperm/mL), and optimal ($>55 \times 10^6$ sperm/mL). Harnessing the centrifugal force generated by an electrically powered engine, Trak propels the sperm cells through the test cartridge (prop), which houses individual test chambers. From the loading of the sample to the production of results, the entire process takes approximately seven minutes [11].

The Trak sperm testing kit contains a uniquely designed collection cup coated with a liquefaction enzyme into which the sample is collected at the time of ejaculation. After liquefaction, 250 µL of the ejaculate is loaded into the prop, which is then mounted to the engine and the lid covering the Trak centrifuge apparatus is sealed shut. Next, a centrifugal force is initiated on the sample and maintained for six to seven minutes [11]. During this process, the sample is driven through the prop, into a series of chambers and finally filters into a collection channel. Once completed, the results of the centrifuged sample can be read as a column appearing at the distal end of the Trak prop. Delineated with white lines accompanied by the text, "Low, Moderate, Optimal", the user can easily analyze their provided results immediately after the conclusion of the test (Figure 3.4) [11]. However, aside from its high cost of $125, a significant

limitation of this home-based device is its inability to measure the multiple standard semen parameters (volume, pH, motility, morphology etc.) besides sperm concentration. This limitation highlights the fact that the results provided by the Trak Sperm Testing System do not fully rule out infertility.

3.4 Limitations of Home Sperm Testing

3.4.1 Availability

One potential limitation of home sperm testing is the lack of availability some patients may experience due to the cost of the device and/or not owning a smartphone.

3.4.2 Lack of Information on All Semen Parameters

Another limitation of these devices is the lack of complete information provided for each semen parameter [10]. Furthermore, while some tests provide multiple data points for various parameters, other devices provide only a single result for one parameter.

3.4.3 Outcome of False Negative Results

As the home sperm testing devices can only measure a portion of the multiple semen parameters available, there exists the possibility of patients receiving a false negative for infertility due to such limited data [10]. Therefore, it must be stressed that normal results obtained by an at-home sperm test are not to be considered a replacement for the more detailed results of tests carried out by trained laboratory professionals [5].

3.5 Pros and Cons of Home Sperm Testing

The use of cellphones around the world has steadily expanded, reaching a global subscription in 2015 of 96.8 percent (www.itu.int/en/ITU-D/Statistics/Pages/facts/default.aspx). Smartphones, in particular, have a unique application in medicine because they are portable, have considerable processing power, contain high resolution cameras and can connect to the Internet [5]. In light of these facts, smartphones are in a unique position to greatly increase medical access in underserved parts of the world where the care of a fertility specialist is not readily available [7].

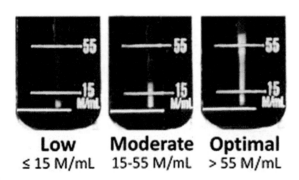

Low
≤ 15 M/mL

Moderate
15-55 M/mL

Optimal
> 55 M/mL

Figure 3.4 Presentation of sperm concentration results from low to optimal.

Increasing access to information, building relationships with medically underserved communities and mitigating a couple's prolonged infertility are just a few ways in which both smartphone-based and non-smartphone-based at-home semen testing benefits patients and physicians alike.

Due to these facts, this proliferation of at-home testing devices has allowed men to check their semen quality in the comfort of their home and contact a fertility specialist, if the results are abnormal [16]. Although at-home sperm tests allow for increased privacy, they are not to be considered a replacement for seeing a fertility specialist. Finally, the results of home-based sperm tests are not a basis for making definitive clinical diagnoses and must be viewed as a preliminary screen to initiate an office visit if abnormal results are observed [5].

3.6 Future of Home Sperm Testing Devices

Infertility is a worldwide problem and, as such, one future application for home sperm testing devices is the use of a simple, low-cost and easy to operate fertility screen for men unable or unwilling to access the care of a fertility specialist. In the United States alone, between 175,000 and 550,000 vasectomies are performed per year [24, 25]. Once the procedure has been completed, it is recommended that a follow-up visit be made between eight and 16 weeks post-vasectomy to ensure surgery success [26]. However, the literature shows that patient follow-up compliance is poor [27]. Considering this, perhaps another future application for the use of home-based sperm tests is to provide a simple, confidential and easy way for patients to confirm sterilization post-operatively [28].

Similarly, the increasing use of private home-based sperm tests could open the door for younger men, who do not regularly see a medical provider, to address their fertility-related concerns. Since this specific population group often neglects seeing a clinician, building this new line of communication between the patient and medical community at large could help diagnose and treat a multitude of otherwise disregarded health problems [5].

3.7 Conclusion

The advancements made in at-home sperm testing over the past two decades have revolutionized the way in which preliminary SA screens can be performed. With the advent and exponential use of the smartphone, the ability to provide infertility-related care for medically underserved populations has become a reality. In addition, the common discomfort many men experience during an office visit to a fertility specialist can now be alleviated by using such novel devices in the privacy of one's home. This benefit has the potential to allow more expedient diagnosis and treatment of male factor infertility. Finally, it must be stated that at-home sperm testing is not to be considered as a replacement for lab-based testing, but as a bridge for patients to receive a properly carried out fertility workup by a trained specialist.

References

1. Katz DJ, Teloken P, Shoshany O. Male infertility - The other side of the equation. *Aust Fam Physician* 2017; **46**: 641–6.

2. Sigman M, Baazeem A, Zini A. Semen analysis and sperm function assays: what do they mean? *Semin Reprod Med* 2009; **27**: 115–23.

3. World Health Organization. (2010) *Laboratory Manual for the Examination and Processing of Human Semen*, 5th ed. Geneva: The WHO Press.

4. Tomlinson MJ. Uncertainty of measurement and clinical value of semen analysis: has standardisation through professional guidelines helped or hindered progress? *Andrology* 2016; **4**: 763–70.

5. Vij SC, Agarwal A. Editorial on "An automated smartphone-based diagnostic assay for point-of-care semen analysis". *Ann Transl Med* 2017; **5**: 507.

6. Datta J, Palmer MJ, Tanton C, Gibson LJ, Jones KG, Macdowall W, Glasier A, Sonnenberg P, Field N, Mercer CH et al. Prevalence of infertility and help seeking among 15 000 women and men. *Hum Repro* 2016; **31**: 2108–18.

7. Sigman M. Cell phone microscope for semen analysis. *Fertil Steril* 2016; **106**: 549.

8. Amann RP, Waberski D. Computer-assisted sperm analysis (CASA): capabilities and potential developments. *Theriogenology* 2014; **81**: 5–17. e11–13.

9. Yoon YE, Kim TY, Shin TE, Lee E, Choi KH, Lee SR, Hong YK, Park DS, Kim DK. Validation of swimcount, a novel home-based device that detects progressively motile spermatozoa: correlation with World Health Organization fifth semen analysis. *World J Mens Health* 2019.

10. Yu S, Rubin M, Geevarughese S, Pino JS, Rodriguez HF, Asghar W. Emerging technologies for home-based semen analysis. *Andrology* 2018; **6**: 10–19.

11. Schaff UY, Fredriksen LL, Epperson JG, Quebral TR, Naab S, Sarno MJ, Eisenberg ML, Sommer GJ. Novel centrifugal technology for measuring sperm concentration in the home. *Fertil Steril* 2017; **107**: 358–64.e354.

12. Coppola MA, Klotz KL, Kim KA, Cho HY, Kang J, Shetty J, Howards SS, Flickinger CJ, Herr JC. SpermCheck Fertility, an immunodiagnostic home test that detects normozoospermia and severe oligozoospermia. *Hum Repro* 2010; **25**: 853–61.

13. Lux L, Boehlecke B, Lohr KN. (2004) *AHRQ Technology Assessments Effectiveness of Portable Monitoring Devices for Diagnosing Obstructive Sleep Apnea: Update of a Systematic Review*. Rockville, MD: Agency for Healthcare Research and Quality.

14. Mao A, Ma X, He Y, Luo J. Highly portable, sensor-based system for human fall monitoring. *Sensors* 2017; **17**.

15. Aggidis AG, Newman JD, Aggidis GA. Investigating pipeline and state of the art blood glucose biosensors to formulate next steps. *Biosens Bioelectron* 2015; **74**: 243–62.

16. Agarwal A, Panner Selvam MK, Sharma R, Master K, Sharma A, Gupta S, Henkel R. Home sperm testing device versus laboratory sperm quality analyzer: comparison of motile sperm concentration. *Fertil Steril* 2018; **110**: 1277–84.

17. Union IT. (2017) *ICT Facts and Figures 2017*. Geneva, Switzerland.

18. Klotz KL, Coppola MA, Labrecque M, Brugh VM, Ramsey K, Kim KA, Conaway MR, Howards SS, Flickinger CJ, Herr JC. Clinical and consumer trial performance of a sensitive immunodiagnostic home test that qualitatively detects low concentrations of sperm following vasectomy. *J Urol* 2008; **180**: 2569–76.

19. Butt A, Chohan MA. Comparative efficacy of density gradient and swim-up methods of semen preparation in intrauterine insemination cycles. *JPMA* 2016; **66**: 932–7.

20. Quinn MM, Jalalian L, Ribeiro S, Ona K, Demirci U, Cedars MI, Rosen MP. Microfluidic sorting selects sperm for clinical use with reduced DNA damage compared to density gradient centrifugation with swim-up in split semen samples. *Hum Reprod* 2018; **33**(8): 1388–93.

21. Tomlinson M, Lewis S, Morroll D. Sperm quality and its relationship to natural and assisted conception: British fertility society guidelines for practice. *Hum Fertil* 2013; **16**: 175–93.

22. Hamilton JA, Cissen M, Brandes M, Smeenk JM, de Bruin JP, Kremer JA, Nelen WL, Hamilton CJ. Total motile sperm count: a better indicator for the severity of male factor infertility than the WHO sperm classification system. *Hum Reprod* 2015; **30**: 1110–21.

23. Castello D, Garcia-Laez V, Buyru F, Bakiricioglu E, Ebbesen T, Gabrielsen A, Meseguer M. Comparison of the swimcount home diagnostic test with conventional sperm analysis. *Adv Androl Gynecol* 2018; 2018.

24. Eisenberg ML, Lipshultz LI. Estimating the number of vasectomies performed annually in the United States: data from the National Survey of Family Growth. *J Urol* 2010; **184**: 2068–72.

25. Kogan P, Wald M. Male contraception: history and development. *Urol Clin North Am* 2014; **41**: 145–61.

26. Sharlip ID, Belker AM, Honig S, Labrecque M, Marmar JL, Ross LS, Sandlow JI, Sokal DC. Vasectomy: AUA guideline. *J Urol* 2012; **188**: 2482–91.

27. Duplisea J, Whelan T. Compliance with semen analysis. *J Urol* 2013; **189**: 2248–51.

28. Kanakasabapathy MK, Sadasivam M, Singh A, Preston C, Thirumalaraju P, Venkataraman M, Bormann CL, Draz MS, Petrozza JC, Shafiee H. An automated smartphone-based diagnostic assay for point-of-care semen analysis. *Sci Transl Med* 2017; **9**(382): eaai7863. doi: 10.1126/scitranslmed.aai7863

Standard Semen Analysis: Leukocytospermia

Renata Finelli, Ralf Henkel

4.1 Introduction

4.1.1 Semen Analysis

The investigation of the male fertility potential starts with the analysis of seminal fluid. The seminal fluid or ejaculate is composed of a heterogeneous water-based solution (seminal plasma) deriving from secretions of prostate, testes, seminal vesicles and bulbourethral glands, and cellular components that include mature spermatozoa and epithelial cells derived from the genitourinary tract as well as the generically defined "round cells" (i.e. leukocytes, Sertoli cells and germ cells) [1]. Hence, the standard semen analysis provides insight into the testicular production of spermatozoa as well as the functionality and secretory activity of the associated sex glands [2]. Moreover, it permits the identification of genetic conditions associated with male infertility, such as azoospermia or globozoospermia, and orientates the choice of treatments or the necessity for further tests and investigations. Currently, semen analysis is performed according to the most recent WHO guidelines [2], which provide instructions for the evaluation of macroscopic (liquefaction, viscosity, appearance, volume, pH) and microscopic (sperm concentration, motility, morphology, vitality, presence of round cells and agglutination zones) seminal characteristics. The lower reference value for each parameter is represented by the fifth percentile, calculated based on a selected population of 1953 recent fathers [2]. However, it should be noted that men having seminal parameters below the reference values provided can still be fertile. On the other hand, men showing seminal parameters above the lower reference values are not necessarily fertile as about 15 percent of the men are reported to be infertile despite having normal semen parameters according to World Health Organization (WHO) criteria [3].

4.1.2 Leukocytes in the Ejaculate

Leukocytes are physiologically present in seminal fluid of all men. Polymorphonuclear (PMN) granulocytes represent 50–60 percent of circulated leukocytes in semen. These cells mainly originate from the prostate and seminal vesicles and have a diameter of 14 µm [1]. In addition to PMN granulocytes, macrophages (20–30 percent) and T-lymphocytes (2–5 percent) are less represented in semen and originate from the epididymis and rete testis, and have a cellular diameter of 16–20 µm and 8–12 µm, respectively [1]. Leukocytes can be differentiated from other round cells through microscopic evaluation at x1000 magnification, as nuclear size and shape can help identifying specific cellular types. More sophisticated techniques are based on an immunocytochemical approach based on the detection of leukocyte antigens such as CD45. However, the most common assay performed in clinics for neutrophils' discrimination is the Endtz test [4], described in detail in the further sections.

4.1.2.1 Function of Leukocytes

Leukocytes are physiologically present in seminal fluid of fertile and infertile men. Their concentration can increase in case of genital tract infection and inflammations and are therefore considered a diagnostic parameter [5, 6]. Generally, leukocytes play an important role in the removal of pathogens, or inflammation. Furthermore, leukocytes are involved in the phagocytosis of defective sperm, reducing the ejaculation of morphologically abnormal and immature sperm. In addition to this elimination of sperm in the male genital tract, leukocytes are also involved in their elimination and selection in the female genital tract. Since spermatozoa have antigenic properties, leukocytes will infiltrate the female genital tract and eliminate defective and moribund spermatozoa from the cervix and uterus. This in turn contributes to the selection of the most competent sperm to further ascent the female genital tract into the fallopian tubes. Different processes characterize this "silent" phagocytosis of male germ cells in the male and female genital tracts where reactive oxygen species (ROS) and pro-inflammatory cytokines play no role [7, 8]. Instead, an intrinsic apoptotic process is triggered by translocating phosphatidylserine from the inner leaflet of the plasma membrane to the out leaflet. Since the male germ cells are transcriptionally and translationally silent, this process needs to be called a regulated cell death rather than programed cell death [9].

By using electron microscopy, it has been observed that the process of the spermatozoa phagocytosis includes a) an increased volume of leukocytes, b) the development of cellular projections to contact the sperm cell, c) the formation of tight adhesions between leukocytes and spermatozoa, followed by d) the engulfment of the cell to the leukocytes' cytoplasm [10]. Simultaneously, leukocytes can also remove damaged and/or immature sperm by forming extracellular structures, which act like a trap. The fusion of extracellular traps formed by different leukocytes has also been observed when leukocytes act close to each other [10]. Once sperm have been phagocytized, ROS are generated by the enzyme peroxidase in the phagosomes and literally destroys the pathogens [11].

4.1.2.2 Occurrence of Leukocytes in the Semen

4.1.2.2.1 Infections

As important components of the immune system, leukocytes are activated in case of infections and involved in the removal of pathogens. The most common pathogens originate from the urinary tract or are sexually transmitted, and include *Escherichia coli*, Proteus spec., Klebsiella spec., Streptococcus spec. and *Chlamydia trachomatis* [11]. Several infections can be asymptomatic, such as urethritis and orchitis, while the symptomatology of prostatitis can vary significantly between patients [12]. Pathogens are eliminated by PMN granulocytes and macrophages by the generation of ROS as well as through phagocytosis. The entire process is orchestrated by cytokines, small (about 5–20 kDa) proteins secreted by leukocytes having pro- or anti-inflammatory effects. These molecules regulate the communication between cells and are further subdivided into interleukins (ILs), chemokines, interferons and tumor necrosis factors (TNFs) [13]. The secretion of cytokines regulates the activation of an inflammatory response as well as its inactivation [11]. The infection and the related tissue damage induce the synthesis of interleukin-1, which, in turn, activates neutrophils and macrophages. In a complex network of cell-to-cell interactions, these leukocytes secrete other molecules (i.e. IL-8, ROS, IL-6 and hepatocyte growth factor - HGF), which regulate their own function, the inflammatory response and aim to remove pathogens [13]. Although the function of cytokines is to control the infection, as a side effect, they can affect the male fertility potential. A negative association between high levels of cytokines (IL-6, IL-8 and TNF) and poor semen quality has been reported in the literature [11, 14, 15]. IL-6 secreted by PMN granulocytes and macrophages is able to induce the synthesis of antibodies by B-lymphocytes, which can have a negative impact on sperm functions [14]. On the other hand, IL-8 and TNF-α increase the level of ROS and lipid peroxidation and negatively affect sperm membranes, sperm morphology, metabolism and thus male reproductive functions [16–18].

4.1.2.2.2 Lifestyle Factors

Besides infections, other conditions related to lifestyle can induce leukocytospermia and/or increase the concentration of ROS released into the semen. Cigarette smoking represents a well-known cell mutagen and carcinogenic factor and its impact on male infertility has been widely investigated. A positive association between smoking habit and seminal leukocytes and ROS concentrations has been reported, with an increase of 48 percent and 107 percent, respectively, observed in smokers in comparison with nonsmoker patients [19]. In addition, the increase in oxidative stress leads to higher levels of 8-oxo-2'-deoxyguanosine, a validated marker of oxidative stress and sperm DNA damage [19]. Moreover, in patients abusing alcohol and/or drugs, poor semen quality has been reported as well as a significant higher percentage of seminal leukocytospermia and oxidative stress [20]. Eating habits also determine the establishment of an oxidative microenvironment in semen as a diet rich in sugars and lipids determines obesity [21], which is characterized by a systemic inflammatory response with high seminal ROS levels [22]. The increased visceral fat causes the systemic release of inflammatory mediators with repercussion on seminal quality and redox balance [23]. Furthermore, semen quality is altered after exposure to air and environmental pollution such as pesticides, plasticizers or heavy metal, as well as radiation. All this is leading to a shift of the redox balance towards an oxidative condition, the increase of inflammatory markers and reduced semen quality [24].

4.1.2.3 Reactive Oxygen Species Production of Leukocytes

Leukocytes produce ROS as a mechanism of defense against the presence of pathogens. ROS are oxygen-based molecules which are, due to the presence of one or more unpaired electrons in the outer orbit, highly reactive, with extremely short half-life times. Molecules exhibiting such unpaired electrons are called radicals and include the superoxide anion ($O_2^{\cdot-}$), hydroxyl radical ($OH^{\cdot}$), peroxyl radicals ($ROO^{\cdot}$) and alkoxyl radicals ($RO^{\cdot}$). On the other hand, ROS also include nonradical oxygen derivatives such as organic hydroperoxides ($ROOH$) and hydrogen peroxide (H_2O_2) [25]. Due to their electronic instability, ROS can interact with lipids, proteins, or the DNA and thereby cause lipid peroxidation of membrane lipids, inactivation of enzymes and sperm DNA damage. In this context, it is important to realize that H_2O_2, compared to other ROS, is relatively stable. However, H_2O_2 is a reactive component of the Fenton and Haber-Weiss reactions where H_2O_2 reacts with ferrous (Fe^{2+}) and ferric (Fe^{3+}) ions to produce $OH^{\cdot}$ and dismutate to superoxide, respectively [26]. In addition, considering that H_2O_2 is not charged, it can penetrate plasma membranes just like water and then react with proteins and DNA inside spermatozoa.

When they are activated, leukocytes can produce 1000 times more the amount of ROS produced by sperm [27]. The generation of ROS by leukocytes starts with the enzyme glucose-6-phosphate dehydrogenase, involved in the hexose monophosphate pathway and responsible for the synthesis of the cofactor nicotinamide adenine dinucleotide phosphate (NADPH). NADPH, in turn, is an electron donor for the enzyme NADPH oxidase, which catalyzes the conversion of oxygen into $O_2^{\cdot-}$ [21].

Generally, there are a number of tests available to identify leukocytes. According to the WHO manual [2], leukocytes should either be determined by their cellular peroxidase content by means of the use of ortho-toluidine [28] or with a more time-consuming and more expensive immunocytochemical test against CD45 [29]. Alternatively, the peroxidase stain using benzidine, the Endtz test [4], is commonly used.

4.2 Principle of the Peroxidase Stain Tests

Leukocytes are selectively differentiated from other round cells on the basis of their enzymatic peroxidase content as tested by the ortho-toluidine and Endtz tests. These tests are based on the histochemical staining of cellular granules containing myeloperoxidase, an enzyme characteristically expressed by granulocytes. Other leukocytes such as lymphocytes, macrophages and monocytes as well as immature germ cells are unstained as they do not express the enzymatic peroxidase activity. This allows the discrimination between granulocytes and other round cells. However, activated granulocytes are also unstained when they have already undergone the exocytosis of their granules before the staining.

4.2.1 Protocol of the Ortho-Toluidine Test

4.2.1.1 Preparation of Stock and Working Solutions

A 67 mmol/L phosphate buffer, pH 6.0, is prepared by dissolving 9.47 g Na_2HPO_4 in 1 L distilled water. In addition, another solution with 9.08 g KH_2PO_4 is also prepared in 1 L distilled water. Then, add 12 mL of the Na_2HPO_4 solution to 88 mL of the KH_2PO_4 solution until the pH is 6.0. Further, a saturated (250 g dissolved in 1 L distilled water) solution of NH_4Cl and a solution of 148 mmol/L of disodium ethylenediamine tetraacetic acid (Na_2EDTA) in phosphate buffer as well as the ortho-toluidine solution (2.5 mg in 10 mL 0.9 percent saline) are prepared.

In order to prepare the working solution, 1 mL of the NH_4Cl solution, 1 mL of Na_2EDTA and 10 μL of 30 percent H_2O_2 are added to 9 mL ortho-toluidine substrate and vortexed. This solution can be used up to 24 hours after preparation

4.2.1.2 Cellular Staining

After liquefaction, the semen sample is mixed well and 0.1 mL liquefied semen is then mixed with 0.9 mL of the working solution and incubated for 20–30 minutes at room temperature. Following another mixing, an aliquot of this suspension is loaded on a hemocytometer, incubated in a humid chamber for 4 minutes and analyzed under phase contrast at ×200 or ×400 magnification.

4.2.1.3 Evaluation of Stained Leukocytes

At least 200 brown (peroxidase-positive) leukocytes in a replicate are counted (peroxidase-negative cells are not stained) and the concentration of peroxidase-positive leukocytes (10^6 cells/mL) is calculated.

4.2.1.4 Quality Control

Reagents should be routinely checked by including a positive control in the analysis.

4.2.2 Protocol of the Endtz Test

4.2.2.1 Preparation of Stock and Working Endtz Solution

The Endtz stock solution is prepared with benzidine (0.125 g), 96 percent ethanol (50 mL) and sterile water (50 mL). It should appear clear and yellow and it is stable for six months after preparation. From this stock solution, the working solution is prepared by mixing 2.0 mL stock solution and 25 µL 3 percent hydrogen peroxide. The working solution should be freshly prepared on a weekly basis. Both solutions should be stored in the dark.

4.2.2.2 Cellular Staining

When liquefaction of the ejaculate is complete, an aliquot of the semen sample is mixed with phosphate buffered saline (PBS) and working Endtz solution (1 : 1 : 2 vol./ vol.) in an amber centrifuge tube. The solution is properly mixed and incubated for five minutes, at room temperature in the dark.

4.2.2.3 Evaluation of Stained Leukocytes

At least 200 brown (peroxidase-positive) leukocytes in a replicate are counted (peroxidase-negative cells are not stained) and the concentration of peroxidase-positive leukocytes (10^6 cells/mL) is calculated.

Quality control: reagents should be routinely checked by including a positive control in the analysis.

4.2.3 Protocol of the Immunocytochemical Staining

Since macrophages or monocytes as well as leukocytes that have already released their peroxisomes cannot be detected by the peroxidase staining techniques, other techniques can be used to determine the seminal leukocyte concentration. One of these techniques is the immunocytochemical staining using anti-CD45 antibodies. Using this technique all classes of leukocytes can be detected as leukocytes express the CD45 antigen.

4.2.3.1 Preparation of Stock and Working Solutions

Dulbecco's phosphate-buffered saline (DPBS), tris-buffered saline (TBS; pH 8.2) and a 1 mol/L tetramisole-HCl are prepared. The substrate solution is then prepared by dissolving 2 mg naphthol AS-MX phosphate in 9.7 mL TBS. Subsequently, 0.2 mL dimethylformamide and 0.1 mL of the tetramisol-HCl solution are added. Finally, just before use, 10 mg Fast Red TR are added, and the solution is filtered through a 0.45 µm pore size filter.

The fixative for the slides is prepared by mixing 95 mL acetone, 95 mL methanol (100 percent) and 10 mL of 37 percent formaldehyde.

Primary (mouse monoclonal anti-CD45) and secondary (alkaline phosphatase labeled anti-mouse rabbit immunoglobulins) antibodies are to be obtained from a relevant company. Harris' hematoxylin is used as counterstain.

4.2.3.2 Cellular Staining

When liquefaction of the ejaculate is complete, 500 µL of the semen sample are mixed with 2.5 mL of DPBS and centrifuged for five minutes at 500×g. Then, the supernatant is discarded, and the pellet resuspended with five times its volume with DPBS and centrifuges again for five minutes at 500×g. After repeating this step again, the pellet is re-suspended in DPBS to an approximate sperm concentration of 50×10^6 sperm/mL. Afterwards, a smear of 5 µL of this suspension is made on a slide, allowed to air-dry and then fixed with the fixative for 90 seconds. Thereafter, the slides are washed twice with TBS, drained and stained with the anti-bodies.

For binding of the primary anti-body, 10 µL of the antibody solution is added in the slide and incubated for 30 minutes at room temperature in a humid chamber. Afterwards, slides are washed twice with TBS and drained. Then, the previously incubated area is covered with 10 µL of the secondary antibody solution and incubated for 30 minutes in a humid chamber at room temperature. This step is followed by two washes with TBS and draining of the slides. Thereafter, the same area is covered with 10 µL alkaline phosphatase–anti-alkaline phosphatase complex

(APAAP) and incubated for one hour in a humid chamber at room temperature, washed twice with TBS, drained and finally incubated with 10 μL naphthol phosphate substrate solution for 20 minutes in a humid chamber at room temperature.

Once slides have developed a reddish color, they are washed once with TBS, counterstained for a few seconds with hematoxylin, washed with tap water and mounted in an aqueous mounting medium.

4.2.3.3 Evaluation of Stained Leukocytes

For evaluation, slides are examined in replicate with bright field optics at $\times 200$ or $\times 400$ magnification. CD45-positive cells appear red. The concentration and total number of CD45-positive cells out of at least 200 cells (sperm and other cells) are then calculated. Calculation of CD45-positive cells is done by calculating them relative to the sperm on the slide.

4.3 Reference Values

In agreement with the previous editions, the most recent WHO guidelines report the reference value of 1.0×10^6 peroxidase-positive cells /mL semen as lower reference limit [2]. Leukocyte concentrations higher than the reference value define a condition named as leukocytospermia.

For immunocytochemical testing using anti-CD45 antibodies, it is important to note that the values cannot be compared with those obtained by the peroxidase tests (ortho-toluidin and Endtz tests). Generally, the values obtained by the immunocytochemical test are higher [30]. Hence, the suggested lower reference value for leukocytospermia from the WHO [2] does not apply.

4.4 When to Perform the Peroxidase Test

The peroxidase test (ortho-toluidine or Endtz test) is usually performed in agreement with a semen analysis when the concentration of round cells is reportedly higher than 0.20×10^6/mL [2].

4.5 Clinical Interpretation of the Test

Leukocytospermia has been associated with male genital tract infections and inflammation [2]. Although many studies failed to identify any association between leukocytospermia and infective diseases [31], leukocytospermia represents a prognostic factor for infertility as it has been correlated with poor semen quality (low sperm count, motility and normal morphologically sperm) [32]. In a recent study, Homa et al. indicated that semen samples with PMN leukocyte counts have significantly higher seminal ROS than those samples having no leukocytes [33]. On the other hand, seminal oxidative stress determined as oxidation-reduction potential (ORP) with the MiOXSYS system and sperm DNA fragmentation were not increased in the leukocyte group. Yet, sperm DNA damage correlated positively with seminal ROS levels and the ORP. Hence, the determination of leukocytospermia in the workup of male infertility has been debated by international Andrology bodies, which have provided contradictory guidelines for leukocyte assessment and relative treatment. According to the American Urological Association (AUA) and the American Society for Reproductive Medicine (ASRM), leukocytospermia significantly contributes to male infertility as it is a manifestation of a genital tract infection [34]. However, its evaluation is suggested only in case of unexplained infertility or in the context of in vitro fertilization and any treatment is recommended. The Canadian Urological Association (CUA) promotes the evaluation of leukocytospermia only in case of symptomatic prostatitis and a antimicrobial therapy, although clinicians can choose the treatment according to their own judgment [35]. Finally, the European Association of Urology (EAU) considers leukocytospermia as a sign of clinical inflammation, but not infection [36]. Moreover, although an antibiotic therapy does not guarantee an increased chance of conception, a therapy is warranted.

4.5.1 Controversy around the World Health Organization Cut-Off of Leukocytospermia

In agreement with the fifth edition of the WHO guidelines [2], leukocytospermia is defined as a seminal leukocyte concentration higher than 1.0×10^6 leukocytes/mL. However, the value of the lower reference value is still under debate as some studies report an impact of ROS on sperm function at leukocytes concentrations as low as 0.1, 0.2 or 0.5×10^6 leukocytes/mL [37–42]. These studies argue that the cut-off set by the WHO for leukocytospermia is too high, hence leading to a misdiagnosis and underestimation of the prevalence and effects of leukocytospermia. Sharma et al. reported high levels of oxidative stress also in patients with leukocytes below the reference value provided, suggesting that any leukocyte concentration can be considered as "safe" for preventing oxidative stress-related damage [38]. Moreover, Henkel et al. observed a positive correlation between leukocytes and extrinsic ROS (leukocyte-derived ROS) in non-leukocytospermic patients and reduced sperm count, motility and morphology [37]. On the other hand, intrinsic (intracellular sperm-derived) ROS are rather correlated with sperm DNA damage. A high reference value for leukocytospermia may determine the exclusion of patients from treatments, which could be beneficial for infertility. Hamada et al. showed that patients with leukocyte concentrations between 0.2 and 1.0×10^6 leukocytes/mL can benefit from doxycycline treatment for three months as they showed higher pregnancy rate than untreated patients [43]. Therefore, further studies are required to analyze the role of seminal leukocytes in male reproduction and for the identification of the most suitable low reference value regarding leukocytospermia.

4.6 Conclusion

The analysis of the seminal leukocyte concentration by a peroxidase test (ortho-toluidine or Endtz test) is of great interest in combination with the standard semen analysis for the evaluation of the male fertility status. On one side, leukocytes are physiologically present in semen fluid as they play a role in phagocytosis and elimination of pathogens and immature sperm cells. On the other hand, leukocytospermia has been associated with male genital tract infections and inflammation, suggesting the importance of a leukocyte evaluation in the workup of male infertility. Although several studies report an association between leukocytospermia and poor semen quality, the reference value for clinics and its diagnostic power is still under debate, supporting the necessity of further studies.

References

1. Johanisson E, Campana A, Luthi R, De Agostini A. Evaluation of "round cells" in semen analysis: a comparative study. *Hum Reprod Update* 2000; **6**: 404–12.

2. World Health Organization. (2010) *WHO Laboratory Manual for the Examination and Processing of Human Semen*, 5th ed. Geneva: The WHO Press.

3. Hamada A, Esteves SC, Nizza M, Agarwal A. Unexplained male infertility: diagnosis and management. *Int Braz J Urol* 2012; **38**: 576–94.

4. Endtz AW. A rapid staining method for differentiating granulocytes from "germinal cells" in Papanicolaou stained semen. *Acta Cytol* 1974; **18**: 2–7.

5. Rowe PJ, Comhaire FH, Hargreave TB, Mahmoud AMA, World Health Organization. (2000) *WHO Manual for the Standardized Investigation, Diagnosis and Management of the Infertile Male.* Cambridge: Cambridge University Press.

6. Pfeifer S, Butts S, Dumesic D et al. Diagnostic evaluation of the infertile male: a committee opinion. *Fertil Steril* 2015; **103**: e18–25.

7. Rossi AG, Aitken RJ. Interactions between leukocytes and the male reproductive system: the unanswered questions. *Adv Exp Med Biol* 1997; **424**: 245–52.

8. D'Cruz OJ, Wang B-L, Haas GG. Phagocytosis of immunoglobulin G and C3-bound human sperm by human polymorphonuclear leukocytes is not associated with the release of oxidative radicals. *Biol Reprod* 1992; **46**: 721–32.

9. Aitken RJ, Baker MA. Oxidative stress, spermatozoa and leukocytic infiltration: relationships forged by the opposing forces of microbial invasion and the search for perfection. *J Reprod Immunol* 2013; **100**: 11–19.

10. Piasecka M, Fraczek M, Gaczarzewicz D et al. Novel morphological findings of human sperm removal by leukocytes in in vivo and in vitro conditions: preliminary study. *Am J Reprod Immunol* 2014; **72**: 348–58.

11. Comhaire FH, Mahmoud AMA, Depuydt CE, Zalata AA, Christophe AB. Mechanisms and effects of male genital tract infection on sperm quality and fertilizing potential: the andrologist's viewpoint. *Hum Reprod Update* 1999; **5**: 393–8.

12. Sandoval JS, Raburn D, Muasher S. Leukocytospermia: overview of diagnosis, implications, and management of a controversial finding. *Middle East Fertil Soc J* 2013; **18**: 129–34.

13. Holdsworth SR, Can PY. Cytokines: names and numbers you should care about. *Clin J Am Soc Nephrol* 2015; **10**: 2243–54.

14. Martínez-Prado E, Camejo Bermúdez MI. Expression of IL-6, IL-8, TNF-α, IL-10, HSP-60, anti-HSP-60 antibodies, and anti-sperm antibodies, in semen of men with leukocytes and/or bacteria. *Am J Reprod Immunol* 2010; **63**: 233–43.

15. Eggert-Kruse W, Boit R, Rohr G, Aufenanger J, Hund M, Strowitzki T. Relationship of seminal plasma interleukin (IL) -8 and IL-6 with semen quality. *Hum Reprod* 2001; **16**: 517–28.

16. Martínez P, Proverbio F, Camejo MI. Sperm lipid peroxidation and pro-inflammatory cytokines. *Asian J Androl* 2007; **9**: 102–7.

17. Mohanty G, Swain N, Goswami C, Kar S, Samanta L. Histone retention, protein carbonylation, and lipid peroxidation in spermatozoa: possible role in recurrent pregnancy loss. *Syst Biol Reprod Med* 2016; **62**: 201–12.

18. Suleiman SA, Elamin Ali M, Zaki ZMS, El-Malik EMA, Nasr MA. Lipid peroxidation and human sperm motility: protective role of vitamin E. *J Androl* 1996; **17**: 530–7.

19. Saleh RA, Agarwal A, Sharma RK, Nelson DR, Thomas AJ. Effect of cigarette smoking on levels of seminal oxidative stress in infertile men: a prospective study. *Fertil Steril* 2002; **78**: 491–9.

20. Close CE, Roberts PL, Berger RE. Cigarettes, alcohol and marijuana are related to pyospermia in infertile men. *J Urol* 1990; **144**: 900–3.

21. Agarwal A, Rana M, Qiu E, AlBunni H, Bui A, Henkel R. Role of oxidative stress, infection and inflammation in male infertility. *Andrologia* 2018; **50**: e13126.

22. Kahn BE, Brannigan RE. Obesity and male infertility. *Curr Opin Urol* 2017; **27**: 441–5.

23. Leisegang K, Bouic PJD, Henkel R. Metabolic syndrome is associated with increased seminal inflammatory cytokines and reproductive dysfunction in a case-controlled male cohort. *Am J Reprod Immunol* 2016; **76**: 155–63.

24. Wright C, Milne S, Leeson H. Sperm DNA damage caused by oxidative stress: modifiable clinical, lifestyle and nutritional factors in male infertility. *Reprod Biomed Online* 2014; **28**: 684–703.

25. Aitken R. Reactive oxygen species as mediators of sperm capacitation and pathological damage. *Mol Reprod Dev* 2017; **84**: 1039–52.

26. Tvrdá E, Massanyi P, Lukáč N. Physiological and pathological roles of free radicals in male reproduction. In Meccariello R, Chianese R, eds. (2017) *Spermatozoa - Facts and Perspectives*. London: IntechOpen.

27. Plante M, De Lamirande E, Gagnon C. Reactive oxygen species released by activated neutrophils, but not by deficient spermatozoa, are sufficient to affect normal sperm motility. *Fertil Steril* 1994; **62**: 387–93.

28. Nahoum CRD, Cardozo D. Staining for volumetric count of leukocytes in semen and prostrate-vesicular fluid. *Fertil Steril* 1980; **34**: 68–9.

29. Wolff H, Anderson DJ. Male genital tract inflammation associated with increased numbers of potential human immunodeficiency virus host cells in semen. *Andrologia* 1988; **20**: 404–10.

30. Villegas J, Schulz M, Vallejos V, Henkel R, Miska W, Sánchez LR. Indirect immunofluorescence using monoclonal antibodies for the detection of leukocytospermia: comparison with peroxidase staining. *Andrologia* 2002; **34**: 69–73.

31. Bachir BG, Jarvi K. Infectious, inflammatory, and immunologic conditions resulting in male infertility. *Urol Clin North Am* 2014; **41**: 67–81.

32. Domes T, Lo KC, Grober ED, Mullen JBM, Mazzulli T, Jarvi K. The incidence and effect of bacteriospermia and elevated seminal leukocytes on semen parameters. *Fertil Steril* 2012; **97**: 1050–5.

33. Homa ST, Vassiliou AM, Stone J et al. A comparison between two assays for measuring seminal oxidative stress and their relationship with sperm DNA fragmentation and semen parameters. *Genes* 2019; **10**: 236.

34. Jarow J, Sigman M, Kolettis PN et al. (2010) *The Optimal Evaluation of the Infertile Male: AUA Best Practice Statement*. American Urological Association Education and Research, Inc., pp. 1–38.

35. Curtis Nickel J. Prostatitis. *Can J Urol* 2011; **5**: 306–15.

36. Jungwirth A, Giwercman A, Tournaye H et al. European Association of Urology guidelines on male infertility: the 2012 update. *Eur Urol* 2012; **62**: 324–32.

37. Henkel R, Kierspel E, Stalf T et al. Effect of reactive oxygen species produced by spermatozoa and leukocytes on sperm functions in non-leukocytospermic patients. *Fertil Steril* 2005; **83**: 635–42.

38. Sharma RK, Pasqualotto FF, Nelson DR, Thomas AJ, Agarwal A. Relationship between seminal white blood cell counts and oxidative stress in men treated at an infertility clinic. *J Androl* 2001; **22**: 575–83.

39. Menkveld R, Kruger TF. Sperm morphology and male urogenital infections. *Andrologia* 1998; **30**: 49–53.

37

40. Punab M, Lõivukene K, Kermes K, Mändar R. The limit of leucocytospermia from the microbiological viewpoint. *Andrologia* 2003; **35**: 271–8.

41. Lackner J, Schatzl G, Horvath S, Kratzik C, Marberger M. Value of counting white blood cells (WBC) in semen samples to predict the presence of bacteria. *Eur Urol* 2006; **49**: 148–53.

42. Thomas J, Fishel S, Hall J, Green S, Newton T, Thornton S. Increased polymorphonuclear granulocytes in seminal plasma in relation to sperm morphology. *Hum Reprod* 1997; **12**: 2418–21.

43. Hamada A, Agarwal A, Sharma R, French DB, Ragheb A, Sabanegh ES. Empirical treatment of low-level leukocytospermia with doxycycline in male infertility patients. *Urology* 2011; **78**: 1320–5.

Chapter 5

Standard Semen Analysis: Morphology

Roelof Menkveld

5.1 Introduction

The evaluation of sperm morphology as a standard procedure to be included in routine semen analysis is under persistent pressure due to several factors relating inter alia to the changing definition and description for a morphological normal spermatozoon. In addition, the description of different methods for the morphology evaluation process [1], the different ways in which the results are reported by different laboratories [2], and the continued lowering of the cut-off, or lower reference value, in the consecutive World Health Organization (WHO) semen analysis manuals published between 1980 and 2010 changed. An additional factor in the demise of sperm morphology evaluation in the routine Andrology laboratory is the continuing trend of non-adherence in many laboratories to the guideline given in the WHO manual(s) [3].

The current 2010 manual [1] provides detailed descriptions for the preparation of the semen smear, the staining of the smears and the methodology for the evaluation process itself. An important aspect for the morphological evaluation of spermatozoa is the criteria for a morphologically normal spermatozoon. In this regard, the 2010 WHO manual now recommends the use of a strict approach based on the (Tygerberg) strict criteria [4]. Due to the stricter criteria and a worldwide decrease in the percentage of morphologically normal spermatozoa, the 2010 WHO manual now proposes a lower reference value of only 4 percent morphologically normal spermatozoa. In a currently published French survey, it was found that many clinicians are regarding sperm morphology of little clinical importance and that even laboratory persons performing sperm morphology assessments regard the procedure as unreliable or the results not very reliable in analytic terms [3]. However, with the stringent application of the current WHO guidelines, sperm morphology can still play a role in the evaluation of a male's fertility potential and clinical treatment.

5.2 Principle of Sperm Morphology Evaluation

The principle of sperm morphology evaluation can be divided into two stages or periods. The first is the early approach, later called the liberal approach [5], which was also the method described in the early WHO manuals (1980–1992). The second is the strict (criteria) approach as introduced by the Tygerberg Hospital team in 1986 and is now the method advocated in the 2010 WHO manual as the method to be followed [6].

5.2.1 Liberal Approach

In contrast to the sperm morphology of domestic animals, showing a very homogeneous picture with very little variation in shape and form, the human sperm morphology is quite different with a very heterogeneous picture showing a wide range of morphological abnormalities. Thus, while in domestic animals it was easy to describe what is a normal spermatozoon, application of this principle was not possible for the human male. Therefore, normality of sperm morphology was reached by describing all types of sperm forms regarded as abnormal. Some investigators identified more than fifty abnormal classes. Sperm normality was therefore determined indirectly or by default. MacLeod made an important contribution by reducing all the different classes of abnormalities to only seven head abnormality classes [7]. In 1971, another important contribution towards standardization of human sperm morphology evaluation was provided by Eliasson, who proposed standard measurements to identify sperm head abnormalities as too small or too large or to be within the normal range [8]. Eliasson also introduced the principle that a spermatozoon should only be regarded as morphologically normal, if the whole spermatozoon was normal, thus including midpiece and tail defects. The spermatozoon should be regarded as normal, unless it fits into an abnormal category.

5.2.2 The Strict Criteria Approach

According to Sigman [6], a major paradigm shift occurred in the late 1980s and early 1990s when a group from South Africa reversed the long-held concept that sperm were normal unless they fit an abnormal category. The Tygerberg Hospital group used the homogeneous appearence of sperm present in the upper endocervical mucus to define morphological normal spermatozoa with precise criteria [6]. Several articles published previously on different aspects of sperm-cervical mucus interaction in vivo and in vitro all reported that there was a strong selection for morphologically normal appearing spermatozoa. However, Menkveld et al. [4] used this observation to describe the appearance of what could be regarded as a morphological normal spermatozoon based on the biological principle of the specific morphological shape being able to penetrate good ovulatory cervical mucus. The spermatozoa population observed in cervical mucus presented a very homologous picture with only small variations in contrast to the very heterogeneous picture seen in the original semen samples.

The basic description for a morphologically normal spermatozoon was primarily based on the work of Eliasson that states the evaluation of the whole spermatozoon and its measurements should be used [8]. However, the strict criteria distinctly differed by stating that the so-called "borderline" normal spermatozoa should be regarded as abnormal. The reasoning behind this was to keep the variations allowed for normality as small as possible. Menkveld et al. [4] also stressed the importance of the WHO manual's guidelines with regard to the making of semen smears, staining of these smears, and the methodology for evaluating the spermatozoa on these smears. Due to these principles, the description by Menkveld [9] and Menkveld et al. [4] is now referred to as the (Tygerberg) strict criteria approach [5].

5.2.3 Classification Criteria for Normal Sperm Morphology

Spermatozoa consist of a head, neck and tail region, with the tail subdivided into the middle, principal and end pieces. For classification purposes, the neck and middle pieces of the spermatozoon are classified together. For a spermatozoon to be considered as morphologically normal, all of the head, neck and tailpieces must be normal. All borderline forms should be considered as abnormal [1, 4].

The head of the spermatozoon must have an oval form with smooth contours. A clearly visible and well-defined acrosome must be present and should cover about 30–60 percent of the anterior part of the sperm head and exhibit a homogeneous light-blue staining indicating an intact acrosome. The generally given measurements for a normal sized spermatozoon of between 3–5 μm and 2–3 μm for length and width, respectively, is probably too long and wide for general purposes as sperm head measurements are staining specific. Several head measurements are available for Papanicolaou stained spermatozoa:

- The WHO 2010 manual [1] provided the following measurements as obtained by a computerized sperm morphology analysis system (CAMA); median length 4.1 μm (95 percent CI 3.7–4.7 μm) and median width 2.8 μm (95 percent CI 2.5–3.2 μm).
- Normal CAMA head measurements (mean and SD) as published by Maree et al. in 2010 [10] are 4.28(0.27) μm for length and 2.65(0.19) μm for width.
- Manual measurement (mean and SD) as published by Menkveld in 2013 [11] are 4.07(0.19) μm for length and 2.98(0.14) μm for width.

The principal piece of the tail should have a uniform calibre along its length, be thinner than the midpiece and should be about 45 μm to 50 μm long and without any sharp bends. A tail looped on itself is regarded as normal. The tail tip is very seldom visible.

No cytoplasmic residues may be present at the neck/midpiece region or on the tail.

5.2.4 Identification Criteria of the Four Abnormal Sperm Morphology Classes

In the literature, four main abnormal sperm morphology classes are distinguished viz. head, neck and midpiece defects, tail defects and the presence of cytoplasmic residues, sometimes also called cytoplasmic droplets [11].

5.2.4.1 Head Defects
5.2.4.1.1 Size

A head is said to be classified as having size defect where the head is too large or too small based on the actual staining method used, but still presenting with an overall oval form.

5.2.4.1.2 Form

This is where the spermatozoa do not present with the classical oval from. This category includes spermatozoa described as elongated forms, tapering forms, and which according to Eliasson (1971) may be smaller or larger than the normal oval form [8], and the so-called pear-shape or pyriform which are usually larger than the normal oval from. Spermatozoa with a V-shaped posterior (post-acrosomal) ends are classified as morphological normal forms on the condition that no elongation is present.

5.2.4.1.3 Acrosomal Defects

Acrosomal defects include size defects, staining defects and structural defects. Size defects are present when an acrosome covers >60 percent or <30 percent of a normal sized head. Acrosome defects can also include staining defects, where the acrosomes do not show the homogeneous light-blue staining when stained according to the Papanicolaou method, or where the acrosome staining in certain areas is absent and the acrosomes show white (patchy) areas. This should not include the presence of (large) vacuoles or cysts. Vacuoles are deemed present when a lighter stained area(s) with well-defined round borders is observed. A cyst is deemed to be present when a lighter stained area(s) with well-defined round borders is present on the outer acrosome area, giving an extruding impression.

5.2.4.1.4 Duplications

Duplications are deemed to be present when usually, two heads are joint together at the neck/midpiece area, but this may also occur at any other part of the sperm structure. When a head duplication is present, this is primarily classified as head abnormality.

5.2.4.1.5 Amorphous

The term amorphous heads includes all other head forms not classified under any of the named abnormal sperm head categories. Spermatozoa with a slight, but definite alternation from the morphological normal forms are considered as borderline and must be classified as an abnormal head form.

5.2.4.2 Neck/Midpiece Defects

As specific neck defects per se are difficult to identify, neck and midpiece defects are considered as one defect type. This includes bend necks, where the neck/midpiece forms a definite angle with the sperm head, an asymmetrical implantation of the neck/midpiece to the posterior region of the sperm head, a thickened neck/midpiece as well as asymmetric bend midpieces. Cases where the mitochondrial material has shifted to the neck or towards the principal tail region showing a very thin midpiece. In these cases, the mitochondrial material present at the neck region must not to be confused with the presence of excessive cytoplasmic material.

5.2.4.3 Tail Defects

Tail defects are present where a definite bend (some definitions specify >90°) is observed at any part of the principal tail piece. Other tail defects are double tails, two or more, extruding from a single sperm head or midpiece, coiled tails or irregular tails or combinations. A bend between the end of the midpiece and beginning of the principal piece of the tail is classified as a tail abnormality and not a neck/midpiece abnormality. A bent tail should not to be confused with a curved tail. Short tails are shorter than tails of the normal specified length and must not be confused with abnormal tails due to the short tail syndrome. Coiled tails are in most cases not due to artifacts, but due to definite abnormalities, as the tails are enclosed in a membrane structure.

5.2.4.4 Cytoplasmic Residues

Although no cytoplasmic material should be present, a small amount of cytoplasmic material, <30 percent of a normal sized sperm head, sometimes occurs and can be regarded as normal. Cytoplasmic material on spermatozoa in stained semen smears are not common and, when present, are usually associated with the occurrence of other sperm defects such as bent necks and elongated spermatozoa. The presence of cytoplasmic material on spermatozoa is associated with the excessive production of reactive oxygen species (ROS).

5.3 Methods for Preparation and Examination of Semen Smears

As part of the standard semen analysis, semen smears are prepared, stained with the Papanicolaou method, and examined for the presence of spermatozoa and round cells. Spermatozoa are then assessed under oil magnification to determine the percentage of morphologically normal spermatozoa for the specific sample.

5.3.1 Preparation of Semen Smears

The identification (ID) information of the semen sample must be noted with pencil on the frosted part of the slide in such a way that, if the slide is kept upright the frosted end is on top and the ID information is upright and readable for easy recovery when stored. Do not use paper labels as the labels may become contaminated when placed in the staining solutions and ID information may therefore not be visible.

Place a drop of 5–15 µL of liquefied semen, depending on the sperm concentration, just under the frosted part of the slide. Another slide is then placed in front of the semen drop, slightly pulled back towards the frosted part so that the semen can spread over the entire width of the slide and the slide is then moved towards the end of the slide, on which the semen is deposited. The speed of the movement and the angle at which the slide is held to draw the semen drop will determine the thickness and number of sperm on the slide. A smaller drop of semen and slow forward movement will provide a thinner smear and less sperm per visual microscopic field, while a bigger angle and a faster forward movement will deposit more sperm in a smaller part of the slide. The smears are slightly air-dried and fixed for at least 10 minutes in an appropriate fixative.

5.3.2 Staining and Mounting of a Semen Smear

Semen smears should be stained with the Papanicolaou method (see WHO 2010 manual, page 62, for details of the staining solutions and procedures) [1].

For mounting of a semen smear, place a small aliquot of mounting medium on a coverslip and place the stained semen smear on top allowing it to spread over the entire cover-slip area. Adjust the cover slip to cover the maximum area of the stained semen smear and remove any air bubbles with the aid of a tweezer.

5.3.3 Examination of the Semen Smear

The first step should be to screen the semen smear with the 10× objective to determine the quality of the smear with regard to quality of staining, the spreading of the spermatozoa on the slide and the presence of any round cells, if any. If round cells are observed, the 400× (HPF) magnification can be used to identify the type of round cells, i.e. white blood cells (WBC) or germinal epithelium cells (precursors) and areas suitable to perform the sperm morphology assessment.

5.3.4 Assessment of Spermatozoa for Morphological Appearance

Evaluate at least 200 spermatozoa using a 1000× or 1500× magnification – ideal is 1250× as found on older microscopes. For greater accuracy, the WHO 2010 manual suggests the evaluation of 2 × 200 spermatozoa.

5.3.5 Evaluation Methodology for Assessment of Morphological Normality

To categorize the spermatozoa as morphologically normal or abnormal, the following simple schedule (algorithm) can be used by asking the following questions while observing a specific spermatozoon [11].

The questions are:

- Is the sperm an oval form with smooth contours? If no = abnormal; if yes – continue
- Is the sperm size normal? If no = abnormal; if yes – continue
- Is an acrosome visible? If no = abnormal; if yes – continue
- Is the acrosome normal in size? If no = abnormal; if yes – continue
- Is the tail inserted correctly? If no = abnormal; if yes – continue
- Is there another neck/midpiece defect? If yes = abnormal; if no – continue
- Is there a tail defect? If yes = abnormal; if no – continue
- Is there a cytoplasmic residue present? If yes = abnormal; if no – a morphological normal spermatozoon is present.

5.4 Reference and Cut-Off Values

Reference values for classifying sperm morphology evaluation results have changed over the years as progress has been made with morphology evaluation techniques, detailed descriptions of the morphology evaluation process have been published and new clinical data have become available [12, 13]. The 2010 WHO manual [1] now uses the term "lower reference limits" to describe normal semen parameter values. The new lower WHO manual reference value of 4 percent for morphologically normal spermatozoa is based on the lower fifth percentile value from data from a combination of several reference populations. The populations were composed of couples with a time-to-pregnancy of ≤12 months of unprotected intercourse. The initial study included about 1600 couples from five centres from three continents but a number of cases were excluded on the basis of certain selection criteria. The criteria included the use of only one sample per father. Where data of several semen samples were available only the data from the first sample was included. Samples had to be complete and produced after an abstinence period of 3–7 days. The laboratories included in the study had to follow the 1999 WHO manual guidelines [14]. Sperm concentrations were determined by the haemocytometer method and sperm morphology evaluation performed according to STRICT CRITERIA [1]. A statement in the manual is included stipulating that men presenting with semen parameter values less than the lower fifth percentile (± 95 percent CI) reference values do not exclude the possibility of an in vivo pregnancy to occur [1].

5.5 Advantages and Disadvantages of Different Sperm Morphology Evaluation Procedures

With the lowering of the normal reference value to 4 percent of morphologically normal spermatozoa in the 2010 WHO manual, much of the potential predictive power of ≥14 percent of morphologically normal spermatozoa originally described has been lost [12, 13].

Several suggestions to overcome this adverse effect have been proposed. In order to obtain a higher cut-off value for normal morphology Rothmann and Bort [15] suggested an algorithm that approached the evaluation process to obtain the percentage of morphologically normal spermatozoa for a semen sample by means of an elimination process of abnormal spermatozoa. The questions are based on known sperm morphology defects included in the four main sperm abnormality classes cited above. By asking a series of very specific questions provided in the algorithm, all spermatozoa with known abnormalities are

excluded. The final conclusion on a sperms morphological normality is based on the outcome of the final question. If a spermatozoon with no abnormality or classification as borderline normal was identified, the spermatozoon is classified as normal. This renders a higher percentage of morphological normal forms. Results obtained using this algorithm showed a predictive value associated with fecundity in the National Institutes of Health Life study [15].

Menkveld [11] suggested that a wider approach should be followed where the type of abnormality or abnormalities should also be included in the final report and not the classification of normal or abnormal only as currently suggested by the 2010 WHO manual. The disadvantage of reporting only the percentage of morphologically normal spermatozoa is that the morphological normality of a spermatozoon is not an indication of a spermatozoon's ability to perform or undergo all the specific steps in the fertilization pathway. However, specific abnormal sperm morphology patterns can be associated with specific abnormal sperm functions [11].

Another disadvantage is that the 2010 WHO manual allows three different staining procedures. Different staining methods may provide different results for the percentage of morphologically normal spermatozoa present. This must be taken into consideration and the staining method reported as this may influence the interpretation and the prognostic value of the sperm morphology evaluation. For instance, Diff-Quik (D-Q) tends to cause some "swelling" of the spermatozoa, which may disguise some abnormalities and may end in identifying a higher percentage of morphologically normal spermatozoa compared to the Papanicolaou method. It is therefore important to use a sperm stain that alters the morphology of the original sperm shape as little as possible, for example the Papanicolaou and possibly the SpermBlue [10] staining. Papanicolaou staining has the advantage that so-called round cells can be recognized or classified as WBC and so-called "precursors", which include several stages of spermatogenetic cells such as the most common spermatids and also the earlier stages like primary and secondary spermatocytes which should normally not be present in a "normal" semen sample. The presence of these cells may indicate an aberration in the process of spermatogenesis due to internal or external stress factors, e.g. presence of WBC can cause excessive production of ROS species [11].

5.6 Clinical Significance of Sperm Morphology

The problem with the semen parameter values provided in the 2010 WHO guideline (Table 5.1) are that they are a single value for each semen parameter. As mentioned, these cut-off values are now referred to as lower reference limits or values based on the lower fifth percentile of a so-called fertile male population. This means that the female partners of the rest of the 5 percent of men included in the study also became pregnant. However, many persons believe that the lower reference values are imperial values and a value under the lower reference value renders the male partner infertile or even sterile. However, it is very important to take note of the fact that semen parameter results must be regarded as an indication of a male's fertility potential and that semen parameter values are largely not interactive or correlated to each other. The fact is, that above a certain numerical level for each semen parameter, there is no corresponding increase in the potential fertility of a male. However, the opposite is also true. The lower the semen parameter values, the lower is the fertility potential of that specific male until such low values are reached for all semen variables that the likelihood of a spontaneous pregnancy becomes very small. Certain of these semen values may be much lower than the values published in the 2010 WHO manual. Therefore, several articles [8, 16, 17] have been published where the semen variables are divided into three groups based on spontaneous pregnancy outcomes in vivo (Table 5.1); these three groups are potential fertile, potential subfertile and potential infertile. It is very important to note that even in the so-called infertile group spontaneous pregnancies are not excluded in cases where the female partner is deemed fertile and intercourse takes place regularly around the ovulation time span of the female partner [18].

5.7 When to Order the Test

The basic sperm morphology evaluation procedure should be regarded as part of the routine semen analysis and when in doubt about the result, the test should be repeated. Since clinical abnormalities are found in cases like a varicocele, especially combined with sperm DNA abnormalities, the test can be re-ordered after treatment, if any, with a clinical investigation. Other indications may be after treatment for male genital tract infections or illnesses combined with high fever for several days. After treatment for a varicocele with a varicocelectomy, a positive response in semen parameters including sperm morphology as well as a correspondent increase in normal sperm DNA content can be expected [19].

5.8 Clinical Case Scenarios

Taking the lower sperm morphology value of ≤ 3 percent normal forms into consideration in place of the normal sperm morphology values as illustrated in Table 5.1, the following theoretical scenarios can be put forward.

In the scenario as presented in Table 5.2, the semen parameters all fall in the potential fertile group. Treatment will depend on several factors such as the age of the couple. In cases of older women, assisted reproductive procedures may be indicated. Couples with a relatively short period of infertility can be advised to wait for some time before starting with

Table 5.1 Classification of Male Fertility Potential According to Classification of Semen Parameters Results Based on Pregnancy Outcome – Tygerberg Hospital Data (1972–1976)

Semen parameter	WHO 2010	Fertility potential classification		
		Infertile	Subfertile	Fertile
Concentration (10^6/ mL)	15.0	<2.0	2.0–9.9	$\geq$10.0
Motility (% progressive)	28.0	<10	10–29	$\geq$30
Morphology (% normal)	4.0	<10	10 –19	$\geq$20
Semen volume (mL)	1.5	<1.0	>6.0	1.0–6.0

Fertile or Normal = Optimal chance for pregnancy
Subfertile or Borderline = Reduced chance for pregnancy
Infertile or Pathological = Small chance for pregnancy

Table 5.2 Theoretical Treatment Options Based on Tygerberg Hospital Semen Classification and World Health Organization Lower Reference Limit Value for Sperm Morphology – Potentially Fertile Males

Semen parameter	Potential fertility classification		
	Infertile	Subfertile	Fertile
Concentration (10^6/ mL)	<2.0	2.0–9.9	≥10.0
Motility (% progressive)	<10	10–29	≥30
Morphology (% normal)	≤3	≤3	≥4
Semen volume (mL)	<1.0	>6.0	1.0–6.0

Table 5.3 Theoretical Treatment Options Based on Tygerberg Hospital Semen Classification and Lower World Health Organization Reference Limit Sperm Morphology Value – Potentially Subfertile Males

Semen parameter	Potential fertility classification		
	Infertile	Subfertile	Fertile
Concentration (10^6/ mL)	<2.0	2.0–9.9	≥10.0
Motility (% progressive)	<10	10–29	≥30
Morphology (% normal)	≤3	≤3	≤3
Semen volume (mL)	<1.0	>6.0	1.0–6.0

Table 5.4 Theoretical Treatment Options Based on Tygerberg Hospital Semen Classification and Lower World Health Organization Reference Limit Sperm Morphology Value – Potentially Infertile Males

Semen parameter	Potential fertility classification		
	Infertile	Subfertile	Fertile
Concentration (10^6/ mL)	<2.0	2.0–9.9	≥10.0
Motility (% progressive)	<10	10–29	≥30
Morphology (% normal)	≤3	≤3	≥4
Semen volume (mL)	<1.0	>6.0	1.0–6.0

the treatment. If a female factor is present, treatment with assisted reproductive technologies is indicated.

In Table 5.3, males who were originally classified as potential fertile are now classified as possible subfertile (due to the presence of ≤3% normal in the fertile classification group) and should now be treated in the same manner as potential subfertile males. Here, two scenarios may be possible. The first is to take the type of sperm abnormality present into consideration. In cases of so-called sterilizing defects like globozoospermia, short tail syndrome or immotile cilia syndrome, the only indication would be to perform intracytoplasmic sperm injection (ICSI). Other cases indicating that ICSI may be the only option will be cases of spermatozoa with small heads and/or small acrosome. In other cases where the extended sperm morphology analysis indicated the presence of mainly large-headed spermatozoa it may be useful to perform a sperm DNA integrity test. It has been reported that males presenting with <5 percent of morphologically normal spermatozoa do not per se present with a poor sperm DNA profile [20]. Using the TUNEL assay two groups of men were identified, those having a sufficient proportion of spermatozoa with normal DNA and those with low proportions of spermatozoa with normal DNA [20]. Where the sperm DNA content is normal and other semen parameters fall in either fertile of infertile group, ICSI or IVF treatment may be indicated. In cases with an abnormal percentage of spermatozoa present with abnormal DNA, the only possibility may be to perform ICSI. Although these cases may show normal fertilization rates, the pregnancy rates are very often low due to the role of the parental DNA in the development of the embryo after the six cell stage.

In scenario three as presented in Table 5.4 where all the semen parameters fall in the infertile group, ICSI will probably be the only treatment option.

References

1. World Health Organization. (2010) *WHO Laboratory Manual for the Examination and Processing of Human Semen*, 5th ed. Geneva: World Health Organization.

2. Van den Hoven L, Hendricks JC, Verbeet JG, Westphal JR, Wetzels AM. Status of sperm morphology assessment: an evaluation of methodology and clinical value. *Fertil Steril* 2015; **103**: 53–8.

3. Gatimel N, Mansoux L, Moreau J, Parinaud J, Léandri RD. Continued existence of significant disparities in the technical practice of sperm morphology assessment and the clinical implications: results of a French questionnaire. *Fertil Steril* 2017; **107**: 365–72.

4. Menkveld R, Stander FSH, Kotze TJW, Kruger TF, van Zyl JA. The evaluation of morphological characteristics of human spermatozoa according to stricter criteria. *Hum Reprod* 1990; **5**: 586–92.

5. Comhaire F, Schoonjans F, Vermeulen L, De Clercq N. Methodological aspects of sperm morphology evaluation: comparison between strict and liberal criteria. *Fertil Steril* 1994; **62**: 857–61.

6. Sigman M. Male reproduction – Semen analysis. *Fertil Steril* 2018; **110**: 278–81.

7. MacLeod J, Gold RZ. The male factor in fertility and infertility. IV. Sperm morphology in fertile and infertile marriage. *Fertil Steril* 1952; **2**: 394–414.

8. Eliasson R. Standards for investigation of human semen. *Andrologie* 1971; **3**: 49–64.

9. Menkveld R. (1987) An investigation of environmental influences on spermatogenesis and semen parameters. Ph.D. dissertation (in Afrikaans). Faculty of Medicine, University of Stellenbosch, South Africa.

10. Maree L, Du Plessis SS, Menkveld R, Van der Horst G. Morphometric dimensions of the human sperm head depends on the staining method used. *Hum Reprod* 2010; **25**: 1369–82.

11. Menkveld R. Sperm morphology assessment using strict (Tygerberg) criteria. *Methods Mol Biol* 2013; **927**: 39–50.

12. Menkveld R. Clinical significance of the low normal sperm morphology value as proposed in the 5th WHO laboratory manual for the examination and processing of human semen. *Asian J Androl* 2010; **12**: 47–58.

13. Menkveld R, Holleboom CAG, Rhemrev JPT. Measurement and significance of sperm morphology. *Asian J Androl* 2011; **13**: 59–68.

14. Cooper TG, Noonan E, von Eckardstein S, Auger J, Baker HWG, Behre HM, Haugen TB, Kruger T, Wang C, Mbizvo MT, Vogelsong KM. World Health Organization reference values for human semen characteristics. *Hum Reprod Update* 2010; **16**: 231–45.

15. Rothmann SA, Bort A-M. Sperm morphology. *Encyclopedia of Reproduction* 2018; **5**: 85–95.

16. Menkveld R. (2007) The basic semen analysis. *In* Oehninger S and Kruger TF, eds., *Male Infertility. Diagnosis and Treatment*. Oxford: Informa Healthcare, pp. 141–70.

17. Björndahl L, Mortimer D, Barratt CLR, Castilla JA, Menkveld R, Kvist U, Alvarez JG, Haugen TB. (2010) *A Practical Guide to Basic Laboratory Andrology*. Cambridge: Cambridge University Press.

18. Van Zyl JA, Menkveld R. Oligozoospermia: recent progress and outcome of 73 pregnancies in oligozoospermic couples. *Andrologia* 2006; **38**: 87–9.

19. Alhathal N, San-Gabriel M, Zini A. Beneficial effects of microsurgical varicocelectomy on sperm maturation, DNA fragmentation, and nuclear sulfhydryl groups: a prospective trail. *Andrology* 2016; **4**: 1204–8.

20. Henkel R, Hoogendijk CF, Bouic PJD, Kruger TF. Differential relationship between P- and G-pattern, normal sperm morphology and DNA fragmentation (Abstract). *J Reproduktionsmed Endokrinol* 2010; **7**: 290–1.

6

Sperm Vitality: Eosin-Nigrosin Dye Exclusion

Rakesh Sharma, Ashok Agarwal

6.1 Introduction/ Background

Assessment of sperm vitality is an important component of semen analysis. It helps to distinguish spermatozoa that are alive and immotile from those that are dead. Sperm vitality can be assessed routinely on all semen samples by assessing the membrane integrity of the cell by identifying the spermatozoa with an intact cell membrane. This can be done by using 1) the dye exclusion test or 2) the hypotonic or hypoosmotic swelling test. Sperm vitality can therefore provide a good comparison with the motility of the sample. Eosin is used as a marker for dead cells because eosin can penetrate the cells when the membrane is damaged, while cells that have an intact membrane remain unstained. Nigrosin is a background stain that increases the contrast to the otherwise faintly stained cells [1, 2, 3, 4]. Both the single step and two-step staining using eosin and nigrosin have been used to assess sperm vitality. Both the wet preparation and the air-dried methods have been compared to study the correlation with motility [5, 6, 7]. The wet preparations evaluated by using either positive or negative phase-contrast microscopy consistently showed higher percentage of nonviable cells compared to the air-dried eosin-nigrosin smears. The air-dried smears have consistently shown that the sum of the motile (viable) and stained (presumed dead) preparations never exceeded 100 percent indicating that the air-dried method is the method of choice for determining vitality. In this chapter, we describe the staining protocols for vitality, the cut-off of motility when vitality must be tested, indications for poor motility and quality control recommended for performing sperm vitality in conjunction with basic semen analysis.

6.2 Principle/Mechanism of Eosin-Nigrosin Test

The dye exclusion or the eosin-nigrosin test or the vitality test is based on the dye exclusion method as a result of structural damage in the sperm plasma membrane. A damaged sperm plasma membrane as in the case of dead cells looses its semi-permeability and forms tiny pores that allow normally membrane-impermeant stains to enter the cell, whereas an intact sperm membrane does not allow the stain to enter [8].

6.2.1 One-Step versus Two-Step Eosin-Nigrosin Test

The one-step eosin-nigrosin stain contains a mixture of eosin (0.67 percent) and nigrosin (10 percent) dissolved in water [3]. This technique was later modified by including 0.9 percent NaCl in distilled water [9]. Equal volumes of liquefied semen and eosin-nigrosin solution are mixed for 30 seconds at room temperature and smears are prepared for assessing vitality.

The two-step eosin-nigrosin technique was introduced by Eliasson in 1971 [13]. In this case, the solution contains 1 percent eosin Y and 10 percent nigrosin. Semen samples are incubated with eosin for 15 seconds and nigrosin for ≤15 seconds. This technique was later modified by Dougherty et al. [14] by incubating 5 percent eosin Y for 15 seconds and nigrosin for ≤15 seconds. Björndahl et al. compared the modified one-step technique with motility and found it to be reliable, easy and simple compared to the one-step eosin alone irrespective of the number of dead cells [9].

6.3 Preparation of Stains for One- and Two-Step Eosin-Nigrosin Technique

Sperm vitality can be measured using the eosin staining either alone or in combination with nigrosin.

6.3.1 One-Step Eosin-Nigrosin Technique

This technique uses nigrosin to increase the contrast between the background and the sperm heads making it easier to visualize [8, 9].

6.3.2 Preparation of the Reagents

6.3.2.1 Eosin Y

1. Dissolve eosin Y (0.67 g; color index 45380) and 0.9 g of sodium chloride in 100 mL of purified water with gentle heating.
2. Eosin-nigrosin solution: add 10 g of nigrosin (color index 50420) to the 100 mL of eosin Y solution.
3. Boil the suspension, allow it to cool to room temperature.
4. Filter the solution through filter paper (90g/m^2) to remove coarse and gelatinous precipitates.
5. Store in sealed dark-glass bottles.
6. After complete liquefaction, mix the semen sample thoroughly.
7. Mix equal volumes of the sample (50 µL) and eosin-nigrosin solution in a porcelain spot plate. Wait for 30 seconds.
8. Mix the sample again before removing another replicate aliquot and repeat step 7 above.
9. Make a smear on a glass slide and allow to air dry.
10. Mount with a cover slip and observe each slide with brightfield optics at 1000× magnification and oil immersion.
11. Evaluate at least 200 spermatozoa in replicate.
12. Calculate and report the average and percentage of vital cells from the replicate slides.
13. Report the percentage of vital spermatozoa to the nearest whole number.

6.3.3 Staining Using Eosin Alone

1. NaCl 0.9 percent (w/v): prepare by dissolving 0.9 g of NaCl in 100 mL of purified water.
2. Eosin Y: 0.5 percent (w/v): prepare by dissolving 0.5 g of eosin Y (color index 45380) in 100 mL of 0.9 percent NaCl.

6.3.4 Procedure for Staining

1. Mix the liquefied semen sample.
2. Mix one volume of the sample with equal volume of eosin Y solution on the microscope slide. Mix well by swirling the sample on the slide.
3. Cover with a 22 mm × 22 mm coverslip and leave for 30 seconds. Remix the sample and remove an aliquot, mix with eosin and repeat steps 2 and 3.
4. Examine each slide under a negative phase contrast optics at 200× or 400× magnification.
5. Evaluate at least 200 spermatozoa in duplicate.

6. Calculate and report the average and percentage of vital cells from the replicate slides.
7. Report the percentage of vital spermatozoa to the nearest whole number.

6.3.5 Two-Step Method (Cleveland Clinic Protocol)

The two-step protocol is described in detail using the eosin-nigrosin staining [10].

6.3.5.1 Eosin-Y 1 Percent Solution (Figure 6.1):

1. Weigh 0.5 g of eosin-Y and add to 50 mL of deionized water.
2. Dissolve this solution using gentle heat.
3. Cool the liquid to room temperature and filter using filter paper.

Note: This reagent is stable for three months at room temperature.

6.3.5.2 Nigrosin 10 Percent Solution (Figure 6.2):

1. Add 5 g of nigrosin to 50 mL of deionized water.
2. Dissolve this solution using gentle heat.
3. Cool the liquid to room temperature and filter using filter paper.

Note: This reagent is stable for three months at room temperature.

6.3.6 Procedure

1. Label two frosted slides with the medical record number, the patient's name, and date.

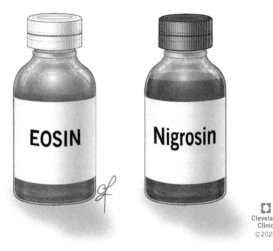

Cleveland Clinic
©2020

Figure 6.1 Eosin-Y 1 percent solution and nigrosin 10 percent solution.

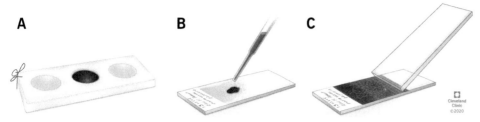

Figure 6.2 Mixing of the stain in (A): a Boerner slide well and (B–C): preparation of the smear.

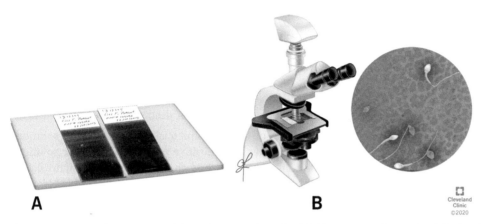

· **Figure 6.3** A): Stained eosin-nigrosin slides with a cover slip; B): brightfield microscope showing live (white) and dead (pink) spermatozoa. 1000x magnification

2. Place one drop of well-mixed semen into Boerner slide well.
3. Add two drops of 1 percent aqueous eosin-Y.
4. Mix well with a wooden stirrer for 15 seconds.
5. Add two drops of 10 percent aqueous nigrosin.
6. Mix well with a wooden stirrer in Boerner slide well (Figure 6.2).
7. Immediately make two thin smears from this mixture by pipetting 10 μL onto each labeled slide (Figure 6.3A). Allow the slides to air dry.
8. Coverslip with Cytoseal mounting media.

6.3.7 Scoring

1. Nigrosin provides a dark background that makes it easier to distinguish faintly stained spermatozoa.
2. Using oil at 1000× magnification, observe spermatozoa under bright field microscopy (Figure 6.3B).
3. Record the percentage of viable sperm.

4. Spermatozoa with pink or dark red heads are considered dead.

Note:

1. Sperm vitality should be tested as soon as possible after liquefaction of the semen sample, preferably within 30 minutes, but no later than one hour after ejaculation. This is important to avoid the deleterious effects of dehydration or changes in temperature on vitality.
2. Once mixed with the stain, smears must be made as soon as possible (within 30 seconds) to avoid over staining.
3. The percentage of viable cells normally exceeds that of motile cells. The vitality should be greater than or equal to the specimen motility.
4. Spermatozoa with a faint pink head are considered as alive. If the stain is only limited to part of the neck region, and the rest of the head area is unstained, this is considered a "leaky neck membrane" and is not a sign of cell death.

6.4 Clinical Interpretation of the Test

Vitality is a confirmatory test of the poor sperm motility. The total number of membrane-intact spermatozoa in the ejaculate is of biological significance.

Semen samples with a large proportion of vital but non-motile cells are indicative of structural defects in the flagellum [11]. The presence of a high percentage of immotile and non-viable cells (necrozoospermia) may be indicative of epididymal pathology [12].

6.5 Advantages and Disadvantages of the Eosin-Nigrosin Test

It is a simple, easy and cost effective test. It does not require any expensive equipment and can be performed in a simple lab setting.

6.6 Clinical Significance of the Eosin-Nigrosin Test

It is important to differentiate between necrozoospermia and asthenozoospermia. Patients with Kartagener syndrome have absence of dynein arms and are characterized by ciliary dyskinesia or defects in the axonemal apparatus that results in immotile sperm.

6.7 When to Order an Eosin-Nigrosin Test

According to WHO's fifth edition [8], vitality slides must be prepared when the total motility is lower than 40 percent. According to WHO's fourth edition [4], the test must be performed when the type "a" motility is less than 25 percent.

6.7.1 Normal Range

The lower reference limit for vitality according to the WHO's fifth edition is 58 percent (fifth centile, 95 percent CI 55–63).

Note: For specimens with <40 percent motility, the vitality should be greater than or equal to the specimen motility.

6.7.2 Clinical Scenario

A patient provides a semen sample with an ejaculate volume of 2.5 mL, sperm concentration of 40×10^6/mL and 6 percent normal morphology. Upon examination, no sperm are displaying any kind of motility.

In this scenario, it is important to know if the non-motile sperm are viable or not. This can be easily confirmed by the eosin-nigrosin test.

6.7.3 Sources of Error or Variation in Assessing Sperm Vitality

I.   Use of incorrect magnification
II. Improper staining
III. Excessive delay in preparation of the smear
IV. Overestimation of dead spermatozoa

Use of some commercially available eosin solutions can give false–positive results because these solutions are hypotonic and these stress the spermatozoa. In such cases it is recommended to add 0.9 g of NaCl to 100 mL of solution in order to increase osmolality of eosin solution [7].

6.8 Quality Control

1. A monthly patient control should be run to check the quality of reagents. The specimen's motility should be assessed prior to the quality control (QC) run.
2. When new reagents are prepared, QC must be performed before they can be used for a new patient specimen.
3. The specimen should be stained with the old lot of reagents as well as the new lot of reagents. Both sets of slides should be scored for the vitality percent results.
4. The comparison of the two lots of reagents should be within 10 percent of each other.
5. If results are not within the acceptable range, repeat using another specimen.

References

1. Blom E. A one-minute live-dead sperm stain by means of Eosin-Nigrosin. *Fertil Steril* 1950; **1**: 176–7.

2. Eliasson R. Supravital staining of human spermatozoa. *Fertil Steril* 1977; **28**: 1257.

3. Mortimer D, Curtis EF, Camenzind AR. Combined use of fluorescent peanut agglutinin lectin and Hoechst 33258 to monitor the acrosomal status and vitality of human spermatozoa. *Hum Reprod* 1990; **5**: 99–103.

4. World Health Organization. (1999) *WHO Laboratory Manual*

for the Examination of Human Semen and Sperm-Cervical Mucus Interactions, 4th ed. Cambridge: Cambridge University Press.

5. Cooper TG, Hellenkemper B. Method-related estimates of sperm vitality. *J Androl* 2009; **30**: 214–18.

6. Moskovtsev SI, Librach CL. (2013) Methods of sperm vitality assessment. In Douglas T. Carrell and Kenneth I. Aston, eds., *Spermatogenesis: Methods and Protocols, Methods in Molecular Biology*, vol. 927. London: Springer Science+Business Media, LLC. doi: 10.1007/978-1-62703-038-0_2

7. Björndahl L, Söderlund I, Johansson S, Mohammadieh M, Pourian MR, Kvist U. Why the WHO recommendations for eosin-nigrosin staining techniques for human sperm vitality

assessment must change. *J Androl* 2004; **25**: 671–8.

8. World Health Organization. (2010) *WHO Laboratory Manual for Examination of Human Semen and Sperm-Cervical Mucus Interaction*, 5th ed. Cambridge: Cambridge University Press.

9. Björndahl L, Söderlund I, Kvist U. Evaluation of the one-step eosin-nigrosin staining technique for human sperm vitality assessment. *Hum Reprod* 2003; **18**: 813–16.

10. Agarwal A, Gupta S, Sharma R. (2016) Eosin-nigrosin staining procedure. In Agarwal A, Gupta S and Sharma R, eds., *Andrological Evaluation of Male Infertility*. London: Springer International Publishing, pp. 73–7.

11. Chemes EH, Rawe YV. Sperm pathology: a step beyond descriptive morphology. Origin,

characterization and fertility potential of abnormal sperm phenotypes in infertile men. *Hum Reprod Update* 2003; **9**: 405–28.

12. Correa-Pérez JR, Fernández-Pelegrina R, Aslanis P, Zavos PM. Clinical management of men producing ejaculates characterized by high levels of dead sperm and altered seminal plasma factors consistent with epididymal necrospermia. *Fertil Steril* 2004; **81**: 1148–50.

13. Eliasson R, Treichl MB. Supravital staining of human spermatozoa. *Fertil Steril* 1971; **22**: 134–7.

14. Dougherty KA, Emilson LB, Cockett AT, Urry RL. A comparison of subjective measurements of human sperm motility and viability with two live-dead staining techniques. *Fertil Steril* 1975; **26**: 700–3.

Sperm Vitality: Hypo-Osmotic Swelling Test

Alexandre Rouen, Rajasingam S Jeyendran

7.1 Physiological Aspects

The hypo-osmotic swelling (HOS) test, introduced in 1987 to assess the functional integrity of the human sperm membrane, appears to have withstood the test of time. Many articles have been published on the subject since its inclusion in the third edition of the World Health Organization (WHO) manual in 1992 [1, 2, 3, 4, 5].

The concept of the HOS test is that only sperm with intact membranes will swell (balloon) when exposed to hypo-osmotic conditions due to the influx of water, thus indicating that the membrane is morphologically intact and physiologically active [6]. A membrane, such as the one used for dialysis, will allow solutes of a certain size to passively pass through it to maintain osmotic equilibrium when exposed to hypo-osmotic conditions, a phenomenon called semi-permeability. A physiologically active membrane, however, will prevent such an osmotic equilibrium until it reaches a critical stage when the osmotic stress cannot be actively managed, resulting in rupture of the membrane. Indeed, physiologically, the osmolarity in the intracellular compartment is higher than that of the extracellular compartment, resulting in an osmotic pressure gradient. This would normally cause an influx of water into the cell, which would in turn cause swelling, if it was not for the presence of active ionic transport processes (physiologically active membrane). The maintenance of cell volume relies heavily on those systems. However, they are only efficient up to a certain point, and in very low osmolarity environment, such as during the HOS test, they can be overwhelmed, leading to cell swelling [7].

The HOS test evaluates different characteristics of the sperm membrane as compared to the dye exclusion test. The dye exclusion test is based on how the living cell membrane acts as a physical barrier to dye penetration, thus, not allowing nuclear staining. When the membrane is damaged, such as that found in non-vital (dead) cells, it allows the entry of dye into the cell. Treatment of sperm with the membrane fixative glutaraldehyde (2 percent) had no significant effect on Eosin Y (0.5 percent) uptake versus non-treated cells. In contrast, almost no swelling was observed in the HOS test after glutaraldehyde treatment [8], suggesting that membrane function, rather than a physically intact membrane, is of critical importance when sperm are subjected to a HOS test. In addition, electron microscopy indicated that the sperm membrane of the tail bulges and swells in response to the hypo-osmotic condition. Bollendorf et al. [9] emphasized this phenomenon, showing that the majority of patients with a subnormal HOS test have a normal vitality based on the dye exclusion test, and that only 12.5 percent of men with a low HOS test exhibit low vitality. It therefore appears that while the dye exclusion test explores the membrane in a structural way, the HOS test is based on its functional capacities, which explains the discrepancy between dye exclusion and HOS tests.

7.2 Technical Aspects

The HOS test is performed by combining 0.1 mL of ejaculate with 1.0 mL of a hypo-osmotic solution prepared by mixing 7.35 g sodium citrate and 13.51 g fructose in 1 L of distilled H_2O. After incubation of the solution for at least 30–60 minutes, but no more than 120 minutes at 37^0C, 100 or 200 spermatozoa are observed with a phase contrast microscope, and the percentage of spermatozoa with tail changes typical of a reaction in the HOS test (swollen, HOS-reactive, or HOS-positive spermatozoa) is determined [6, 10]. No additional equipment is required. The spermatozoa can be fixed with formaldehyde (18.5 percent, 0.1 mL) or ethanol/acetic acid (3:1), which retains the shape of the spermatozoa, so that they can be stored and observed at a later date [11]. A longitudinal study evaluating the semen quality monthly over nine months from 45 men revealed a mean of 64.08 percent HOS-positive with a median fluctuating only 7 percent over that period, which highlights the precision and reproducibility of the HOS test as compared to sperm motility [12].

7.3 Hypo-Osmotic-Swelling-Positive Spermatozoa Evaluation as a Diagnostic Tool

Ejaculates are classified as normal if they contain 60 percent or more HOS-positive spermatozoa and are regarded as abnormal if fewer than 50 percent of the spermatozoa are HOS-positive. The 50–59 percent range is considered "equivocal" [11]. The large majority (96 percent) of the ejaculates from 1890 participants who requested a vasectomy gave more than 60 percent HOS-positive spermatozoa [13]. Additional studies have confirmed the validity of these cut-off values, based on outcomes such as pregnancy rates or embryo implantation rates [14, 15, 16, 17, 18].

A physiologically active membrane is a prerequisite for sperm motility, capacitation, acrosome reaction and binding of the spermatozoon to the oolemma. The HOS test may detect subtle injury or incompetence of the sperm plasma membrane, which may be responsible for the reduced fertilizing potential of the sperm that results in non-viable embryos, low pregnancy rates, or miscarriages. Thus, the assessment of the sperm membrane may prove valuable in routine semen analysis, especially when the value of conventional semen analysis is the subject of debate [19].

Although significant, the correlation between the dye exclusion test and the HOS test results is surprisingly low with a correlation coefficient of r = 0.52 [6], even though the HOS test had initially been thought to evaluate sperm vitality, similarly to the dye exclusion test. In addition, the correlation coefficients between the HOS test results and several standard sperm parameters are generally so low that the outcome of the HOS test cannot be accurately predicted from these other observations [20]. However, the correlation between the HOS test results and the zona-free hamster egg penetration (Sperm Penetration Assay; SPA) as well as in vitro fertilization outcome is very high [6, 11, 21, 22, 23, 24, 25, 26]. Multiple studies have reported on the ability of the HOS test to predict in vivo and in vitro

pregnancies [2, 17, 26, 27, 28, 29] as well as recurrent pregnancy loss [30, 31, 32].

Using the HOS test as an independent variable for sperm function and the IVF outcome (fertile/infertile) as the dependent variable in a forward logistic regression analysis, the HOS test could correctly predict the IVF outcome in 88.4 percent of the cases with 12.0 percent false positive and 7.7 percent false negative rate [23](Jeyendran et al., 1989).

Check et al. [2, 15] concluded that the results of the HOS test are significantly more reliable than the results of the standard semen analysis as a predictor of conception. These investigators found that no couple, regardless of the standard semen analysis results, achieved a pregnancy when the HOS test was abnormal. By contrast, even if the semen analysis was abnormal, the large majority of men were able to fertilize their partners' oocytes as long as the HOS test was normal or equivocal (i.e., ≥ 50 percent reactive spermatozoa). Comparing the HOS test with normal sperm morphology, SPA, and IVF, Coetzee et al. [22] concluded that an abnormal HOS test was the most reliable indicator of a male factor infertility.

Incidentally, the HOS test has also been effectively used to evaluate spermicidal effects of chemotherapeutic agents [33, 34], pesticides [35] and to screen potential contraceptive agents [36, 37]. Polystyrene and polypropylene specimen containers affect the HOS test response as compared to glass containers [15]. Moreover, common laboratory treatment procedures may also influence the hypo-osmotic swelling responses [38]. Finally, the HOS test also appears to be useful as a measure of cryosurvival [16, 39, 40].

7.4 A Further Look: The Hypo-Osmotic Swelling Classification

The different types of tail swelling that can be observed under hypo-osmotic condition are: no tail swelling (a), swelling present only at the tip of the tail (b and c), bending at the hairpin curvature of the tail (d and e), shortened and thickened tail (f), and swelling of the entire tail (g), as described by Jeyendran et al. [6] (Figure 7.1). With regard to this classification, sperm that were formerly classified as "HOS-positive" are sperm that exhibit a flagellar swelling, that is to say a swelling of the "b" to "g" categories. Continuous monitoring of tail swelling changes of individual sperm revealed several subsets of sperm

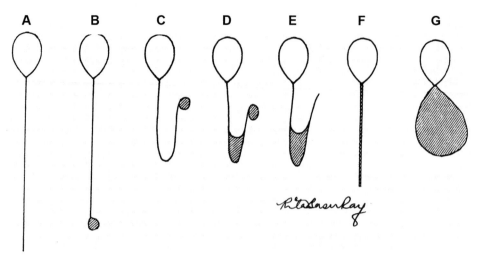

A   B   C   D   E   F   G

Figure 7.1 Schematic representation of typical morphological changes in human spermatozoa subjected to hypo-osmotic stress. (A) No change, (B)–(G) various types of tail changes. Swelling in tail is indicated by the hatched area.

populations within an ejaculate that respond differently to hypo-osmotic stress [41]. It has been proposed that the differential analysis of the various types of tail curling may aid in minimizing false positives [42]. For instance Bassiri et al. [43] compared different types of sperm swelling under hypo-osmotic conditions and concluded that the sperm with the tail tip swelling were the most competent based on analysis of head morphology, DNA fragmentation, protamine deficiency (nuclear immaturity marker) and Annexin V expression (apoptotic marker). Stranger et al. [44] had previously confirmed the DNA competency of the sperm with tail tip swelling.

In that study, looking at the different HOS classes, the HOS test morphology exhibited a stronger association with DNA fragmentation than with the presence of head vacuoles, suggesting that membrane alteration is an earlier phenomenon than vacuole formation in sperm physiology. They showed that abnormal sperm samples (based on routine semen analysis) exhibited a higher proportion of HOS test-positive "a" spermatozoa, and a lower proportion of HOS test "d/e" and "f" spermatozoa, suggesting that the latter are associated with normal fertility potential. Similar results were obtained with regards to DNA fragmentation, with the "d/e" and "f" classes carrying the lowest DNA fragmentation rate. Bassiri et al. [43] showed similar results, this time suggesting that the "b" and "d" classes were associated with the most fertile sperm in terms of DNA fragmentation,

protamine deficiency, and externalization of phosphatidylserine. These two studies were performed not at the sperm level, but at the global level, looking at the aforementioned quality parameters globally, and correlating them to the respective proportion of each HOST class.

7.5 Hypo-Osmotic Swelling Test-Based Sperm Selection

As opposed to those two studies, the following were performed "cell by cell", looking at each cell individually based on their HOST class, suggesting the HOS test could be used to select spermatozoa during intra-cytoplasmic sperm injection (ICSI). Pang et al. [5] showed that HOS can allow for the selection of sperm with a lower rate of aneuploidy in patients with a normal karyotype, with 17 times less aneuploid sperm in the "b", "c", and "d" types as compared to the rate observed prior to the HOS test. Rouen et al. [45] evidenced that the HOS test could be used to select chromosomally balanced spermatozoa in chromosomal rearrangement carriers (reciprocal and Robertsonian translocations, pericentric inversions), describing a new HOS test class termed "b+". These results on normal karyotype aneuploidy and abnormal segregation in chromosomal rearrangement carriers suggest that membrane integrity can be viewed as a reflection of nuclear balance and organization. Rouen et al. hypothesized that an abnormal chromosomal content would prevent full nuclear condensation, and, in turn, might initiate an early apoptosis process, altering the sperm membrane. This membrane alteration would consequently alter the sperm response to hypo-osmolarity, and affect the tail conformation when incubated in a hypo-osmotic solution. These studies conclude that the HOS test may aid in selecting chromosomally balanced spermatozoa in patients with high aneuploidy rates or chromosomal rearrangement carriers, and selecting spermatozoa with high nuclear and membrane quality. Recent studies by Rouen et al. (to be published) suggest that in patients with a normal karyotype, b+ spermatozoa might be associated with significantly lower rates of DNA fragmentation and DNA decondensation and a more normal nuclear architecture. This suggests that b+ spermatozoa would be the most competent.

Since the HOS test identifies sperm with intact functional membranes without altering them, it has been effectively utilized to select sperm for ICSI from a population of non-motile sperm [3, 4, 46, 47, 48, 49, 50, 51, 52]. Indeed, according to the WHO guidelines [53], it is possible and safe to perform HOS prior to ICSI, in order to select viable spermatozoa. Recent studies suggest that this could also be used to select highly competent spermatozoa in a way to optimize reproductive outcome.

7.6 Conclusion

The HOS test is of particular interest for routine semen analysis because it measures an entirely different entity than the already existing sperm parameters. Compilation of all the data that have been published so far, and reanalysis, where appropriate and possible, leads to the conclusion that the HOS test provides additional information not obtained by conventional semen analysis. An abnormal HOS test is often associated with poor results in the SPA and unsuccessful IVF, and in-vivo fertilization rarely occurs when the HOS test is abnormal and is independent of the other semen parameters. Thus, an abnormal HOS test provides reasonable certainty that the ejaculate is infertile [54]. Furthermore, it has been suggested that response to hypo-osmolarity not only reflects membrane integrity, but also spermatic nuclear organization. On this basis, it can be concluded that the HOS test is a useful adjunct to existing sperm assays and could be included as a standard test during routine semen analysis. In addition, the HOS test can be used to monitor other sperm procedures, such as sperm selection for ICSI, sperm processing, sperm cryosurvival, and the effect of toxins on sperm. Finally, HOS can also be used to inject highly competent spermatozoa prior to ICSI, in patients with high aneuploidy rates, in patients with chromosomal rearrangements, or even in the global infertile population.

References

1. World Health Organization. (1992) *WHO Laboratory Manual for the Examination of Human Semen and Semen-Cervical Mucus Interaction*. Cambridge: Cambridge University Press.

2. Check JH, Epstein R, Nowroozi K, Shanis BS, Wu CH, Bollendorf A. The hypoosmotic swelling test as a useful adjunct to the semen analysis to predict fertility potential. *Fertil Steril* 1989; **52**(1): 159–61

3. Casper RF, Meriano JS, Jarvi KA, Cowan L, Lucato ML. The hypo-osmotic swelling test for selection of viable sperm for intracytoplasmic sperm injection in men with complete

asthenozoospermia. *Fertil Steril* 1996; **65**(5): 972–6.

4. Ahmadi A, Ng SC. The single sperm curling test, a modified hypo-osmotic swelling test, as a potential technique for the selection of viable sperm for intracytoplasmic sperm injection. *Fertil Steril* 1997; **68**(2): 346–50.

5. Pang MG, You YA, Park YJ, Oh SA, Kim DS, Kim YJ. Numerical chromosome abnormalities are associated with sperm tail swelling patterns. *Fertil Steril* 2010; **94**: 1012–20.

6. Jeyendran RS, Van der Ven HH, Perez-Pelaez M,Crabo BG, Zaneveld LJD. Development of an assay to assess the functional integrity of the human sperm membrane and its relationship to

other semen characteristics. *J Reprod Fertil* 1984; **70**: 219–28.

7. Cheng X, Pinsky PM. The balance of fluid and osmotic pressures across active biological membranes with application to the corneal endothelium. *PLOS ONE* 2015; **10**: e0145422.

8. Schrader SM, Platek SF, Zaneveld LJD, et al. Sperm viability: a comparison of analytical methods. *Andrologia* 1986; **18**: 530–8.

9. Bollendorf A, Check JH, Kramer D. The majority of males with subnormal hypoosmotic test scores have normal vitality. *Clin Exp Obstet Gynecol* 2012; **39**(1): 25–6.

10. Ramu S, Jeyendran RS. The hypo-osmotic swelling test for evaluation of sperm membrane

integrity. *Methods Mol Biol* 2013; **927**: 21–5.

11. Van der Ven HH, Jeyendran RS, Al-Hasani S, Perez-Pelaez M, Diedrich K, Zaneveld LJD. Correlation between human sperm swelling in hypoosmotic medium (hypoosmotic swelling test) and in vitro fertilization. *J Androl* 1986; **7**: 190–6.

12. Schrader SM, Turner TW, Breitenstein MJ, Simon SD. Longitudinal study of semen quality of unexposed workers. I. Study overview. *Reprod Toxicol* 1988; **2**(3–4): 183–90.

13. de Castro M, Jeyendran RS, Zaneveld LJD. Hypoosmotic swelling test: analysis of prevasectomy ejaculates. *Arch Androl* 1990; **24**: 11–16.

14. Van Kooij RT, Balerna M, Roatti A, Campana Z. Oocyte penetration and acrosome reactions of human sperms. II: Correlation with other seminal parameters. *Andrologia* 1986; **18**: 503–8.

15. Check JH, Nowroozi K, Wu CH, Bollendorf A. Correlation of semen analysis and hypoosmotic swelling test with subsequent pregnancies. *Arch Androl* 1988; **20**: 257–60.

16. Check ML, Check JH. Poor hypo-osmotic swelling test results from cryopreserved sperm despite preservation of sperm motility. *Arch Androl* 1991; **26**(1): 37–41.

17. Tartagni M, Cicinelli E, Schonauer MM, Causio F, Petruzzelli F, Loverro G. Males with subnormal hypo-osmotic swelling test scores have lower pregnancy rates than those with normal scores when ovulation induction and timed intercourse is used as a treatment for mild problems with sperm count, motility, or morphology. *J Androl* 2004; **25**(5): 781–3.

18. Check JH, Aly J. Sperm with an abnormal hypo-osmotic swelling test – normal fertilization, normal embryo development, but implantation failure. *Clin Exp Obstet Gynecol* 2016; **43**(3): 319–27.

19. De Jonge C. Semen analysis: looking for an upgrade in class. *Fertil Steril* 2012; **97**: 260–6.

20. Jeyendran RS, Van der Ven HH, Zaneveld LJD. The hypoosmotic swelling test: an update. *Arch Androl* 1992; **29**: 105–16.

21. Wang C, Chan SYW, Ng M, So WWK, Tsoi W, Lo T, Leung A. Diagnostic value of sperm function test and routine semen analysis in fertile and infertile men. *J Androl* 1988; **9**: 384–9.

22. Coetzee K, Krunger FT, Menkveld R, Lombard CJ, Swanson RJ. Hypoosmotic swelling test in the prediction of male fertility. *Arch Androl* 1989; **23**: 131–8.

23. Jeyendran RS, Van der Ven HH, Rachagan SP, Perez-Plaeaz M, Zaneveld LJD. Semen quality and in-vitro fertilization. *Aust NZ J Obsetet Gynecol* 1989; **29**: 168–72.

24. Check JH, Stumpo L, Lurie D, Benfer K, Callan CA. Comparative prospective study using matched samples to determine the influence of subnormal hypo-osmotic test scores of spermatozoa on subsequent fertilization and pregnancy rates following in-vitro fertilization. *Hum Reprod* 1995; **10**(5): 1197–200.

25. Mladenović I, Mićić S, Genbaćev O, Papić N. Hypoosmotic swelling test for quality control of sperm prepared for assisted reproduction. *Arch Androl* 1995; **4**(3): 163–9.

26. Tartagni M, Schonauer MM, Cicinelli E, Selman H, De Ziegler D, Petruzzelli F, D'Addario V. Usefulness of the hypo-osmotic swelling test in predicting pregnancy rate and outcome in couples undergoing intrauterine insemination. *J Androl* 2002; **23**(4): 498–502.

27. Datta S, Giri A, Datta AK. Role of hypo-osmotic sperm swelling test in assisted reproduction. *J Indian Med Assoc* 1996; **94**(12): 440–2.

28. Kiefer D, Check JH, Katsoff D. The value of motile density, strict morphology, and the hypoosmotic swelling test in in vitro fertilization-embryo transfer. *Arch Androl* 1996; **37**(1): 57–60.

29. Jedrzejczak P, Taszarek-Hauke G, Hauke J, Pawelczyk L, Duleba AJ. Prediction of spontaneous conception based on semen parameters. *Int J Androl* 2008; **31**(5): 499–507.

30. Patankar SS, Deshkar AM, Sawane MV, Mishra NV, Kale AH, Gosavi GB. The role of hypo-osmotic swelling test in recurrent abortions. *Indian J Physiol Pharmacol* 2001; **45**(3): 373–7.

31. Saxena P, Misro MM, Chaki SP, Chopra K, Roy S, Nandan D. Is abnormal sperm function an indicator among couples with recurrent pregnancy loss? *Fertil Steril* 2008; **90**(5): 1854–8.

32. Bhattacharya SM. Hypo-osmotic swelling test and unexplained repeat early pregnancy loss. *J Obstet Gynaecol Res* 2010; **36**(1): 119–22.

33. Kohn FM, Schuppe HC, Schill WB, Jeyendran RS. Hydrogen hexachloroplatinate induces the acrosome reaction in human spermatozoa. *Int J Androl* 1995; **18**(6): 321–5.

34. Reiter WJ, Tomek S, Zielinski CC, Marberger M. Effect of carboplatin on the functional integrity of the human sperm membrane in vitro. *J Androl* 2002; **23**(3): 338–40.

35. Ratcliffe JM, Schrader SM, Steenland K, Clapp DE, Turner T, Hornung RW. Semen quality in papaya workers with long term exposure to ethylene dibromide. *Br J Ind Med* 1987; **44**(5): 317–26.

36. Ratnasooriya WD, Jayawardena KGI, Wadsworth RM. Effects of enalapril on human sperm motility. *Contracept* 1990; **41**(2): 213–19.

37. Ratnasooriya WD, Premakumara GAS. Effects of the prostanoid receptor antagonist, di-4-phloretin phosphate, upon human sperm motility. *Contracept* 1992; **45**(3): 239–48.

38. Hossain AM, Selukar R, Barik S. Differential effect of common laboratory treatments on hypoosmotic swelling responses of human spermatozoa. *J Assist Reprod Genet* 1999; **16**(1): 30–4.

39. Jeyendran RS, Van der Ven HH, Perez-Pelaez M, Zaneveld LJD. Nonbeneficial effects of glycerol on the oocyte penetrating capacity of cryopreserved and incubated human spermatozoa. *Cryobiology* 1985; **22**(5): 434–7.

40. Bachtell NE, Conaghan J, Turek PJ. The relative viability of human spermatozoa from the vas deferens, epididymis and testis before and after cryopreservation. *Hum Reprod* 1999; **14**(12): 3048–51.

41. Hossain AM, Rizk B, Barik S, Huff C, Thorneycroft IH. Time course of hypo-osmotic swellings of human spermatozoa: evidence of ordered transition between swelling subtypes. *Hum Reprod* 1998; **13**: 1578–83.

42. Chan SW, Wang C, Ng M, et al. Evaluation of computerized analysis of sperm movement characteristics and differential sperm tail swelling patterns in predicting human sperm in vitro fertilizing capacity. *J Androl* 1989; **10**: 133–8.

43. Bassiri F, Tavalaee M, Shiravi AH, Mansouri S, Nasr-Esfahani MH. Is there an association between HOST grades and sperm quality? *Hum Reprod* 2012; **27**(8): 2277–84.

44. Stranger JD, Vo L, Yovich JL, Almahbobi G. Hypo-osmotic swelling test identifies individual spermatozoa with minimal DNA fragmentation. *Reprod Biomed Online* 2010; **21**: 474–84.

45. Rouen A, Carlier L, Heide S, Egloff M, Marzin P, Ader F, Schwartz M, Rogers E, Joyé N, Balet R, Lédée N, Prat-Ellenberg L, Cassuto NG, Siffroi JP. Potential selection of genetically balanced spermatozoa based on the hypo-osmotic swelling test in chromosomal rearrangement carriers. *Reprod Biomed Online* 2017; **35**(4): 372–8.

46. Liu J, Tsai YL, Katz E, Compton G, Garcia JE, Baramki TA. High fertilization rate obtained after intracytoplasmic sperm injection with 100% nonmotile spermatozoa selected by using a simple modified hypo-osmotic swelling test. *Fertil Steril* 1997; **68**(2): 373–5.

47. Vandervorst M, Tournaye H, Camus M, Nagy ZP, Van Steirteghem A, Devroey P. Patients with absolutely immotile spermatozoa and intracytoplasmic sperm injection. *Hum Reprod* 1997; **12**: 2429–33.

48. Ved S, Montag M, Schmutzler A, Prietl G, Haidl G, van der Ven H. Pregnancy following intracytoplasmic sperm injection of immotile spermatozoa selected by the hypo-osmotic swelling-test: a case report. *Andrologia* 1997; **29**(5): 241–2.

49. Sallam H, Farrag A, Agameya A, Ezzeldin F, Eid A, Sallam A. The use of a modified hypo-osmotic swelling test for the selection of viable ejaculated and testicular immotile spermatozoa in ICSI. *Hum Reprod* 2001; **16**(2): 272–6.

50. Westlander G, Barry M, Petrucco O, Norman R. Different fertilization rates between immotile testicular spermatozoa and immotile ejaculated spermatozoa for ICSI in men with Kartagener's syndrome: case reports. *Hum Reprod* 2003; **18**(6): 1286–8.

51. Peeraer K, Nijs M, Raick D, Ombelet W. Pregnancy after ICSI with ejaculated immotile spermatozoa from a patient with immotile cilia syndrome: a case report and review of the literature. *Reprod Biomed Online* 2004; **9**(6): 659–63.

52. Sallam HN, Farrag A, Agameya AF, El-Garem Y, Ezzeldin F. The use of the modified hypo-osmotic swelling test for the selection of immotile testicular spermatozoa in patients treated with ICSI: a randomized controlled study. *Hum Reprod* 2005; **20**(12): 3435–40.

53. World Health Organization. (2010) *WHO Laboratory Manual for the Examination of Human Semen and Semen-Cervical Mucus Interaction*. Cambridge: Cambridge University Press.

54. Jeyendran RS, Zaneveld LJD. Controversies in the developments and validation of new sperm assays. *Fertil Steril* 1993; **59**: 726–8.

57

Determination of Mitochondrial Membrane Potential by Flow Cytometry in Human Sperm Cells

Nicolas Germain, Nathalie Jouy, Carole Marchetti, Philippe Marchetti

8.1 Introduction

8.1.1 Sperm Mitochondria and Male Fertility

Mitochondria are crucial organelles of eukaryotic aerobic cells (somatic and germ cells) because they produce adenosine triphosphate (ATP) and are modulators of ion homeostasis, generators of free radicals and regulators of cell death. Numerous studies reported that mitochondrial functionality was associated with sperm quality. Indeed, mitochondrial activities regulate many important sperm functions including sperm motility, hyperactivation, capacitation, acrosome reaction, and fertilization [1]. The exact mechanisms that link mitochondrial activities and sperm functions are often poorly understood or remain debated. Sperm mitochondria are arranged in the midpiece close to the flagellar. It seemed obvious that mitochondrial injuries can result in decreased sperm motility since motility is an ATP-dependent process, thus reliant on the energetic function of mitochondria for powering the flagellar motion. However, increasing evidence suggests that the dependence on mitochondria-derived ATP for human sperm motility is not unique and that glycolysis may replace mitochondrial oxidative phosphorylation [2]. Furthermore, spermatozoa can adapt their metabolic pathways depending on the availability of substrates. This is feasible since sperm mitochondria possess specific enzyme isoforms with distinct kinetics [2]. In addition to their role as an ATP producer, mitochondria regulate the lifespan of spermatozoa. Reduction in mitochondrial activities judged by the drop in the mitochondrial membrane potential ($\Delta\psi$m) has been regarded as an early cell death event [3]. The relevance of sperm mitochondria in fertility may also be associated with their role in the intermediate metabolism as producer of reactive oxygen species (ROS) or as regulator of intracellular calcium homeostasis, which are known to regulate proper sperm functions [4].

Irrespective of these mechanistic considerations, numerous clinical studies indicate that the determination of mitochondrial function constitutes a proper method for evaluating sperm quality and therefore male fertility.

8.1.2 Mitochondrial Functionality and the Inner Mitochondrial Membrane Potential ($\Delta\psi$m) in Spermatozoa

In the mitochondrial matrix, the oxidization of substrates leads to the transport of electrons along the electron transport chain complexes of the inner mitochondrial membrane resulting in the extrusion of protons across the inner membrane to generate the proton-motive force. The proton-motive force consists of two components, the transmembrane proton gradient (ΔpH) and the inner membrane potential ($\Delta\psi$m). The electrical gradient, $\Delta\psi$m (around 150 mV, negative inside) makes a larger contribution than the pH gradient (0.5 pH units, inside alkaline). The proton-motive force drives ATP synthesis. Thus, the $\Delta\psi$m is considered as the driving force for mitochondrial ATP production [5]. According to recent findings, $\Delta\psi$m also regulates other non-energetic mitochondrial functions including mitochondrial Ca2+ sequestration, ROS production, and regulation of cell death. Thus, the $\Delta\psi$m can be viewed as a general indicator of mitochondrial functionality, which reflects sperm cell health. That is why the assessment of mitochondrial functionality can be performed by estimating the $\Delta\psi$m in spermatozoa.

For over 30 years, many clinical and research studies have been published unveiling a link between

$\Delta\psi$m and sperm motility (for recent review see [2]). One of the first publications reported a positive correlation between $\Delta\psi$m and sperm motility in ejaculates from patients with fertility problems [6]. This result was later validated in a larger cohort of infertile patients [7]. Moreover, it was demonstrated that the detection of $\Delta\psi$m is an effective test to assess sperm quality in the preparatory steps before IVF [7, 8, 9]. There is a significant correlation with $\Delta\psi$m in both neat semen and prepared sperm. Interestingly, $\Delta\psi$m can predict the success of an IVF [8, 9]. The limits in most of these related studies are the recruitment of infertile patients, constituting a selection bias. More recently, analysis of $\Delta\psi$m in men from the general population confirmed the previous data linking $\Delta\psi$m and sperm motility. Overall, these results underline the relevance of using $\Delta\psi$m as a mitochondrial biomarker in male fertility [10].

Interestingly, mitochondrial functionality is also involved in other steps that are required to render sperm competent to fertilize oocytes. Thus, mitochondrial functions are associated with sperm capacitation, sperm acrosin activity and the acrosome reaction [11]. Accordingly, using cell sorting showed that sperm mitochondria with high $\Delta\psi$m constituted a subpopulation prone to undergo calcium ionophore-induced acrosome reaction [12].

In conclusion, the determination of mitochondrial functionality by the assessment of $\Delta\psi$m provides useful information on the overall quality and the fertilizing capacities of human spermatozoa.

8.1.3 Methods to Detect the Inner Membrane Potential in Spermatozoa

The use of different fluorochromes on living spermatozoa allows the detection of $\Delta\psi$m by fluorometric methods including flow cytometry. These fluorochromes have in common the fact that they are lipophilic and cationic. These characteristics make them permeable to the hydrophobic plasma membrane and allow their accumulation into the mitochondrial matrix (cations are attracted to the negative potential) in viable cells depending on the value of the $\Delta\psi$m. According to the Nernst equation, there is a tenfold increase in the concentration of fluorochrome within mitochondrial matrix for every 61.5 mV increase in $\Delta\psi$m. For these reasons, fluorochromes that detect $\Delta\psi$m are known as potentiometric dyes and the fluorescence intensity of the accumulated fluorochromes is

correlated to $\Delta\psi$m. Sperm mitochondria accumulating high concentrations of fluorochromes correspond to polarized mitochondria (with $\Delta\psi$m high) whereas mitochondria accumulating lower concentrations of fluorochromes are depolarized (and have a low $\Delta\psi$m) (see Figure 8.1). All of these probes need a minute attention to technical details and adequate controls to allow for a correct analysis. To ascertain that the fluorochrome behavior is related to $\Delta\psi$m in sperm cells, it is important to perform control experiments in which protonophores such as Cl-CCP and FCCP or the K+ ionophore valinomycin are used to depolarize the inner mitochondrial membranes. The incubation of sperm cells with Cl-CCP or valinomycin should result in a drop in the incorporation of the fluorochrome (about 1–1.5 log fluorescence). This highlights that the potentiometric dye incorporation is indeed driven by the mitochondrial membrane potential (see Figure 8.1).

In past decades, we have observed the availability of new potentiometric dyes that allow for more reliable and accurate measurements of $\Delta\psi$m. Potential sensitive dyes are either rosamines, rhodamines or carbocyanine derivatives. The dyes' behavior may be influenced by environmental events independent of the $\Delta\psi$m. For instance, some of the potentiometric dyes undergo self-quenching upon overaccumulation in the mitochondrial matrix distorting the $\Delta\psi$m detection. The other major problem of these fluorochromes is the occurrence of non-specific accumulation within spermatozoa independently of the $\Delta\psi$m. These issues must be taken into account when developing any new experiments and require the use of depolarization control (e.g. with Cl-CCP) for each experimental series (see protocol 8.2.3). The main potentiometric probes used in spermatozoa are listed in Table 8.1 with their specific fluorescence characteristics.

Rhodamine 123 (Rh123) was the first fluorescent probe used to assess $\Delta\psi$m in spermatozoa [6] then widely used in other studies. However, the use of Rh123 is often delicate given major drawbacks such as the existence of non-specific Rh123-binding sites, a risk of self-quenching as well as high photo-instability [5]. For these reasons, we do not recommend its use especially for inexperienced technicians.

The carbocyanine derivative 3,3'-dihexyloxacarbocyanine iodide [DiOC6(3)] was extensively used to detect mitochondrial membrane depolarization preceding nuclear apoptosis. DiOC6(3) bears the major

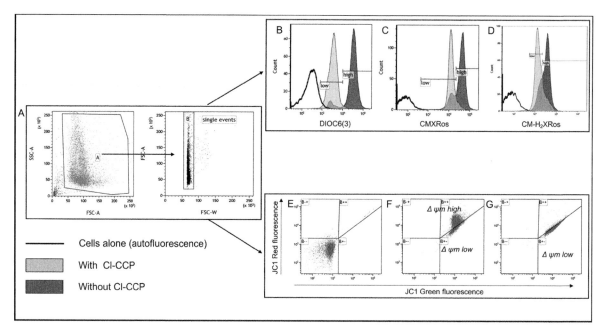

Figure 8.1 Gating strategy and representative cytofluorometric histograms of spermatozoa stained with potentiometric dyes. Figure 8.1A: Left) SSC-A versus FSC-A density plot. Each dot represents an individual sperm cell that has passed through the laser. A gate has been applied to identify spermatozoa (Gate A), and to remove debris (on the lower left corner); (Figure 8.1A: Right). FSC-A versus FSC-W plot. This plot is used to discriminate doublets from single cells. Events out of the Gate B are considered as doublets; Figure 8.1B–D. Analysis of histograms of spermatozoa from one sample. Spermatozoa are stained with the following potentiometric dyes: DIOC6(3) (B), CMXRos (C) and CM-H$_2$XRos (D). Unlabeled cells are represented by dark lines, labeled cells incubated with Cl-CCP as control by light gray profile and labeled cells without Cl-CCP by dark gray profile; Figure 8.1E–G. Two-parameter (dual color fluorescence) JC-1 dot plot. Unlabeled cells are represented in Figure 8.1E (as negative control), JC-1 stained cells in Figure 8.1F and JC-1 stained cells incubated with Cl-CCP (as positive control) in Figure 8.1G.

advantage of having a limited self-quenching effect. However, some disadvantages with the use of DiOC6 (3) staining were reported at high concentrations such as a mitochondrial uptake also dependent on the plasma membrane potential and a lack of mitochondrial specificity [5]. Thus, DiOC6(3) is also a valuable dye to assess Δψm by flow cytometry in sperm samples when used in low concentrations (<40 nM) [7, 8].

Several potentiometric dyes, including the rhodamine derivatives tetramethylrhodamine ethyl ester (TMRE) and tetramethylrhodamine methyl ester (TMRM), have been developed in the past decades. There are also potential problems with TMRM/TMRE, specifically self-quenching when used at high concentrations [5]. Nevertheless, TMRM/TMRE represent one of the most efficient fluorochromes for Δψm measurements in living cells including spermatozoa [8]. Particularly, the analysis of TMRE/TMRM staining is uncomplicated compared to the analysis of JC-1, which emits a double fluorescence that could be affected by potential-independent parameters.

Chloromethyl-X-rosamine (CMXRos) dye (AKA MitoTrackerRed) and its reduced form CM-H$_2$XRos are more photostable than Rh123 and were suggested to accurately evaluate changes in Δψm [8]. CMXRos contains a thiol-reactive chloromethyl moiety that reacts with mitochondrial thiol groups and therefore CMXRos yields a potential advantage of being fixable [13]. However, the fixation step can potentially disturb CMXRos staining and we recommend comparing results with and without fixation to unsure that CMXRos remains a reliable marker of Δψm after sperm fixation with formaldehyde. More recently, a series of chloromethyltetramethylrosamine analogs (MitoTracker dyes) that differ in their excitation/emission wavelengths were introduced as new potentiometric probes. However, their use in sperm samples has yet to be fully validated.

In clinical studies, the carbocyanine fluorescent probe 5,5' ,6,6'-tetrachloro-1,1' ,3,3'-tetraethylbenzimidazolyl-carbocyanine iodide (JC-1) was extensively used to accurately evaluate changes in Δψm [14, 15]. JC-1 selectively labels sperm mitochondria depending

Table 8.1 Main characteristics of Δψm-sensitive probes

Probe name	Dye family	Maximum absorption	Laser	Maximum emission	Filter band pass	Estimated threshold for self quenching	Characteristics	Cautions
CMH2XRos CMXRos	Rosamines	579 nm	561 nm	585/15	610/20	>100nm	- Contain a thiol-reactive chloromethyl moiety retaining the probe by mitochondria after formaldehyde fixation (to be tested)	- Analysis often difficult - Unreliable results when used with antioxidants

JC-1		514 nm monomer form 585 nm J-aggregate form	488nm	529 nm monomer form 590 nm J-aggregate form	525/30 610/20	>2nm	- High sensitivity
							- Ratiometric dye
							- 2 emissions spectra:
							  - green = monomeric state = invariant with mitochondrial membrane potential
							  - red = aggregate state = sensitive to mitochondrial membrane potential	

DIOC6(3)	Carbocyanines	484 nm	488nm	501 nm	525/30	>40nm	- Not specific to mitochondria - Inhibit mitochondrial respiration - Sensitive to plasma membrane potential	- Use the lowest concentrations - Adapt number of sperm cells/dye ratio
TMRE TMRM	Rhodamines	540 nm 548 nm	488 nm / 561 nm	595 nm 574 nm	585/15	>500nm	- Label specifically mitochondria	- Reversible staining
Rhodamine 123		507 nm	488nm	529 nm	525/30	ND	- Lack of specificity	- Contradictory data
Live/Dead blue	Amine fixation	350 nm	405 nm	450 nm	450/50	ND	- Used to determine the viability of cells prior to the fixation and permeabilization - The dye reacts with free amines both in the cell interior and on the cell surface - Excitation by UV laser	- Always use buffer protein and tris free

on the $\Delta\psi$m and is considered as one of the most sensitive and specific fluorochrome for the detection of $\Delta\psi$m. Unlike other potentiometric dyes, after excitation at 488 nm, JC-1 emits fluorescence in two different wavelengths according to its aggregation state. Cells with high $\Delta\psi$m accumulate in their mitochondrial matrix high concentrations of JC-1 that aggregate and fluoresce orange/red (590 nm) while cells with low $\Delta\psi$m contain less JC-1 that stay at a monomeric state and fluoresce green (527 nm). Due to its dual emission wavelengths, JC-1 has been labeled as more reliable than other potentiometric dyes for monitoring $\Delta\psi$m. Typically, $\Delta\psi$m depolarization leads to a shift from red to green fluorescence. However, the intensity of the green fluorescence emitted by the JC-1 monomer form can be dependent on $\Delta\psi$m-insensitive parameters. Furthermore, the presence of antioxidants provides unreliable results in human sperm labeled with JC-1 [16]. In spermatozoa, dissipation of $\Delta\psi$m with valinomycin or Cl-CCP used as control (see protocol) does not always increase the green fluorescence. Thus, in our study we found that it is better to rely on the red-orange fluorescence emission of JC-1 aggregates to assess changes in $\Delta\psi$m in sperm samples [8]. Interestingly, depending on sperm samples, the resolution between the two fluorescence peaks ($\Delta\psi$m low and $\Delta\psi$m high) of JC-1 aggregates can be weak thus rending the analysis of JC-1 aggregate histograms more subjective [8]. Subsequently, the analysis of the percentage of $\Delta\psi$m high-stained with JC-1 can be more subjective than with other potentiometric dyes. For these reasons, sperm staining with potentiometric dyes that emit in single-fluorescence should be preferred to the use of JC-1.

In conclusion, fluorochromes TMRM/TMRE, CMXRos, DiOC6(3) and JC-1 are adequate for reliable $\Delta\psi$m evaluation in sperm samples. All of these fluorochromes stain mitochondria of live spermatozoa and allow for accurate cytofluorometric analysis. CMXRos is potentially fixable. TMRM/TMRE is simple to use and can accurately monitor $\Delta\psi$m without JC-1 limitations. The choice of the fluochrome will depend on their fluorescence spectra in order to use them in combination with other fluorescent markers.

8.1.4 Flow Cytometric Detection of the Inner Membrane Potential in Spermatozoa

Flow cytometry constitutes a powerful semi-quantitative method to investigate $\Delta\psi$m in spermatozoa. One of the main advantages of flow cytometry is the large number of spermatozoa (thousands of cells) that can be estimated in a few seconds thus increasing the reliability of the results. Flow cytometric $\Delta\psi$m assays can be of great interest in the assisted reproductive technology (ART) laboratory. Their automatic analysis can rapidly determine sperm quality with great accuracy. Flow cytometric $\Delta\psi$m assays give reliable information on sperm cell populations and thus could represent an interesting alternative to the visual estimation of motility, which is particularly time-consuming and remains subjective.

Flow cytometry is especially suited to detect heterogeneity within the sperm cell population. Flow cytometric $\Delta\psi$m determination can be used to discriminate sperm cells with active ($\Delta\psi$m high) and non-active ($\Delta\psi$m low) mitochondria. Flow cytometric analysis of spermatozoa stained with the fluorochromes described above revealed in each case two cellular subpopulations corresponding to two fluorescence peaks with different intensities (see Figure 8.1). One subset of spermatozoa that incorporates more fluorochrome (about 1–1.5 log more) corresponds to spermatozoa with high $\Delta\psi$m ($\Delta\psi$m high cells). The other subset of spermatozoa is less fluorescent and corresponds to $\Delta\psi$m low spermatozoa.

Flow cytometry also allows for the simultaneous evaluation of $\Delta\psi$m in individual spermatozoa along with other sperm parameters. This is why it is important to have a large panel of reliable potentiometric probes emitting in different fluorescence channels, thus increasing the choice of excitation or emission wavelengths. These potentiometric dyes such as CMXRos, DiOC6(3), TMRE/TMRM emit single fluorescent peak and can be used simultaneously in combination with other fluorochromes evaluating other sperm features. JC-1 because of its dual emission wavelengths is much more difficult to use in combination with other dyes in a single laser cytometer. Since they emit a single fluorescence peak, CMXRos, DiOC6(3) and TMRE allow the combination with different supravital fluorochromes. Here, we developed a double-staining protocol dedicated to the simultaneous evaluation of $\Delta\psi$m and cell viability after staining with CMXRos and Live/Dead blue, respectively (see protocol 8.2.3.5).

Interestingly, flow cytometry can be proposed to detect $\Delta\psi$m in conjunction with the acrosome reaction in spermatozoa. Evaluation of acrosome membrane integrity constitutes an important parameter to evaluate semen quality and male fertility. Several fluorescence techniques are available in flow cytometry to determine acrosome integrity. Spontaneous acrosome reaction (acrosomal status) can be assessed by using fluorescein isothiocyanate conjugate–anti CD46 monoclonal antibody [12] or Lectin-FITC staining [17]. In these conditions, acrosome reaction and the $\Delta\psi$m can be measured simultaneously using Lectin-FITC and chloromethyl-X-rosamine (CMXRos) staining, respectively (see protocol).

Overall, the simultaneous detection of several sperm parameters on individual spermatozoa contributes to a better estimation of the fertilizing potential of semen samples.

This chapter gives essential information about flow cytometric methods used for the appropriate assessment of $\Delta\psi$m in spermatozoa. Some details and critical steps are presented to highlight the risks of pitfalls in $\Delta\psi$m determination.

8.2 Determination of Mitochondrial Membrane Potential in Human Sperm Cells by Flow Cytometry

8.2.1 Materials

⚠ **CAUTION** Wearing personal protective equipment is strongly recommended during all following steps with, at a minimum, gloves, lab coat or disposable Tyvek gown and eye protection.

8.2.1.1 Reagents

- Cells. The staining is performed on purified sperm.
  - o For the two-layer density gradient: ISolate® 90 percent and 50 percent (purchased from Irvine Scientific, now Fujifilm)
  - o For washing: Sperm Washing Medium (purchased from Irvine Scientific, now Fujifilm)
  - o For re-suspension: Ferticult™ Flushing Medium (purchased from FertiPro)
- Phosphate-buffered saline (PBS) (prepared in-house or purchased, e.g. from Gibco). Store at 4 °C.
- Serum free media (purchased, e.g. from Sigma-Aldrich or Thermo-Fisher). Store at 4°C.
- Dimethylsulfoxide (DMSO; Sigma-Aldrich). Store at room temperature. ⚠ **CAUTION** DMSO is

toxic; avoid contact with skin, eyes or mucous membrane; harmful if inhaled or swallowed. Use gloves when handling.
- 5,5',6,6'-Tetrachloro-1,1',3,3'-tetraethylbenzimidazolcarbocyanine iodide (JC-1; Sigma-Aldrich). Store at -20 °C. ⚠ **CAUTION** JC-1 is toxic; avoid contact with skin, eyes or mucous membrane; harmful if inhaled or swallowed. Use gloves when handling.
- MitoTracker™ CMXRos (purchased from Invitrogen). Store at -20 °C.
- MitoTracker™ CM-H_2XRos (reduced form of CMXRos) (purchased from Invitrogen). Store at -20 °C. ⚠ **CAUTION** Reduced forms of the MitoTracker™ probes are sensitive to oxidases in serum, it is thus important to use serum free media.
- Tetramethylrhodamine ethyl ester perchlorate (TMRE, purchased, e.g. from Invitrogen or Sigma-Aldrich). Store at 4°C.
- Tetramethylrhodamine methyl ester perchlorate (TMRM, purchased, e.g. Invitrogen or Sigma-Aldrich). Store at 4°C.
- 3,3'-Dihexyloxacarbocyanine Iodide (DIOC6(3), purchased, e.g. Invitrogen or Sigma-Aldrich). Store at room temperature.
- 2-(6-Amino-3-imino-3H-xanthen-9-yl) benzoic acid methyl ester (Rhodamine 123, purchased, e.g. Invitrogen or Sigma-Aldrich). Store at -20°C
- LIVE/DEAD™ Fixable Blue Dead Cell Stain Kit, for UV excitation (purchased from Invitrogen). Store at -20 °C. ⚠ **CAUTION** LIVE/DEAD™ Fixable Blue Dead Cell is toxic; avoid contact with skin, eyes or mucous membrane; harmful if inhaled or swallowed. Use gloves when handling.
- Lectin from *Pisum sativum* FITC conjugate (pea, purchased from Sigma-Aldrich). Store at -20°C. ⚠ **CAUTION** Lectin from *Pisum sativum* FITC conjugate is toxic; avoid contact with skin, eyes or mucous membrane; harmful if inhaled or swallowed. Use gloves when handling.
- Carbonyl cyanide 3-chlorophenylhydrazone (Cl-CCP, CCCP, purchased, e.g. from Sigma-Aldrich). Store at 4°C. ⚠ **CAUTION** Cl-CCP is very toxic; avoid contact with skin; harmful if inhaled or swallowed. Use gloves when handling.
- Carbonyl cyanide 4-(trifluoromethoxy) phenylhydrazone (FCCP, purchased, e.g. from Sigma-Aldrich). Store at 4°C. ⚠ **CAUTION**

FCCP is very toxic; avoid contact with skin; harmful if inhaled or swallowed. Use gloves when handling.

- Valinomycin (Sigma-Aldrich). Store at 4 °C. ⚠ **CAUTION** Valinomycin is very toxic; avoid contact with skin; harmful if inhaled or swallowed. Use gloves when handling.

8.2.1.2 Equipment

- Cell culture equipment.
- Plastic tubes for flow cytometry analysis
- 4 and −20°C refrigerators.
- Centrifuge.
- Flow cytometer (see Equipment Setup)

8.2.1.3 Equipment Set-up

The aforementioned dyes can be detected by a BD LSRFortessa™ X-20 flow cytometer (from BD Biosciences-US) equipped with a solid-state blue laser (488 nm, 50 mW), a red laser diode (638 nm, 100 mW), a violet laser diode (403 nm, 50 mW), a yellow green laser diode (561 nm, 50 mW) and a Ultraviolet (UV) laser (355 nm, 15 mW). Other flow cytometers equipped with blue, red, violet, yellow green lasers, and a UV laser (such as for example the melody and FACSAria from BD Biosciences, Cytoflex and Astrios from Beckman Coulter, Attune from Thermo-Fisher) can be used as well. The software for the acquisition is FACS DIVA software 7.0 from BD Biosciences and Kaluza v2.1 software from Beckman Coulter for analysis. Laser and filters used for each probe are shown in Table 8.1. In addition, FSC and SSC are measured using 488/10 nm band pass filter and Lectin-FITC using 529/24 nm band pass filter following excitation with the blue laser (488 nm). Further information on the characteristics of the dyes, the suggested lines of excitation and filters can be found at www.thermofisher.com/fr/fr/home/life-science/cell-analysis/labeling-chemistry/fluorescence-spectraviewer.html or www.biolegend.com/en-us/spectra-analyzer [last accessed October 1, 2020].

8.2.2 Sperm Sample Preparation

- Place sperm on the gradient surface: ideally 1 mL.
- Centrifuge at 300 g for 10 minutes.
- Using a 2 mL or 5 mL pipette with a suction system, gently aspirate the seminal fluid and the 50 percent phase, then part of the 90 percent phase, until a small distance from the pellet if it is visible, otherwise leave the last 500 μL of the fraction 90 percent in case of non-visible pellet.
- Homogenize the pellet or the last 500 μL of the 90 percent phase and transfer the sperm suspension into a tube containing 2 mL of Sperm Washing Medium, homogenize well.
- Centrifuge for 10 minutes at 200 g.
- Remove the supernatant with a 2- or 5-mL pipette.
- Resuspend the final pellet in Ferticult® Flushing medium:

   o If the pellet is not visible, take up 0.1 mL.

   o If the pellet is visible, take up to 1 mL.

- After adding Ferticult® Flushing medium, mix well.

8.2.3 Flow Cytometry Preparation

8.2.3.1 Preparation of Samples

- Recover 5×10^5 spermatozoa from gradient and adjust total volume to 100 μL with pre-warmed (37°C) serum free media.
- Prepare a positive control, in which sperm mitochondria have been depolarized (see preparation of positive control 8.2.3.2).

TIPS:

- Prepared spermatozoa stored at room temperature or at 37°C maintains a constant proportion of Δψm high cells at least for the first 60 minutes.
- ⚠ **CAUTION** Do not refrigerate samples. Spermatozoa stored at 4°C undergo a decrease in the percentage of Δψm high cells irrespective of the Δψm -dependent dye used.

8.2.3.2 Preparation of Positive Control

- To provide the positive control, add mitochondrial uncoupler/ionophore in one of the samples to desired final concentration (see Table 8.2) and incubate at 37°C for 30 minutes before staining (one hour before flow cytometry assay).
- For example, add 10 μL of 10 μM of Cl-CCP (1 μM final concentration).

8.2.3.3 Preparation of Probes Working Solution

- Warm the serum free media to 37°C.
- Prepare a probe working solution by diluting the probe stock solution with pre-warmed serum-free media according to Table 8.2.

Table 8.2 Concentrations of fluorescent probes, uncouplers and ionophore used

	Fluorescent probes								Viability	Uncouplers/ionophore		
	Mitochondrial membrane potential							Acrosomal membrane integrity				
Probe name	CM-H$_2$XRos	CMXRos	JC-1	TMRE	TMRM	Rhodamine 123	DIOC6(3)	Lectin from *Pisum sativum*	Live Dead Blue	Cl-CCP	FCCP	Valinomycin
Solvent for stock solution	DMSO			Ethanol				PBS	DMSO	DMSO		
Stock solution concentration	1 mmol/L	1 mmol/L	2.5 mmol/L	1 mmol/L	1 mmol/L	1 mmol/L	4 mmol/L	1 mg/mL	NA	100 µmol/L		
Working solution concentration (pre-warmed medium)	1 µmol/L	1 µmol/L	25 µmol/L	10 µmol/L	10 µmol/L	100 µmol/L	1 µmol/L	0,1 mg/mL	NA	10 µmol/L	10 µmol/L	1 µmol/L
Final concentration	50 nmol/L	50 nmol/L	1 µmol/L	250 nmol/L	250 nmol/L	5 µmol/L	20 nmol/L	0,5 µg/mL	1 µL	1 µmol/L	1 µmol/L	100 nmol/L

- For example, add 2 μL JC-1 stock to 198 μL of pre-warmed medium. 4 μL of JC-1 working solution is required for each sample (100 μL with 5×10^5 spermatozoa). Therefore, 200 μL of JC-1 working solution would be enough for 50 flow cytometry samples.
- Vortex the probe working solution thoroughly.
- The probe working solution must be used immediately after preparation proceeding to the staining in next section.

TIPS:

- Do not store working solutions that have been used.
- Stock solution concentration may be adjusted to your use to avoid waste.
- Always do final dilutions of stock solution in pre-warmed serum free media; DMSO can be harmful for spermatozoa.
- ⚠ CAUTION Store stock solution in the dark.
- ⚠ CAUTION Avoid repeated freeze/thaws of stock solution vials as this may compromise their integrity.
- After vortexing, aggregates may be present for JC-1 dye but should not interfere with flow cytometry.

8.2.3.4 Basic Protocol for Staining with TMRE, TMRM, JC-1, DIOC6(3), Rhodamine 123, CMXRos and CM-H₂XRos

- Add desired probe working solution to samples and positive control.
- Gently resuspend cells in the probe working solution.
- Incubate at room temperature or 37°C for 30 minutes in the dark.

TIPS:

- 20-minute period of incubation is enough for DiOC6, CMXRos and TMRE to equilibrate into the cells.
- ⚠ CAUTION For JC-1 staining, a 30-minute period of incubation is needed and allows a better separation of the high fluorescence peak of JC-1 red-orange.

8.2.3.5 Advanced Protocol 1 for Simultaneous Determination of Sperm Mitochondrial Membrane Potential and Cell Viability

Sperm mitochondrial potential and viability can be determined at the same time:

- Add proper Live/Dead Blue viability dye concentration (see Table 8.2) and membrane potential probe at the same time.
- Incubate at room temperature or 37°C for 30 minutes in the dark.
- Wash cells with 2 mL of PBS and pellet by centrifugation at 300 g for five minutes at room temperature. Discard supernatant and repeat once.
- Discard supernatant and resuspend cells in 100 μL PBS.

TIPS:

- For viability assays based on amine fixation (like Live/Dead) be careful to use protein- and tris-free buffer.

8.2.3.6 Advanced Protocol 2 for Simultaneous Determination of Sperm Mitochondrial Membrane Potential and Acrosome Membrane Integrity

Sperm mitochondrial potential and acrosomal integrity can be determined at the same time:

- Add proper Lectin from *Pisum sativum* concentration (see Table 8.2).
- Incubate at room temperature or 37°C for 30 minutes in the dark.
- Add proper membrane potential probe concentration (see Table 8.2).
- Incubate at room temperature or 37°C for 30 minutes in the dark.

TIPS:

- Lectin from *Pisum sativum* results in aggregation, we therefore recommend cytometry analysis of the two combined parameters without any washing that could result in aggregation modification.

8.2.4 Flow Cytometry Analysis

8.2.4.1 Standard Protocols

8.2.4.1.1 Gating Strategies

Gates have to be applied to exclude unwanted populations and therefore to select only sperm cells for further Δψm determination.

The first step in gating is the selection of sperm cells based on their forward (FSC) and side scatter (SSC) properties. Classically, FSC and SSC represent an estimation of size and granularity of the cells, respectively. This method allows to remove dead cells and debris. Standard results from a purified sperm sample are shown in Figure 8.1A. Gate A has been applied to select sperm population and to remove debris (Figure 8.1A left panel; debris are outside Gate A on the left corner). This principle of gating can be applied again to perform doublet discrimination (Figure 8.1A, Gate B right panel). It selects only single sperm cells (Gate B on the dot-plot FSC-Area versus FSC-Width) and remove sperm cell aggregates (doublets) that emit "false" high fluorescence (Figure 8.1A, right panel). It is to note that gating sperm cells can be complex for neat semen samples where there are other cell types (such as round cells, leukocytes). Thus, spermatozoa within the Gates A and B can be further analyzed for correct $\Delta\psi$m determination.

8.2.4.1.2 Determination of Inner Membrane Potential Subpopulations

Figure 8.1B–D represent some examples of typical single parameter histograms obtained for $\Delta\psi$m detection after staining with the following potentiometric probes DiOC6(3), CMXRos, CM-H$_2$XRos. As shown, there are two peaks which are interpreted as $\Delta\psi$m high (high fluorescence) and $\Delta\psi$m low (low fluorescence) within sperm cells. In order to accurately identify the $\Delta\psi$m low subpopulation, flow cytometric analysis should be repeated in the presence of appropriate control of depolarization after incubation with uncouplers such as FCCP/Cl-CCP or with valinomycin. Figure 8.1B–D shows control histograms (in this case after incubation with Cl-CCP), in light gray, overlaid onto the dataset, in black, allowing the accurate discrimination of $\Delta\psi$m low and high subpopulations. It is to note that autofluorescence of unlabeled sperm cells is minimal (Figure 8.1B–D).

Figure 8.1E–G refer to the dual color fluorescence dot plot of JC-1 staining. JC-1 possess two fluorescence emission peaks: at high $\Delta\psi$m the fluorescence emission is mostly orange-red, whereas at low $\Delta\psi$m it shifts to green fluorescence. The typical JC-1 dot-plot indicates that sperm cells (Figure 8.1F) emit high levels of both green and orange-red fluorescence. Pre-treatment with Cl-CCP results in a significant drop in the orange-red fluorescence without change in the green fluorescence pattern (Figure 8.1G). This procedure is used to discriminate the low and high $\Delta\psi$m subpopulations.

TIPS:

- Using analytical software, measurements and statistics can be obtained for many parameters including the number of cells and percentage of cells within the gates. Alternatively, median and/or mean fluorescence intensity (MFI) can be used.
- Use unlabeled cells to adjust voltage settings that place autofluorescence peak within the first decade. Using the same settings, confirm that labeled fluorescence of sperm cell population is within the last decade. If not, it may be necessary to adjust the experimental conditions. One must be careful to avoid detector saturation.

8.2.4.1.3 Critical Parameters and Troubleshooting

8.2.4.1.3.1 Control Experiments – The most useful agents for control experiments are the uncouplers (Cl-CCP, FCCP) and the ionophore Valinomycin. They dissipate the mitochondrial membrane potential and are used to validate the experimental conditions. The conditions of their use are summarized in Table 8.2.

TIPS:

- The effects of Cl-CCP and Valinomycin seem to be more efficient than FCCP in dissipating $\Delta\psi$m in spermatozoa.
- ⚠ **CAUTION** We have observed that some patients present decreased sensitivity to the uncouplers and Valinomycin. Cl-CCP and Valinomycin concentrations should be titrated to evaluate the optimum concentration for maximum effect.

8.2.4.1.3.2 Dye Concentration – To produce accurate and reliable results, the potentiometric probes and the cell concentrations should be monitored with care. As shown in Figure 8.2, when sperm mitochondria are stained with low concentrations (20–40 nM) of DiOC6(3), the probe reaches equilibrium in the mitochondria with low quenching effects. The use of lower concentrations results in incomplete staining whereas concentrations higher than 40 nm can induce non-mitochondrial staining and fluorescence quenching.

8.2.4.1.3.3 Dye Characteristics – Each fluorescent probe possesses specific fluorescence characteristics (Table 8.1) that determine the choice of the laser wavelength and of the proper fluorescence combinations.

TIPS:

- DiOC6(3), CMXRos and TMRE patterns of cell fluorescence are stable and remain unchanged for at least 120 minutes of incubation in the medium at 37°C.

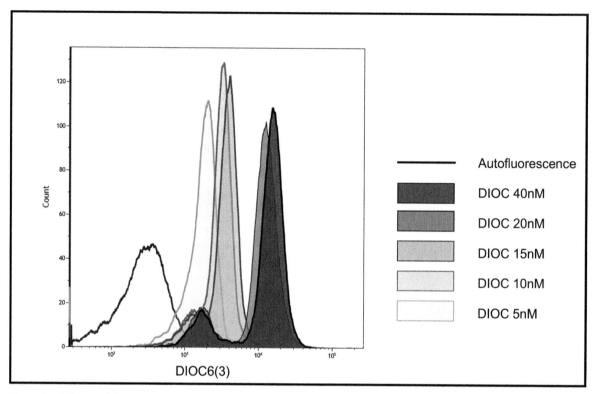

Figure 8.2 Influence of the DiOC6(3) concentration on the distribution of fluorescence and cytofluorometric histograms of spermatozoa (see text for details).

- Patterns of cell fluorescence are stable and remain unchanged if the staining is done at 37°C or at room temperature

8.2.4.1.3.4 Acquisition Speed and Number of Events – Although Flowcytometry settings are instrument-specific, several parameters may provide general insights to other users. Speed at which cells pass in front of the laser may have an impact on the sensitivity of the fluorescence detection and high speed may alter the discrimination between $\Delta\psi$m low and high (Figure 8.3B). For this reason, we recommend a flow speed around 15 μL/s (low speed) for better results (Figure 8.3A). Typically, a minimum of events is needed to achieve proper determination of $\Delta\psi$m subpopulations. Therefore, we recommend acquiring a minimum of 10,000 events per sample.

8.2.4.2 Simultaneous Determination of Sperm Mitochondrial Membrane Potential and Acrosome Membrane Integrity or Viability by Flow Cytometry

Figures 8.4 and 8.5 refer to the simultaneous determination of mitochondrial membrane potential and

other functional parameters such as viability or acrosome membrane integrity.

TIPS: Before starting with dual fluorescence analysis, stain samples with single fluorochromes to properly set up the fluorescence levels and reveal the amount of spectral overlap. If required, apply fluorescence compensation.

8.2.4.2.1 Sperm Inner Membrane Potential and Acrosome Membrane Integrity

8.2.4.2.1.1 Gating – Linear scales are more effective than logarithmic scales for displaying datasets with values spread. Lectin-FITC labeling can induce modifications in size and structure of spermatozoa. Therefore, we recommend gating on FSC and SSC parameters in logarithmic scale (Figure 8.4).

8.2.4.2.1.2 Results – As shown in Figure 8.4E, spermatozoa sample contains two distinct CMXRos subpopulations. In the CMXRos low subpopulation (i.e. $\Delta\psi$m low) the intensity of Lectin-FITC fluorescence is higher (Figure 8.4F) than that observed in the $\Delta\psi$m high subpopulation (CMXRos high) (Figure 8.4G),

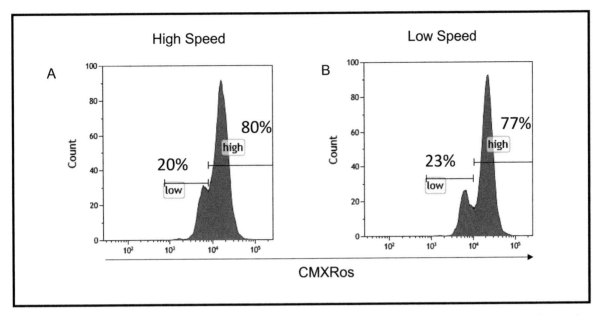

Figure 8.3 Impact of acquisition speed on the sensitivity of the CMXRos fluorescence detection and discrimination between the Δψm low and high peaks. Sperm cells are stained with CMXRos then analyzed by flow cytometry. Speed at which cells pass in front of the laser is around 60 μL/min (high speed) (Figure 8.3A) or 15 μL/min (low speed) (Figure 8.3B).

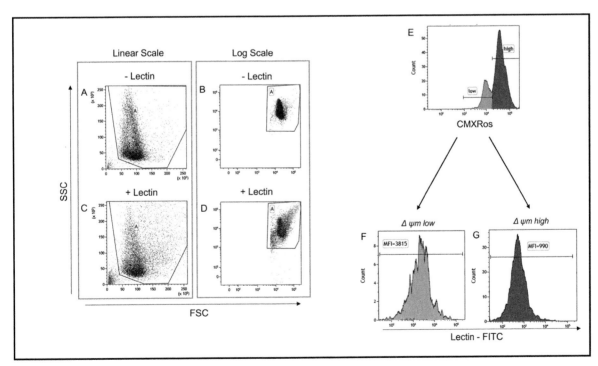

Figure 8.4 Simultaneous determination of sperm mitochondrial membrane potential and acrosomal membrane integrity in spermatozoa. Figure 8.4A–D: Gating strategy: Sperm cells are stained with CMXRos for Δψm determination and with (Figure 8.4C and 8.4D) or without Lectin-FITC for detection of acrosomal membrane integrity (Figure 8.4A and 8.4B) then analyzed in the FSC/SSC plot represented in linear scale (Figure 8.4A and 8.4C) or in logarithmic scale (Figure 8.4B and 8.4D); Representative distribution of CMXRos fluorescence in spermatozoa attained simultaneously with CMXRos and Lectin-FITC (Figure 8.4E). Δψm low and high gates are set based on this profile. Using these gates, the typical distribution of Lectin-FITC fluorescence and mean fluorescence intensity (MFI) are determined in the Δψm low (Figure 8.4F) and Δψm high (Figure 8.4G) subpopulations of spermatozoa.

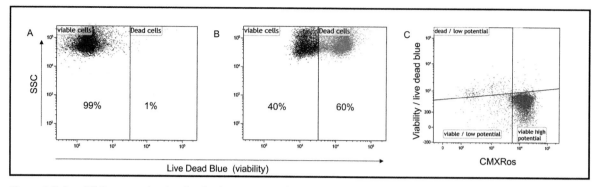

Figure 8.5 A and B: Representative dot plots for determination of spermatozoa viability, SSC is in log scale to avoid the spread of cell population. Sperrmatozoa were incubated with (8.5B, as positive cell death control) or without (8.5A) DMSO before Live/Dead staining. C: Representative dot plot for simultaneous determination of sperm mitochondrial membrane potential and viability in spermatozoa. Spermatozoa are stained with CMXRos and Live/Dead blue (see text for details).

indicating that loss of acrosomal membrane integrity (lectin-FITC positive) is higher spermatozoa with low $\Delta\psi$m. This result confirms the correlation between mitochondrial activity and acrosomal membrane integrity.

- ⚠ **CAUTION** Analysis of Lectin from *Pisum sativum* FITC conjugate has to be conducted rapidly after incubation; if not, sample aggregation may continue.

8.2.4.2.2 Sperm Inner Membrane Potential and Viability

A double staining procedure using CMXRos and Live/Dead blue in order to have compatible wavelengths allows us to assess $\Delta\psi$m and sperm cell viability simultaneously (Figure 8.5). All dead spermatozoa (Live/Dead blue positive spermatozoa) has low $\Delta\psi$m (CMXRos low). Conversely the population of viable spermatozoa (Live/Dead-negative) contains two subpopulations, one that exhibited a reduction in $\Delta\psi$m comparable with dead spermatozoa and one with high $\Delta\psi$m (Figure 8.5).

8.3 Conclusion: Relevance for Assisted Reproductive Technologies

An important feature of proper $\Delta\psi$m determination in spermatozoa is that it should provide relevant indications to the clinician, and pertinent information for the individual follow-up of patients.

The determination of $\Delta\psi$m in combination with classic parameters of semen quality might be helpful for the diagnosis of male infertility. We and others have shown that the percentage of $\Delta\psi$m high is a more discriminative criterion than sperm motility to detect male fertility [7, 8, 10]. $\Delta\psi$m determination via flow cytometry could be used as a routine screening test for male infertility. However, it requires the determination of cut-off values that clearly discriminate normal from asthenozoospermia patients.

We also propose to use $\Delta\psi$m as a biomarker to identify the most appropriate ART treatment for an individual infertile patient. Indeed, the main result of our clinical study is that IVF represents a rational first-line therapy for infertile men presenting >64 percent of $\Delta\psi$m high spermatozoa while another therapeutic option like ICSI instead of IVF should be proposed to patients with <64 percent of $\Delta\psi$m high spermatozoa [9]. Therefore, $\Delta\psi$m determination may help identify the most appropriate ART treatment for infertile patients.

Inner membrane potential can also be relevant in assessing the quality of cryopreserved sperm by evaluating the effects of toxin or environmental pollutants on sperm [10].

In conclusion, the determination of $\Delta\psi$m in human sperm cells represents a proper test to measure sperm quality, to evaluate the fertilizing ability of sperm and for diagnosing male infertility.

References

1. Moraes CR, Meyers S. The sperm mitochondrion: organelle of many functions. *Anim Reprod Sci* 2018; **194**: 71–80.

2. Piomboni P, Focarelli R, Stendardi A, Ferramosca A, Zara V. The role of mitochondria in energy production for human sperm motility. *Int J Androl* 2012; **35**: 109–24.

3. Ramalho-Santos J, Varum S, Amaral S, Mota PC, Sousa AP, Amaral A. Mitochondrial

functionality in reproduction: from gonads and gametes to embryos and embryonic stem cells. *Hum Reprod Update* 2009; **15**: 553–72.

4. Amaral A, Lourenço B, Marques M, Ramalho-Santos J. Mitochondria functionality and sperm quality. *Reprod* 2013; **146**: R163–74.

5. Perry SW, Norman JP, Barbieri J, Brown EB, Gelbard HA. Mitochondrial membrane potential probes and the proton gradient: a practical usage guide. *BioTechn* 2011; **50**: 98–115.

6. Evenson DP, Darzynkiewicz Z, Melamed MR. Simultaneous measurement by flow cytometry of sperm cell viability and mitochondrial membrane potential related to cell motility. *J Histochem Cytochem* 1982; **30**: 279–80.

7. Marchetti C, Obert G, Deffosez A, Formstecher P, Marchetti P. Study of mitochondrial membrane potential, reactive oxygen species, DNA fragmentation and cell viability by flow cytometry in human sperm. *Hum Reprod* 2002; **17**: 1257–65.

8. Marchetti C, Jouy N, Leroy-Martin B, Defossez A, Formstecher P, Marchetti P. Comparison of four fluorochromes for the detection of the inner mitochondrial membrane potential in human spermatozoa and their correlation with sperm motility. *Hum Reprod* 2004; **19**: 2267–76.

9. Marchetti P, Ballot C, Jouy N, Thomas P, Marchetti C. Influence of mitochondrial membrane potential of spermatozoa on in vitro fertilisation outcome. *Andrologia* 2011; **44**: 136–41.

10. Zhang G, Wang Z, Ling X, Zou P, Yang H, Chen Q, Zhou N, Sun L, Gao J, Zhou Z, et al. Mitochondrial biomarkers reflect semen quality: results from the MARCHS study in Chongqing, China. *PLOS ONE* 2016; 11: e0168823.

11. Zhang G, Yang W, Zou P, Jiang F, Zeng Y, Chen Q, Sun L, Yang H, Zhou N, Wang X, et al. Mitochondrial functionality modifies human sperm acrosin activity, acrosome reaction capability and chromatin integrity. *Hum Reprod* 2019; **34**: 3–11.

12. Gallon F, Marchetti C, Jouy N, Marchetti P. The functionality of mitochondria differentiates human spermatozoa with high and low fertilizing capability. *Fertil Steril* 2006; **86**: 1526–30.

13. Peña FJ, Ball BA, Squires EL. A new method for evaluating stallion sperm viability and mitochondrial membrane potential in fixed semen samples. *Cytometry B Clin Cytom* 2018; **94**: 302–11.

14. Donnelly ET, O'Connell M, McClure N, Lewis SE. Differences in nuclear DNA fragmentation and mitochondrial integrity of semen and prepared human spermatozoa. *Hum Reprod* 2000; **15**: 1552–61.

15. Piasecka M, Laszczyńska M, Gaczarzewicz D. Morphological and functional evaluation of spermatozoa from patients with asthenoteratozoospermia. *Folia Morphol* 2003; **62**: 479–81.

16. Uribe P, Villegas JV, Boguen R, Treulen F, Sánchez R, Mallmann P, Isachenko V, Rahimi G, Isachenko E. Use of the fluorescent dye tetramethylrhodamine methyl ester perchlorate for mitochondrial membrane potential assessment in human spermatozoa. *Andrologia* 2017; **49**: 1–7.

17. Farlin ME, Jasko DJ, Graham JK, Squires EL. Assessment of Pisum sativum agglutinin in identifying acrosomal damage in stallion spermatozoa. *Mol Reprod Dev* 1992; **32**: 23–7.

Capacitation and Acrosome Reaction: Fluorescence Techniques to Determine Acrosome Reaction

Raúl Sánchez, Fabiola Zambrano, Pamela Uribe

9.1 Introduction

The acrosome reaction (AR) is an essential process of spermatozoa for fertilization and is characterized by the exocytosis of the acrosomal content and the release of hybrid membrane vesicles formed by patches of the outer acrosomal membrane and the plasma membrane. Through acomplex membrane fusion process, which exposes the inner acrosomal membrane, both the morphology of the plasma membrane and the distribution of proteins involved in sperm–egg interaction are changed [1, 2]. AR also modifies sperm function, since acrosome-reacted sperm are no longer able to bind to the zona pellucida, but to the oolemma [3].

Given the biological importance of the acrosome reaction, several techniques to assess this exocytotic process have been developed. Determination of the ability of spermatozoa to undergo the acrosome reaction has turned out to be a useful parameter in order to evaluate male infertility [4]. The difference between spontaneous and induced acrosome reaction, i.e. the inducibility of acrosome reaction, is of prognostic value for the sperm fertilizing capacity [5]. For diagnostic purposes, it is important that the results from different laboratories are comparable. This is only possible if the methods equally detect acrosomal events and result in comparable percentages of acrosome reaction. Dyes and fluorescein-conjugated lectins bind to different structures of the acrosome [6]. Staining protocols and assays based on lectins labeled with fluorescent dyes are easy to perform, relatively inexpensive and frequently used to quantify sperm acrosome reaction [7]. More sophisticated methods such as immune cytochemistry with monoclonal antibodies or electron microscopy are not available in all laboratories [8]. Recently, the incorporation of flow cytometry into these protocols has led to new, easy, reproducible, reliable and fast protocols for the determination of this important sperm function [9].

9.1.1 Sperm Function

Prior to fertilization, spermatozoa must undergo a series of physiological changes before being able to fertilize an oocyte. These changes occur in the female reproductive tract, where spermatozoa interact with the microenvironments in the female genital tract during their journey to meet the oocyte in the ampulla of the fallopian tube. Finally, the spermatozoon binds to the oocyte, triggers acrosome reaction and hypermobility, a movement that facilitates the penetration of oocytes' covering [2].

The support of this structure is obtained by the cytoskeleton, constituting the plasma membranes and acrosome membranes. The main element of the cytoskeleton of the sperm head is the perinuclear theca, a rigid capsule that covers the nucleus and that once the fusion of plasmatic membrane and outer acrosome membranes occurs with the acrosome reaction, must preserve the integrity of the DNA.

The equatorial segment corresponds to the area where the inner and outer acrosomal membranes converge and fuse, and contains the receptors involved in the sperm binding. The post acrosome sheath is associated with the oocyte activation [10, 11].

9.1.2 Acrosome Reaction

This species-specific process implies the existence of molecules for recognition between male and female gametes and is triggered by the presence of oviductal fluid factors that aid in extracellular signaling and recognition of the oocyte [12, 13]. The AR can occur spontaneously and can also be induced in vitro. It is indispensable for the fertilization process and is generated as a result of the action of suitable inductors (reviewed by [8]).

The acrosome is derived from the Golgi apparatus during spermiogenesis and because of its origin, structure and cellular function, it is comparable to a lysosome. Unlike normal lysosomal exocytosis, acrosome reaction is regulated by a complex mechanism involving phosphoinositide, interaction of endogenous and exogenous nucleotides, Ca^{2+}, calmodulin, microtubules and microfilaments. In the initial steps of acrosome reaction, outer acrosomal membrane and plasma membrane fuse at various sites forming so-called hybrid-membrane vesicles, a process leading to a fenestration of the acrosome with eventual complete acrosomal loss and the release of the acrosomal contents. As a result, instead of exposing the outer acrosomal membrane, the internal acrosomal membrane is exposed as a new rostral surface membrane. The vesicles release their content of hydrolytic enzymes, as the sperm penetrates through the zona pellucida, allowing the spermatozoon to bind to the oolemma and eventually enter the oocyte.

In vivo, the acrosomal reaction begins with the stimulation of a natural agonist such as progesterone or the zona pellucida. This stimulus causes an entry of Ca^{2+} into the spermatozoa, which involves ATPases whose function is to maintain low levels of Na^+ and Ca^{2+} and high levels of K^+. The entry of Ca^{2+} causes the deactivation of ATPases, in addition to an increase in intracellular Na^+ with a H^+ output and consequently, an increase in intra-acrosomal pH, which induces the activation of enzymes such as acrosin. The increase in intracellular Ca^{2+} induces the formation of second messengers, which are incorporated into a cascade of events that occurs during the acrosome reaction and the activation of enzymes such as phospholipase A2 generating lyso-phosphatidylcholine and arachidonic acid that are both necessary for the fusion of membranes needed in the acrosomal reaction (review by Beltrán et al., [14]). The specific recognition of gametes, the sperm binding with its acrosome intact to zona pellucida, the induction of the acrosomal reaction and the prevention of polyspermia are related to the zona pellucida protein ZP3. ZP3 is the protein involved in the sperm binding and induction of acrosome reaction. This process is referred to as primary binding. Subsequently, the sperm can start penetrating the zona and interact with another zona protein, ZP2 [15]. This binding is stronger and is referred to as secondary binding [16].

9.1.3 Factors to Induce Acrosome Reaction

Acrosome reaction can be induced under artificial conditions (in vitro) with Test-Yolk buffer, albumin addition, zona pellucida, follicular fluid, calcium ionophore, prolonged incubation times, low incubation temperatures and hypertonic media among others [17, 18]. The determination of the ability of spermatozoa to perform AR is used as a test to evaluate sperm function since it correlates with the results of in vitro fertilization [8]. The three most commonly used inducers of AR are (a) low temperature, (b) calcium ionophore and (c) progesterone, with the latter inducer being considered physiological.

9.1.3.1 Low Temperature

The AR is induced by low temperature according to **Sanchez et al** [19]. After swim-up, sperm suspensions are treated in two different ways: (i) Control group: 24 hours at room temperature, additional incubation at 37°C for 3 hours; (ii) Experimental low temperature: 24 hours at 4°C, additional incubation at 37°C for 3 hours. Following the experimental procedures, slides with spermatozoa are prepared to determine the acrosomal status of spermatozoa. This method correlates well with in vitro fertilization, and a total AR <13 percent and inducibility of AR <7.5 percent is associated with low number of oocyte fecundation in in vitro fertilization [5].

9.1.3.2 Calcium Ionophore

The AR is induced by calcium ionophore according to Ozaki et al. [20]. A stock solution of calcium ionophore A23187 (9.55×10^{-3} M in 100 percent DMSO) is prepared and stored at −20°C. Working solutions are prepared by diluting the thawed stock of ionophore 1:10 in modified human tubular fluid 30 minutes before stimulation of the AR. Aliquots of the working solutions are added to the samples to achieve concentrations of 10 μM ionophore (0.1 percent v/v DMSO). Control samples are treated simultaneously under the same conditions, except that only 0.1 percent DMSO is added without ionophore. An infertile male shows a significantly reduced number of acrosome-reacted spermatozoa [21]. The difference between complete acrosome-reacted spermatozoa with and without treatment is determined. A percentage difference of ≤ 5 percent indicates male infertility [22].

9.1.3.3 Progesterone

Spermatozoa (10^7 cells/mL) are prepared in Biggers, Whitter and Whittingham medium (BWW, pH 7.2; Genmed Scientifics Inc., USA) and incubated for 3 hours at 37°C and 0.5 percent CO_2 (sperm viability is more than 95 percent after incubation). Afterwards, an aliquot of capacitated spermatozoa is incubated with progesterone (P4; final concentration of 40 μM) according to Chen et al. [23]. The P4-induced AR should be more than 24 percent and is significantly correlated to good in vitro fertilization rate [23, 24].

9.1.4 Tests Used to Measure Acrosome Reaction

Several techniques have been proposed to differentiate acrosome-intact from acrosome-reacted human sperm with different staining techniques; light and electron microscopic examination, indirect immunofluorescence using polyclonal and monoclonal antibodies and labeling with fluorescein-conjugated lectins.

9.1.4.1 Direct Tests

The direct method to evaluate the AR is transmission electron microscopy. Considered the most accurate to detect the AR, both for clinical practice and for research, its use is limited, especially due to the requirement of very costly equipment and specialized personnel for the preparations and analysis. It is also a laborious method and determines only a limited number of cells.

9.1.4.2 Indirect Tests

These tests are the most commonly used and can be based on histochemical methods with different stains using light microscopy, such as the triple stain technique or antibodies and lectins that are labeled with fluorescent molecules that can be determined with immunofluorescence microscopy or flow cytometry. Since fluorescence techniques are more cited protocols, these techniques have been selected for discussion in this chapter.

9.2 Fluorescence Detection of the Acrosome

9.2.1 Principle of Hoechst 33258/FITC-*Pisum sativum* Agglutinin (PSA-FITC) Staining in Simultaneous Assessment of Viability and Acrosome Reaction Rate of Human Sperm

9.2.1.1 Principle

The PSA-FITC lectin is a dimeric lectin, consisting of two ab monomers with high affinity for α-D-mannose and α-D-glucose residues of glycoproteins present in the plasma membrane of the acrosomal domain of the sperm head. This technique is a negative staining technique that stains the acrosomal area of acrosome-reacted sperm, thus those sperm that lost their acrosome [25]. The PSA-FITC has been extensively used to assess AR in fixed human sperm [20].

9.2.1.2 Protocol

Supravital nuclear staining with bis-benzimide (Hoechst 33258; Sigma) is used to identify dead sperm cells. The dye is added to the sperm suspensions (approximately 1×10^6 spermatozoa) one minute before the final washing prior to preparation of the sperm smear. To permeabilize the sperm membrane, the slides are treated with 100 percent methanol for 30 seconds, followed by incubation for 30 minutes in a moisture chamber at room temperature in phosphate-buffered salt (PBS) containing 50 mg/mL *Pisum sativum* agglutinin conjugated with fluorescein isothiocyanate, pH 7.4, (FITC-PSA; Sigma) according to [26]. The smears are washed for at least 15 minutes in distilled water, air-dried and examined under an epifluorescence microscope (excitation filter 450–490 nm, dichroic mirror 510 nm, barrier filter 520 nm). For assessment of viability and acrosomal status, 200 spermatozoa are examined in randomly selected fields according to the fluorescence pattern of their acrosomes.

9.2.1.3 Interpretation of Results

The following criteria are used to evaluate the acrosomal status and viability of spermatozoa.

(i) A spermatozoon showing the region of the nucleus marked with Hoechst 33258 (blue) is considered dead.

(ii) A spermatozoon showing the acrosomal region totally or partly marked with PSA-FITC (yellow-green) is considered to be acrosome-reacted.

(iii) Live spermatozoa showing more than 2/3 of the acrosome with fluorescence are considered acrosome-reacted.

9.2.2 Principle of FITC-Concanavalin A (FITC-ConA) Staining in Simultaneous Assessment of Viability and Acrosome Reaction Rate of Human Sperm

9.2.2.1 Principle

Concanavalin A binds specifically to α-mannose and α-glucose residues on the inner acrosomal membrane of the head area of human sperm that will be exposed in only acrosome-reacted sperm [27].

9.2.2.2 Protocol

Supravital nuclear staining is determined with Hoechst 33258 (stock solution: 1 mg/mL) dissolved in Dulbecco buffer phosphate, added to a final concentration of 1 µg/mL and co-incubated with sperm for 10 minutes. The samples are centrifuged twice at $300 \times$ g for 10 minutes and the pellet resuspended in 500 µL of human tubular fluid medium. Spermatozoa are fixed in 10 percent formalin solution (neutral buffered) for at least 60 minutes at room temperature and centrifuged at $300 \times$ g for 10 minutes. Most of the supernatant is removed, and the sperm pellet is resuspended in the remaining solution. A 200 µL aliquot of the fixed sperm suspension is smeared and air-dried on a glass slide coated with 0.05 percent poly-L-lysin solution (5 µL). The slide is rinsed with 0.2 M glycine solution and washed with 10 mM PBS. Spermatozoa are labeled with 25 µL of FITC-ConA 100 µg/mL in 10 mM PBS, pH 7.4) for 25 minutes at room temperature according to Holden et al. [27].

Afterwards, the slides are rinsed with an excess of 10 mM PBS and mounted. At least 200 sperm are examined and scored per slide using a fluorescence microscope (magnification is $1000\times$).

9.2.2.3 Interpretation of Results

The following criteria are used to evaluate the acrosomal status.

(i) Sperm with positive fluorescence in the acrosomal region are scored as acrosome-reacted.

(ii) Sperm without fluorescence in the acrosomal region are considered as acrosome-intact.

(iii) A spermatozoon showing the region of the nucleus marked with Hoechst 33258 (blue) is considered dead.

9.2.3 Principle for FITC-Peanut Agglutinin (FITC-PNA) Staining in Simultaneous Assessment of Viability and Acrosome Reaction Rate of Human Sperm

9.2.3.1 Principle

FITC-PNA binds specifically to the outer acrosomal membrane. In sperm with an intact acrosome, the acrosomal region of the sperm head exhibits a uniform apple-green fluorescence. In acrosome-reacted sperm, only the equatorial segment of the acrosome is stained [28]. This is a method used in our laboratory (Figure 9.1).

9.2.3.2 Protocol

For this assay, sperm are pelleted at $300 \times$ g for five minutes and resuspended in 2 µg/mL Hoechst-33258 solution (Hoechst 33258 is prepared as a 1000x stock solution by dissolving 1 mg H33258 in 1 mL Dulbecco's phosphate-buffered saline. The stock solution is frozen at $-20°C$ (protected from light). The sperm suspensions are incubated for 10 minutes in the dark. Spermatozoa are then washed in PBS solution by centrifugation at $300 \times$ g for five minutes to remove excess stain. Subsequently, the pellet is resuspended in 100 µL of BWW. Twenty microliters of this solution are then smeared on a slide and allowed to dry. In case of problems with labeling or scoring, at least three slides of each sample are prepared. The slides are then immersed in ice-cold methanol for 30 seconds to permeabilize the sperm membranes and allowed to air dry. The fixed smears are immersed in a 40-µg/mL FITC-PNA solution and are covered in foil and incubated at room temperature for 20 minutes. According to Esteves et al. [29], slides are then gently washed in PBS to remove the excess label.

Slides are then rinsed with an excess of 10 mM PBS and mounted. Finally, 200 sperm per slide are examined in a fluorescence microscope (magnification is $1000\times$).

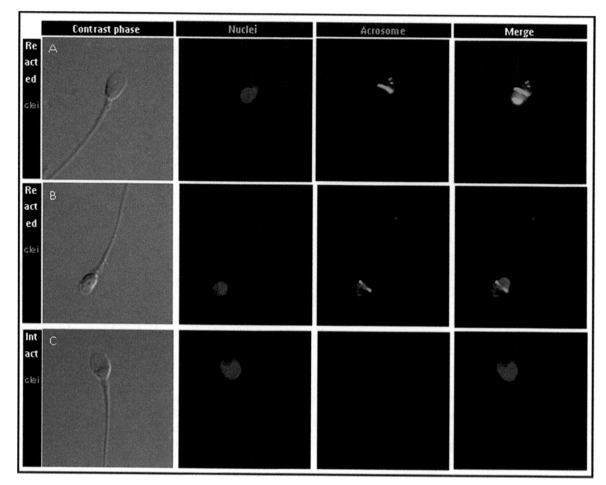

Figure 9.1 Acrosomal status of sperm cells according to PNA labeling and classified as: **A** and **B,** acrosome reacted or **C,** intact acrosome (unlabeled acrosome). Blue stain shows nucleus, green stain shows PNA/FITC. Magnifications 100x.

9.2.3.3 Interpretation of Results

The following criteria are used to evaluate the acrosomal status.

(i) Sperm without fluorescence in the acrosomal region and only in the equatorial segment are scored as acrosome-reacted.

(ii) Sperm without fluorescence in the acrosomal region are considered as acrosome-intact.

(iii) A spermatozoon showing the region of the nucleus marked with Hoechst 33258 (blue) is considered dead.

9.2.4 Reference Values

9.2.4.1 Spontaneous Acrosome Reaction

The percentage AR in control sperm after 3 hours incubation should not be appreciably different from 0 hours control sperm.

9.2.4.2 Induced Acrosome Reaction

- **Low Temperature.** An induced AR less than 20 percent is associated with a low number of fertilized oocytes in in vitro fertilization
- **Calcium Ionophore.** A difference between maximum induced AR and spontaneous AR of less or equal 5 percent indicates male infertility.
- **Progesterone.** An induced AR of more than 24 percent is significantly associated with high fertilization rates in in vitro fertilization.

9.2.5 Advantages/Disadvantages of the Test

FITC-PSA and FITC-ConA staining for detection of acrosome-reacted sperm provide similar results [20].

The advantages of the lectin-based technique are that it is fast, simple, easy to perform, and repeatable.

In contrast, the disadvantages of these tests are: (a) the specimens cannot be preserved under optimal conditions for a long time; (b) the method is expensive compared to histochemical stain techniques, because both fluorescent techniques require lectins and an epifluorescence microscope.

9.2.6 Clinical Significance

The employment of these techniques continues to be useful for the evaluation of infertile patients, especially in cases of unexplained infertility or before starting intrauterine insemination cycles, where it is necessary to investigate whether the sperm produced by the male partner is functional. Likewise, although a large number of fertility centers perform intracytoplasmic sperm injection (ICSI) as standard assisted reproductive technology (ART) procedure, however AR testing may be of value prior to conventional in vitro fertilization as it has a direct correlation with the fertilization outcome.

9.3 Flow Cytometry Detection of Acrosome Reaction

9.3.1 Principle for Anti-CD-46 Staining and Propidium Iodide (Anti-CD-46-PI) in Simultaneous Assessment of Viability and Acrosome Reaction Rate of Human Sperm

9.3.1.1 Principle

The antibody anti-CD-46 is conjugated to a fluorochrome. This staining is positive after sperm lose their acrosome because the CD46 protein is located only on the inner acrosomal membrane [30].

9.3.1.2 Protocol

Approximately 1×10^6 spermatozoa are incubated for 30 minutes at room temperature with human IgG (MiltenyuBistec GMBH, BergischGladbach, Germany) to block binding to Fc receptors. After washing the samples twice with PBS at $250 \times g$ for eight minutes, 10 µL of mouse FITC-conjugated IgG anti-body against human CD46 (BD PharMingen, San Diego, USA) are added. The samples are incubated protected from light at ambient temperature and washed with PBS. Afterwards, 2.5 µg/mL of propidium iodide (Sigma Chemical Company, St Louis, MO, USA) are added to assess sperm viability [31]. Finally, an aliquot of this preparation is analyzed (10,000 events are counted) in a FACSAria cytometer (Becton, Dickinson and Company). The data are analyzed by FACSDiva software (Becton, Dickinson and Company).

9.3.2 Principle for *Pisum sativum* Agglutinin Staining and Propidium Iodide (PSA-PI) in Simultaneous Assessment of Viability and Acrosome Reaction Rate of Human Sperm

9.3.2.1 Principle

Pisum sativum agglutinin is a dimeric lectin, consisting in two ab monomers with high affinity for α-D-mannose and α-D-glucose. This lectin conjugated with fluorescein isothiocyanate (PSA-FITC) recognizes highly glycosylated proteins present in the acrosome. It has also been used to determined acrosomal and plasma membrane integrity in unfixed sperm.

9.3.2.2 Protocol

Spermatozoa (5×10^6 cells/mL) are incubated at 37°C in HTF-BSA supplemented with 0.5 mg/mL PI, 5 mg/mL PSA-FITC [32]. The preparation is analyzed (10,000 events are counted) in a FACSAria cytometer (Becton Dickinson). The data are analyzed by FACSDiva software (Becton Dickinson).

9.3.2.3 Interpretation of Results

The fact that PSA-FITC is incorporated during acrosomal exocytosis in live sperm indicates that the percentage of sperm undergoing AR during the incubation can be assessed by counting cytometry.

Live spermatozoa undergoing exocytosis during incubation remain fluorescent for an extended period of time to analyze this population by flow cytometry.

By using the FITC and PI labeling, four sperm populations can be distinguished:

(i) Unreacted dead sperm (Q1)
(ii) Reacted dead sperm (Q2)
(iii) Unreacted live sperm (Q3)
(iv) Reacted live sperm (Q4)

The population of dead sperm is less than 8 percen [32].

9.3.3 Principle for FITC-Peanut Agglutinin and Propidium Iodide (PNA-PI) in Simultaneous Assessment of Viability and Acrosome Reaction Rate of Human Sperm

9.3.3.1 Principle

PNA-FITC has been described as being a good marker of the external acrosomal membrane and especially of the acrosomal vesicles [9]. This technique is accepted to evaluate the first steps of the AR, characterized by the appearance of vesicles within the acrosome content in human spermatozoa [33].

9.3.3.2 Protocol

The evaluation of the acrosome is performed by incubating sperm with PNA-FITC (300 µg/mL) and propidium iodide (PI) (0.75 µmol/L) for 10 minutes at 37°C in darkness. PI is added at a concentration of 0.75 µmol/L and incubated for 10 minutes. The sperm are washed by centrifugation at 500 × g for five minutes and re-suspended in 300 µL PBS. Samples are analyzed by flow cytometry with a BD FACS Canto II® Flow Cytometer (Becton Dickinson and Company; BD Biosciences, San Jose, CA, USA) and by confocal microscopy (FV 1000® Olympus, Miami, FL, USA) at 520 nm of SYBR-14, and 550 and 610 nm emissions of PNA-FITC and PI, respectively.

9.3.3.3 Interpretation of Results

Live spermatozoa with intact acrosome remain no fluorescence on the sperm head. In contast reacted acrosome sperm show fluorescence

By using the FITC and PI labeling, four sperm populations can be distinguished (Figure 9.2):

(i) Non-viable spermatozoa with intact acrosomes (PNA-/PI+) (Q1)

(ii) Non-viable spermatozoa with reacted acrosomes (PNA+/PI+) (Q2)

(iii) Live spermatozoa with intact acrosome (PNA−/PI−) (Q3)

(iv) Live spermatozoa with reacted acrosome (PNA+/PI−) (Q4).

9.3.4 Advantages/Disadvantages of the Test

The evaluation of the AR by means of flow cytometry determines functional aspects of the sperm cells and can be carried out in a short period of time. Moreover, by using flow cytometry, a high number of cells can be evaluated, which makes this method an ideal method for research and clinical diagnostic.

The disadvantage is the high cost of the flow cytometer and that it requires experienced staff to operate the equipment.

9.3.5 Clinical Significance

Although the use of acrosome evaluation by flow cytometry is more accurate because of the high numbers of cells that are evaluated, its use is limited in clinical practice. However, it has been a valuable contribution for research, not only when acrosomal damage should be evaluated, but also when the effect of new therapies that may increase or inhibit

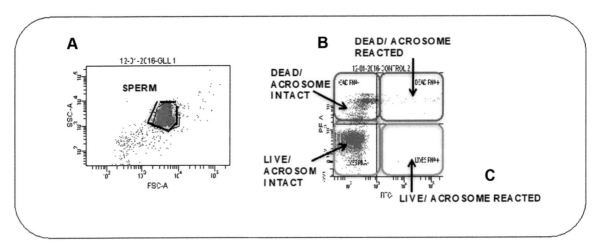

Figure 9.2 Flow cytometry diagrams showing acrosome reaction in human spermatozoa. A) Dot-plot graphs of the FSC channel to measure size versus the SSC channel to measure cell complexity; the areas outlined in black correspond to the population of human spermatozoa evaluated in the membrane integrity and acrosome reaction tests. B): the top left quadrant (red population) shows non-viable spermatozoa with intact acrosomes (PNA-/PI+), the top right quadrant shows non-viable spermatozoa with reacted acrosomes (PNA+/PI+), the bottom left quadrant (green population) shows live spermatozoa with intact acrosome (PNA-/PI-) and the bottom right quadrant contains live spermatozoa with reacted acrosome (PNA+/PI-).

AR are developed. Such therapies include the use of antioxidants or contraceptives. Furthermore, flow cytometry has been proven useful when the effect of chemicals, drugs or treatments such as cryopreservation on sperm, especially on the acrosome are evaluated.

9.4 Conclusion

Since the advent of assisted reproduction techniques and particularly of ICSI, where all-natural physiological steps such as capacitation or AR are circumvented, the inducibility of the AR remains an important test for the evaluation of sperm fertilizing ability. The use of flow cytometry to evaluate thousands of cells simultaneously has allowed its application in research, not only to evaluate the acrosome, but also to determine the mechanisms that modulate this essential physiologic function. Furthermore, it is a valuable tool to evaluate the effects of clinical or laboratory procedures on sperm cells. Finally, the induction of AR remains a good mechanism that allows us to assess the state of sperm capacitation indirectly, and further to provide information on the maintenance of adequate sperm function that is associated with optimal levels of fertilization of the oocyte.

References

1. Mack S, Bhattacharyya AK, Joyce C, van der Ven H, Zaneveld LJ. Acrosomal enzymes of human spermatozoa before and after in vitro capacitation. *Biol Reprod* 1983; **28**: 1032–42.

2. Yanagimachi R. (1988) Mammalian fertilization. In Knobil E, Neill J, eds., *The Physiology of Reproduction*. New York: RavenPress, pp. 135–85.

3. Liu DY, Baker HW. Acrosome status and morphology of human spermatozoa bound to the zona pellucida and oolemma determined using oocytes that failed to fertilize in vitro. *Hum Reprod* 1994; **9**: 673–9.

4. Schill WB, Topfer-Petersen E, Heissler E. The sperm acrosome: functional and clinical aspects. *Hum Reprod* 1993; **3**: 412–15.

5. Henkel R, Muller C, Miska W, Gips H, Schill WB. Determination of the acrosome reaction in human spermatozoa is predictive of fertilization in vitro. *Hum Reprod* 1993; **8**: 2128–32.

6. Cross L, Meizel S. Methods for evaluating the acrosomal status of mammalian sperm. *Biol Reprod* 1989; **41**: 635–41.

7. Kohn FM, Mack SR, Schill WB, Zaneveld LJD. Detection of human sperm acrosome reaction: comparison between methods using double staining, *Pisum sativum* agglutinin, concavalin A and transmission electron microscopy. *Hum Reprod* 1997; **12**: 714–21.

8. Zeginiadou T, Papadimas J, Mantalenakis S. Acrosome reaction: methods for detection and clinical significance. *Andrologia* 2000; **32**: 335–43.

9. Cooper TG, Yeung CH. A flow cytometric technique using peanut agglutinin for evaluating acrosomal loss from human spermatozoa. *J Androl* 1998; **19**: 542–50.

10. Fraser RL. Sperm capacitation and the acrosome reaction. *Hum Reprod* 1998; **13**(1): 9–19.

11. Kupker W, Diedrich K, Edwards RG. Principles of mammalian fertilization. *Hum Reprod* 1998; **13**: 20–32.

12. Issarman PM. Gamete interactions during mammalian fertilization. *Theriogenology* 1994; **41**: 31–44.

13. Fehl P, Miska W, Henkel R. Further indications of the multi component nature of the acrosome reaction-inducing substance of human follicular fluid. *Mol Reprod Dev* 1995; **42**: 80–8.

14. Beltrán C, Treviño CL, Mata-Martínez E, Chávez JC, Sánchez-Cárdenas C, Baker M, Darszon A. Role of ion channels in the sperm acrosome reaction. *Adv Anat Embryol Cell Biol* 2016; **220**: 35–69.

15. Gupta SK. The human egg's zona pellucida. *Curr Top Dev Biol* 2018; **130**: 379–411.

16. Hunnicutt GR, Primakoff P, Myles DG. Sperm surface protein PH-20 is bifunctional: one activity is a hyaluronidase and a second, distinct activity is required in secondary sperm-zona binding. *Biol Reprod* 55: 80–6.

17. Liu DY, Baker HW. Tests of human sperm function and fertilization in vitro. *Fertil Steril* 1992; **58**: 465–83.

18. Oehninger S, Franken DR, Ombelet W. Sperm functional tests. *Fertil Steril* 102: 1528–33.

19. Sanchez R, Topfer-Petersen E, Aitken RJ, Schill WB. A new method for evaluation of the acrosome reaction in viable human spermatozoa. *Andrologia* 1991; **23**: 197–203.

20. Ozaki T, Takahashi K, Kanasaki H, Miyazaki K. Evaluation of acrosome reaction and viability of human sperm with two fluorescent dyes. *Arch Gynecol Obstet* 2002; **266**: 114–17.

21. Xu F, Zhu H, Zhu W, Fan L. Human sperm acrosomal status, acrosomal responsiveness, and acrosin are predictive of the

outcomes of in vitro fertilization: a prospective cohort study. *Reprod Biol* 2018; **18**: 344–54.

22. Ryu BY, Kim SH, Park SY, Jee BC, Jung BJ, Kim HS, et al. Efficacy of acrosome reaction after ionophore challenge (ARIC) test in evaluation of fertilization capacityof human spermatozoa. *Korean J Obstet Gynecol* 1988; **41**: 2562–70.

23. Chen X, Zheng Y, Zheng J, Lin J, Zhang L, Jin J. The progesterone-induced sperm acrosome reaction is a good option for the prediction of fertilization in vitro compared with other sperm parameters. *Andrologia* 2019; **51**: e13278.

24. Krausz C, Bonaccorsi L, Maggio P, Luconi M, Criscuoli L, Fuzzi B, et al. Two functional assays of sperm responsiveness to progesterone and their predictive values in in-vitro fertilization. *Hum Reprod* 1996; **11**: 1661–7.

25. Cross NL, Morales P, Overstreet JW, Hanson FW. Two simple methods for detecting acrosome-reacted human sperm. *Gamete Res* 1986; **15**: 213–26.

26. Mendoza C, Carreras A, Moos J, Tesarik J. Distinction between true acrosome reaction and degenerative acrosome loss by a one-step staining method using Pisum sativum agglutinin. *J Reprod Fertil* 1992; **95**: 755–63.

27. Holden CA, Hyne RV, Sathananthan AH, Trounson AO. Assessment of the human sperm acrosome reaction using concanavalin A lectin. *Mol Reprod Dev* 1990; **25**: 247–57.

28. Mortimer D, Curtis EF, Miller RG. Specific labeling by peanut agglutinin of the outer acrosomal membrane of the human spermatozoon. *J Reprod Fertil* 1987; **81**: 127–35.

29. Esteves SC, Sharma RK, Thomas AJ Jr, Agarwal A. Evaluation of acrosomal status and sperm viability in fresh and cryopreserved specimens by the use of fluorescent peanut agglutinin lectin in conjunction with hypo-osmotic swelling test. *Int Braz J Urol* 2007; **33**: 364–74.

30. Tao J, Du J, Critser ES, Critser JK. Assessment of the acrosomal status and viability of human spermatozoa simultaneously using flow cytometry. *Hum Reprod* 1993; **8**: 1879–85.

31. Carver-Ward JA, Moran-Verbeek IM, Hollanders JM. Comparative flow cytometric analysis of the human sperm acrosome reaction using CD46 antibody and lectins. *J Assist Reprod Genet* 1997; **14**: 111–19.

32. Zoppino FC, Halón ND, Bustos MA, Pavarotti MA, Mayorga LS. Recording and sorting live human sperm undergoing acrosome reaction. *Fertil Steril* 2012; **97**: 1309–15.

33. Fierro R, Foliguet B, Grignon G, Daniel M, Bene MC, Faure GC, Barbarino-Monnier P. Lectin-binding sites on human sperm during acrosome reaction: modifications judged by electron microscopy/flow cytometry. *Arch Androl* 1996; **36**: 187–96.

Chapter 10

Capacitation and Acrosome Reaction: Histochemical Techniques to Determine Acrosome Reaction

Brett Nixon, Shenae L. Cafe, Elizabeth G. Bromfield, Geoffry N. De Iuliis, Matthew D. Dun

10.1 Introduction

Fertilization is an exceptionally specific cell recognition event that represents the culmination of a complex sequence of morphological and functional maturational events. In the case of the male gamete, this process is initiated by the commitment of spermatogonial stem cells to differentiate, sequentially forming spermatogonia, spermatocytes and eventually spermatozoa that are released into the lumen of the seminiferous tubules [1]. In addition to meiotic divisions, this process encompasses extensive cytoplasmic, organelle and nuclear remodeling events, thus establishing the unique and highly polarized architecture of the mature spermatozoon. A key aspect of this phase of development is the modification and repositioning of the Golgi apparatus to form a highly specialized secretory organelle, known as the acrosome, overlying the anterior aspect of the sperm head. Upon release from the testes the functionally immature spermatozoa enter the epididymis where they are progressively remodeled and acquire both motility and the potential to fertilize an oocyte [2]. This potential is eventually realized after passage through the female reproductive tract whereupon the ejaculated cells complete a suite of biochemical and biophysical changes known as capacitation [3]. These successive phases of functional maturation culminate in the acquired ability to release the acrosomal contents, during an event known as the acrosome reaction. This unique exocytotic event facilitates sperm passage through the outer vestments of the oocyte and is essential for successful in vivo fertilization in all mammalian species, including the human [4]. Consequently, failure of acrosomal exocytosis represents a common etiology in defective spermatozoa of male infertility patients that have failed in vitro

fertilization (IVF) in a clinical setting; accounting for as much as 29 percent of unexplained male infertility cases [5, 6]. Much of our current mechanistic understanding of the acrosome reaction is grounded in the ability to stimulate this process in vitro using simple chemically defined media and the application of pharmacological interventions, and/or transgenic mouse models. Here, we discuss the biological significance of the acrosome reaction and the application of histochemical techniques that have been developed to study the progression and completion of this critical physiological event.

10.1.1 The Sperm Acrosome

10.1.1.1 Biogenesis and Structure of the Acrosomal Vesicle

The term "acrosome" was introduced by Lenhossek in 1898 and literally translates as "tip body" or "apical body". Over time, we have come to appreciate that the acrosome is a discrete lysosome-like membranous organelle that is indeed positioned overlying the nucleus within the anterior region of the sperm head. The acrosome is unique to the male gamete and, notwithstanding considerable variation in size and shape between species, this organelle originates from the Golgi apparatus during the remodeling of early spermatids that accompanies spermiogenesis (Figure 10.1) [1]. Acrosomal biogenesis is initiated by the formation of pro-acrosomic vesicles that are generated within, and actively trafficked by, the Golgi apparatus. These entities eventually fuse giving rise to a single, dense, acrosomal vesicle that extends to cover approximately two-thirds of the nuclear surface [1]. This structure is delimited by both inner and outer acrosomal membranes, and, through its association with the overlying acroplaxone (consisting of

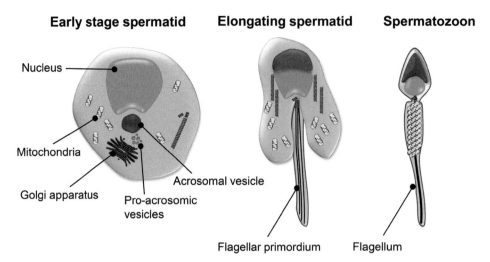

Figure 10.1 Biogenesis of the human sperm acrosome. Schematic diagram depicting the cytodifferentiation of the developing germ cell during spermiogenesis. Formation of the acrosomal vesicle is initiated in early stage spermatids as pro-acrosomic vesicles generated by the Golgi apparatus fuse giving rise to a single, highly specialized secretory organelle that extends to cover approximately two-thirds of the nuclear surface.

actin and keratin fibers) and manchette complex, the acrosomal vesicle becomes anchored to the nuclear envelope and participates in the sculpting of the sperm head during spermiogenesis [1].

In the mature spermatozoon, the acrosomal vesicle incorporates a myriad of structural and enzymatic components that are compartmentalized into either soluble or insoluble fractions. The latter of these consists of particulate material termed the acrosomal matrix; a structure that resists detergent solubilization and has properties consistent with those of functional amyloids [7]. Indeed, the core of the acrosomal matrix is known to comprise several amyloidogenic proteins, as well as other proteins predicted to self-assemble into amyloid [7]. Accordingly, the acrosomal matrix has been postulated to function as a stable scaffold for interactions between the sperm and oocyte and to allow the controlled and sequential release of matrix associated proteins necessary for fertilization during the acrosome reaction. Thereafter, proteases activated by the increased intra-acrosomal pH that results from the induction of the acrosome reaction have been postulated to promote the disassembly of the acrosomal matrix, culminating in the complete loss of the acrosomal cap [7].

Owing to its essential role during fertilization, considerable effort has been devoted to the characterization of the acrosomal contents. Among the dominant proteins identified by biochemical means residing in the acrosomal matrix are acrosin, acrosin binding protein, zona pellucida binding protein, zona pellucida-3 receptor, and zonadhesin. However, the recent application of advanced mass spectrometry analyses has expanded the curated inventory of acrosomal matrix associated proteins to excess of 1,000 candidates [8]. Notably, approximately half of the proteins represented in the acrosomal matrix had not been previously identified in proteomic analyses of spermatozoa, suggesting that the composition of this organelle differs substantially from that of other sperm domains [8]. Moreover, the acrosomal matrix is enriched in proteins classified as having cytoskeletal, oxidoreductase, and hydrolase functions, as well as ancillary proteins categorized as enzyme modulators, proteases, transporters, transferases, nucleic acid binding proteins, chaperones, transfer/carrier proteins, structural proteins, and kinases. Of interest, the proteomic composition of the acrosomal matrix differs between the populations of sperm entering (i.e. caput spermatozoa) and leaving the epididymis (i.e. cauda spermatozoa) raising the prospect that this specialized vesicle may undergo maturational changes during epididymal transit in preparation for downstream functions during fertilization [8]. These findings confirm that the acrosome is a dynamic functional structure comprising an abundance of fertilization-associated proteins; many of which have the potential to be exploited as biomarkers capable of discriminating the acrosomal status and/or fertilization competence of human spermatozoa [9].

10.1.1.2 Physiology of the Acrosome Reaction

In all mammalian species including the human, the completion of an acrosome reaction is a prerequisite for successful fertilization in vivo [10]. Indeed, the importance of the acrosome for human fertilization is evidenced by a rare congenital condition in which spermatozoa are produced with a small spherical head lacking an acrosome [11]. These acrosome-less spermatozoa are unable to bind to or penetrate the zona pellucida (ZP) and accordingly, men with this condition are universally sterile and unable to produce pregnancies via natural conception or standard IVF procedures [4]. This condition can be treated by intracytoplasmic sperm injection (ICSI) [11], albeit with variable success in terms of fertilization rates and pregnancies; depending on whether or not the sperm heads are capable of decondensing normally within the ooplasm [12]. Similarly, the inability to complete an acrosome reaction represents a relatively common etiology in the defective spermatozoa of idiopathic male infertility patients that have failed standard IVF [6], accounting for as much as 29 percent of unexplained male infertility cases [5]. Such defects often manifest in a failure of sperm-zona pellucida penetration, occurring downstream of zona pellucida binding; a condition referred to as disordered zona pellucida-induced acrosome reaction

(DZPIAR), and one that has been associated with severe chronic infertility [4]. It follows that the proportion of sperm with intact acrosomes in the insemination medium is positively correlated with fertilization rates in vitro, thus emphasizing the utility of diagnostic assays that enable determination of sperm competence to complete an acrosome reaction before commencing assisted reproductive technologies (ART).

The acrosome reaction is a distinctive exocytotic process that is initiated by multiple fusion events and subsequent vesiculation occurring between the outer acrosomal membrane and the overlying plasma membrane (Figure 10.2). As this wave of vesiculation radiates across the anterior region of the sperm head, it leads to the destabilization of the acrosomal structure, formation of hybrid membrane vesicles and the concomitant release of the soluble acrosomal contents [10]. The dispersion of the acrosomal contents, which includes a number of powerful hydrolytic enzymes, enables sperm penetration of the tenacious investments surrounding the ovulated oocyte. This, in turn, provides the fertilizing spermatozoon with access to the oocyte plasma membrane beneath, and ultimately secures cytoplasmic continuity between the gametes. Recent work has drawn into question the long-held view that the acrosome reaction proceeds in an "all or none" manner, with accumulating evidence suggesting that the process may instead comprise several intermediate phases, each with their own set of

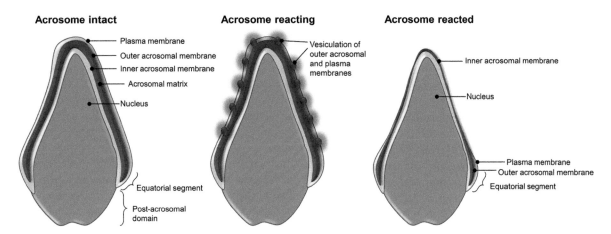

Figure 10.2 Human sperm acrosome reaction. Schematic diagram depicting the progression of the acrosome reaction within the head of a mature human spermatozoon. After initiation of the acrosome reaction, multiple fusion foci form between the outer acrosomal membrane and overlying plasma membrane. As the acrosome reaction proceeds a wave of vesiculation propagates across the anterior region of the sperm head, facilitating the loss of the acrosomal contents and exposure of the inner acrosomal membrane; except in the region of the equatorial segment where the outer acrosomal membrane and the plasma membrane retain their integrity.

functional consequences [13]. In keeping with this model, several features of acrosomal exocytosis, including the relatively slow kinetics at which it proceeds, underscore the highly specialized nature of this secretory process and the prospect that is governed by complex molecular mechanisms [13].

The ability to undergo a physiological acrosome reaction necessitates that spermatozoa have first completed a process of functional maturation, known as capacitation, during their transit of the female reproductive tract [13]. Among the many biochemical and biophysical changes that accompany capacitation, the sperm membrane becomes increasingly fusogenic, owing to alterations in its lipid architecture and the release of decapacitation factors [14]. These combined events serve to modulate intracellular ion concentrations leading to hyperpolarization of the sperm plasma membrane and triggering complex signaling cascades that prime the cell for completion of an acrosome reaction. The precise physiological stimulus that acts downstream of capacitation to induce acrosomal exocytosis remains a matter of some controversy [15]. Indeed, notwithstanding a wealth of evidence that adhesion to zona pellucida ligands act as the key stimulus for induction of acrosomal exocytosis, particularly in the human, alternative models based on studies of transgenic mice now suggest that the timing of the acrosomal exocytosis may actually precede that of zona adhesion [15]. Consistent with this notion, it has been shown that a significant proportion of mouse spermatozoa initiate acrosomal exocytosis in the upper segments of the oviductal isthmus [16], prior to engaging zona pellucida ligands. Moreover, mouse spermatozoa that have undergone an acrosome reaction retain the ability to bind and penetrate the zona pellucida [17].

Such experimental models appear at odds with human studies in which the induction of an acrosome reaction in the in vitro insemination medium actually reduces or prevents sperm from subsequently binding to the zona pellucida [4, 18]. Nevertheless, these data could help account for the ability of agonists, such as follicular fluid and progesterone that sperm encounter within the oviduct prior to zona adhesion, to induce acrosomal exocytosis in the spermatozoa of several species, including the human [9]. The steroidal hormone progesterone reportedly acts by modulating an increase in cytosolic Ca^{2+} levels, an event that can be recapitulated using nonphysiological pharmacological reagents, such as the divalent cation ionophore, A23187. Indeed, by directly facilitating Ca^{2+} influx, the A23187 ionophore obfuscates the need for the intracellular signaling mechanisms and effector pathways that otherwise regulate the progression of the acrosome reaction. It is therefore not surprising that the processes of acrosomal exocytosis driven by calcium ionophore proceed differently from those occurring in response to physiological stimuli such as solubilized zonae pellucidae. Thus, the spatial profile of an ionophore-induced acrosomal reaction is random, with no obvious preference for initiation in the anterior, middle or posterior acrosomal regions [19]. By contrast, solubilized zonae pellucidae exclusively stimulate a slower and more orderly loss of acrosomal components; beginning at the posterior zone of the acrosome and progressing in an anterograde direction [19]. Whilst these data lend support to the notion of receptor-mediated events controlling membrane fusion and release of acrosomal components, the limited availability of human zonae pellucidae prevents this resource being widely used as physiological stimuli in assisted reproductive settings. Thus, despite its limitations, monitoring of the ability of spermatozoa to undergo an ionophore-induced acrosome reaction has become an important diagnostic criterion of human sperm function testing in clinical ART laboratories.

10.1.2 Histochemical Methods for Detection of Acrosome Reaction

The frequency with which spermatozoa undergo an acrosome reaction represents an important parameter in the evaluation of sperm function as it provides a reliable indication of the likely success of standard IVF and artificial insemination [20]. The impetus to analyze acrosomal exocytosis in human spermatozoa is further emphasized by the fact that a failure to complete this event represents a relatively common etiology associated with the defective spermatozoa of male infertility patients. In a majority of these cases, males present with isolated lesions in sperm penetration of the zona pellucida and either no, or low, rates of fertilization, without any attendant reduction in other semen parameters or levels of sperm–zona pellucida binding [20]. Thus, the diagnostic criterion of DZPIAR is that very low proportions of sperm undergo the acrosome reaction (<16 percent) after binding to the zona pellucida; with estimates suggesting that >25 percent of men seeking recourse to assisted reproductive programs due to idiopathic infertility might be afflicted by this condition [5]. Although these patients commonly have a long duration of unexplained infertility, it is encouraging that they routinely achieve high fertilization and pregnancy rates with ICSI [20]. It is therefore important to diagnose patients with defects in acrosomal responsiveness before commencing ART treatment in order to avoid failure of fertilization with standard IVF. Such diagnoses rely on the application of accurate methodology for monitoring acrosomal status and the establishment of clinical reference ranges for acrosome reaction rates achieved using different stimuli (i.e. ionophore versus progesterone versus zona pellucidae) [21].

As discussed previously, the completion of an acrosome reaction leads to the loss of the acrosomal cap overlying the anterior domain of the sperm head. In species that possess large acrosomes (e.g. the guinea pig and hamster), this phenomenon can be observed directly by either light or phase-contrast microscopy. However, by comparison, the acrosome of human spermatozoa is relatively small and thus very difficult to visualize at the level of resolution afforded by standard light microscopy. As a consequence, alternative protocols have been developed for monitoring the progression of an acrosome reaction and/or evaluating the acrosomal status within a given population of human spermatozoa, with these protocols being broadly divided into four categories and each having its own inherent advantages and disadvantages (Table 10.1).

The most widely used methods to determine acrosome reaction incorporate the use of fluorescently conjugated reagents (most commonly plant lectins or antibodies) that selectively bind to glycoproteins residing in the acrosomal matrix or acrosomal membranes [4]. It follows that the release of these glycoproteins during the course of the acrosome reaction can be detected using fluorescence microscopy or by assaying the supernatant using ELISA-based detection protocols. The application of the former technique is described by Sánchez Gutiérrez and colleagues in Chapter 4.1. Accordingly, here we discuss alternative histochemical approaches that exploit the use of various non-fluorescent chromogens to label the protein-rich contents of the acrosome and/or acrosomal membranes. Examples of such cytochemical techniques include the use of single (Coomassie blue),

double (Giemsa stain and Trypan blue) and triple stain (Bismarck brown, Rose bengal, and Trypan blue) protocols, the latter of which permit simultaneous evaluation of sperm viability and acrosomal status and are thus capable of distinguishing a physiological acrosome reaction from that of a false/spontaneous acrosome reaction. Although histochemical techniques may lack the inherent sensitivity achieved using fluorophore conjugated reagents, they nonetheless have several advantages, including that they are relatively inexpensive and easy to perform, utilize stains that are stable (thus avoiding issues of photo-bleaching and deterioration of signal intensity that are common to fluorescent reagents), and the labeled spermatozoa can be readily visualized using standard light microscopy, infrastructure that is commonly available in clinical laboratories (as opposed to expensive specialist fluorescence instrumentation).

10.1.2.1 Triple Stain Method

10.1.2.1.1 Principle/Mechanism

The triple-stain technique was originally developed by Talbot and Chacon [22] to simultaneously evaluate the proportion of viable, acrosome-reacted human spermatozoa in fixed smears. This protocol centers on the application of the cell viability stain, Trypan blue, to discriminate live and dead spermatozoa. Spermatozoa are then fixed in glutaraldehyde, dried onto slides, and the post-acrosomal region and acrosome are differentiated via labeling with Bismarck brown and Rose bengal (stains the acrosomal matrix in acrosome intact spermatozoa), respectively. It is recommended that slides are examined at 1000× magnification with a bright-field microscope and assessed for the percentage of spermatozoa that were alive at the time of fixation and had undergone normal acrosome reactions.

10.1.2.1.2 Brief Methods/Protocol

Spermatozoa may be prepared using standard swim-up or density gradient centrifugation protocols. Owing to the necessity for capacitation before undergoing a physiological acrosome reaction, these cells must be capacitated using standard protocols [23], and thereafter induced to undergo an ionophore [24], progesterone [9] or zona pellucida-induced [21] acrosome reaction. Following the induction of acrosomal exocytosis, sperm suspensions (4×10^6 cells/mL; 200 μL) are mixed 1:1 with 2 percent w/v Trypan blue (T6146, Merck, Darmstadt, Germany)

Table 10.1 Methods Utilized for Detection of the Acrosome Reaction in Human Spermatozoa

Method	Advantages	Disadvantages
1. Light microscopy (bright field or fluorescence) This technique exploits the use of various chromogenic dyes to label the protein-rich contents of the acrosome/acrosomal membranes. Enhanced sensitivity can be achieved via staining of spermatozoa with specific fluorophore conjugated reagents (e.g. plant lectins: *Pisum sativum* agglutinin, peanut agglutinin, concanavalin A, Ricinus communis agglutinin, wheat germ agglutinin; or anti-acrosome antibodies).	Can discriminate progression of spermatozoa through different stages of acrosome reaction.	These methods require counting of hundreds of spermatozoa from each sample and results may be influenced by observer-dependent subjectivity.
2. Transmission electron microscopy This technique uses electrons in place of light to visualize cell structures in fine detail. As the wavelength of electrons is much smaller than that of light, the resolution attainable is many orders of magnitude better than that of a light microscope.	Delivers detailed information on the ultrastructure of the sperm acrosome.	Requires expensive specialized equipment, as well as skilful, trained staff. Is laborious and time-consuming and results are prone to fixation and post-fixation handling artefacts.
3. Fluorescence-activated cell sorting Spermatozoa are separated based on prior staining with fluorescently conjugated antibodies or lectins.	Permits rapid and objective assessment of large numbers of spermatozoa.	This method requires expensive equipment and expertise that may not be readily available within clinical laboratories.
4. Biochemical methods Based on measurement of the enzymatic activity of acrosin, or other enzymes released from the acrosomal vesicle during the acrosome reaction.	Provides objective measurement of acrosome reaction and enzymatic activity of released proteins.	This method is time-consuming and necessitates the use of relatively large numbers of spermatozoa. Does not provide information on the percentage of sperm that have completed an acrosome reaction.

for assessment of viability (noting that dead cells are labeled dark blue), before being pelleted by gentle centrifugation (400 × g for five minutes). The resultant pellet is fixed in 100 μL of 3 percent glutaraldehyde in human tubal fluid (HTF) and incubated at 37°C for 20 minutes. The glutaraldehyde is removed by centrifugation (400 × g for five minutes) and the pellet resuspended in distilled water (1 mL). Aliquots (25 μL) of spermatozoa are placed on a slide, air-dried at room temperature for 30 minutes and sequentially stained with 0.8 percent w/v Bismarck brown Y (cat # 861111, Merck) for five minutes at 40°C, followed by three washes with distilled water and incubation in 0.8 percent w/v Rose bengal (cat #

198250, Merck) prepared in 0.1 M Tris for 40 minutes at room temperature. Slides are then washed in distilled water, dehydrated in graded ethanol (50, 70, 96 percent), cleared in xylene, and mounted with a coverslip. For assessment of the percentage of acrosome reaction in viable spermatozoa, a minimum of 200 cells are examined in randomly selected fields under oil-immersion brightfield optics at 1000× magnification.

10.1.2.1.3 Laboratory and Clinical Interpretation

Four patterns of sperm labeling are anticipated (Figure 10.3) with their clinical interpretation being [22]:

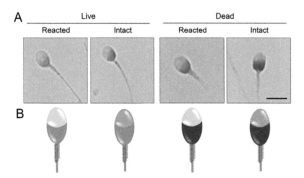

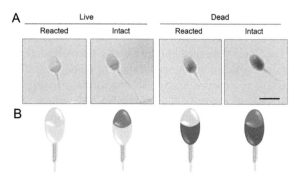

Figure 10.3 Triple-stain technique. (**A**) Representative images and (**B**) corresponding schematic diagrams of human spermatozoa depicting the four categories detected after sequential labeling with Trypan blue, Bismark brown and Rose bengal. Viable spermatozoa are identified on the basis of light brown staining within the post-acrosomal domain, whilst non-viable cells feature dark blue staining of this domain. Spermatozoa with an intact acrosome feature light pink labeling within the apical region of the sperm head, whereas those that have lost their acrosomal contents, either through physiological (live cells) or degenerative (dead cells) acrosome reaction, are demarcated by an unstained (white/clear) apical region. Scale bar = 10 μm.

Figure 10.4 Double-stain technique. (**A**) Representative images and (**B**) corresponding schematic diagrams of human spermatozoa depicting the four categories detected after sequential labeling with Trypan blue and Giemsa stain. Viable spermatozoa are identified on the basis of faint blue/no staining within the post-acrosomal domain, whilst non-viable cells feature dark blue staining of this domain. Spermatozoa with an intact acrosome feature purple labeling within the apical region of the sperm head, whereas those that have lost their acrosomal contents, either through physiological (live cells) or degenerative (dead cells) acrosome reaction, are demarcated by an unstained (white/clear) apical region. Scale bar = 10 μm.

(i) Dead spermatozoa with an intact acrosome = dark blue post-acrosomal domain and light pink acrosomal domain

(ii) Degenerative acrosome reaction of dead spermatozoa = dark blue post-acrosomal domain and an unstained (clear/white) acrosomal domain

(iii) Viable spermatozoa with intact acrosome = light brown post-acrosomal domain and a pink acrosomal domain

(iv) Viable spermatozoa with reacted acrosome = light brown post-acrosomal domain and an unstained (clear/white) acrosomal domain

10.1.2.2 Double Stain Method

10.1.2.2.1 Principle/Mechanism

Similar to the triple stain method described above, the double stain technique is also permissive of simultaneously evaluating sperm viability and acrosomal status [25], but is based on the application of Trypan blue in concert with Giemsa, a solution comprising methylene blue, azure and eosin that selectively labels the outer acrosomal membrane.

10.1.2.2.2 Brief Methods/Protocol

Sperm preparation is equivalent to that outlined in the triple stain protocol above until the point of Trypan blue staining. Thereafter, 25 μL aliquots of the sperm suspension are placed on a slide and air-

dried at room temperature for 20 minutes. The spermatozoa are subsequently stained for 40 minutes with a 10 percent w/v solution of Giemsa stain (cat #G4507, Merck) prepared in distilled water immediately before use. After staining, the slides are washed in distilled water, air-dried at room temperature for 30 minutes and mounted with a coverslip. For assessment of the percentage of acrosome reaction in viable spermatozoa, a minimum of 200 cells are examined in randomly selected fields under oil-immersion brightfield optics at 1000× magnification.

10.1.2.2.3 Laboratory and Clinical Interpretation

Four patterns of sperm labeling are anticipated (Figure 10.4), with their clinical interpretation being [25]:

(i) Dead spermatozoa with intact acrosome = dark blue post-acrosomal domain and purple acrosomal domain

(ii) Degenerative acrosome reaction of dead spermatozoa = dark blue post-acrosomal domain and an unstained (clear/white) acrosomal domain

(iii) Viable spermatozoa with intact acrosome = light blue or unstained post-acrosomal domain and purple acrosomal domain

(iv) Viable spermatozoa with reacted acrosome = light blue or unstained post-acrosomal domain and unstained (clear/white) in the acrosomal domain

10.1.2.3 Single Stain Method

10.1.2.3.1 Principle/Mechanism

The single stain method represents a simple and rapid protocol based on the application of Coomassie Blue G-250 to produce intense labeling of the protein rich acrosomal contents [26]. Although this single step protocol is not capable of discriminating live spermatozoa (and therefore completion of a physiological acrosome reaction), this important objective can be achieved by performing Coomassie Blue labeling in concert with the hypo-osmotic swelling test, the principles of which are described by Jeyendran in Chapter 2.

10.1.2.3.2 Brief Methods/Protocol

Capacitated and acrosome reacted populations of human spermatozoa prepared as described above are first subjected to the hypo-osmotic swelling test to differentiate viable (curled tails) from non-viable cells (straight tails). Spermatozoa are then fixed with 4 percent paraformaldehyde solution for 10 minutes at room temperature before being centrifuged and washed twice using 1.5 mL of 100 mM ammonium acetate (pH 9.0). The resultant sperm pellet is resuspended in 1 mL of 100 mM ammonium acetate and 50 μL of this sperm suspension is then smeared onto glass microscope slides using another glass slide. After air-drying, the slides are incubated in freshly prepared Coomassie stain (comprising: 0.22 percent Coomassie Brilliant Blue G-250 (cat # B0770, Merck), 50 percent methanol, 10 percent glacial acetic acid, 40 percent water) for 2 minutes. Slides are then thoroughly washed using distilled water to remove excess stain prior to being air-dried and mounted with coverslips. Stained sperm are subsequently assessed for the percentage of viable acrosome reacted cells; counting a minimum of 200 cells in randomly selected fields under oil-immersion brightfield optics at 1000× magnification.

10.1.2.3.3 Laboratory and Clinical Interpretation

Four patterns of sperm labeling are anticipated (Figure 10.5), with their clinical interpretation being [26]:

(i) Dead spermatozoa with intact acrosome = dark blue acrosomal domain and straight tail
(ii) Dead spermatozoa with reacted acrosome = light blue/clear acrosomal domain and straight tail
(iii) Viable spermatozoa with intact acrosome = dark blue acrosomal domain and curled tail

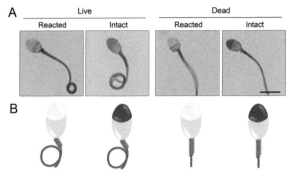

Figure 10.5 Single stain technique. (A) Representative images and **(B)** corresponding schematic diagrams of human spermatozoa depicting the four categories detected after Coomassie Blue G-250 labeling of cells subjected to a hypo-osmotic swelling test. Viable spermatozoa are identified on the basis of a tightly curled tail, whereas non-viable cells possess a straight/curved tail. Spermatozoa with an intact acrosome feature intense dark blue labeling within the apical region of the sperm head, whereas those that have lost their acrosomal contents, either through physiological (live cells) or degenerative (dead cells) acrosome reaction, are distinguished by a light blue/unstained apical region. Scale bar = 10 μm.

(iv) Viable spermatozoa with reacted acrosome = light blue/clear acrosomal domain and curled tail

10.1.2.4 Reference Values and How to Calculate Cut-Off Values

The normal range of acrosome reaction rates detected using the histochemical approaches described above are expected to vary in accordance with the nature of the agonist used for induction of this event. Thus, studies using intact human zonae pellucidae (which is arguably the most physiologically relevant stimuli) have reported an average acrosome reaction rate of 48 percent among the spermatozoa of fertile donors [21]. Notably, however, considerable excursions around this mean value have been witnessed across cohorts of fertile males, with levels of zona pellucida-induced acrosome reaction ranging from 20–98 percent in these individuals [21]. Despite this relatively high degree of variability, the zona pellucida-induced acrosome reaction has been significantly correlated with other indicators of male fertility. Indeed, the rate of zona pellucida-induced acrosome reaction is significantly lower in men with sperm concentrations of $\leq 60 \times 10^6$/mL compared to those with sperm concentrations of $>60 \times 10^6$/mL. Similarly, men with normal sperm morphology of ≥ 15 percent have significantly higher zona pellucida-induced acrosome reaction than men with normal morphology of <15 percent [21].

By comparison, studies on the spermatozoa of infertile patients with consistently low or zero fertilization rates after standard IVF, reported an average zona pellucida-induced acrosome reaction rate of only 6 percent (range 0–16 percent) [5, 6]. In a similar context, normozoospermic men with <16 percent zona pellucida-induced acrosome reaction had <20 percent of the zona pellucida penetrated by sperm, and those with <10 percent zona pellucida-induced acrosome reaction had zero sperm–zona pellucida penetration in vitro [21]. It follows that prospective studies have revealed a significant positive correlation between fertilization rates and the levels of acrosome reaction induced using intact zona pellucida. Illustrative of this, idiopathic infertility patients with <16 percent zona pellucida-induced acrosome reaction and otherwise normal semen analyses have been reported to have an average fertilization rate of only 25 percent following standard IVF [5, 6]. Consistent with these findings, independent studies suggest that patients with normal semen analysis but <15 percent acrosome reaction induced by solubilized zonae pellucidae are also afflicted by poor fertilization results following standard IVF [27]. Taken together, this collective evidence indicates that male factor fertility may be compromised if the zona pellucida-induced acrosome reaction rate falls below 20 percent. This clinical reference has been promulgated in the diagnosis of patients with disordered zona pellucida-induced acrosome reaction (DZPIAR) that are unlikely to achieve fertilization using conventional IVF [5, 6]. However, these data also highlight a wide range for the zona pellucida-induced acrosome reaction among individual fertile men (i.e. reference values of between 20–98 percent). The influence of such variability on the clinical interpretation and diagnostic performance of this bioassay should encourage ART laboratories to pay regard to validating their own optimal procedures.

Aside from the use of intact/solubilized zonae pellucidae, the divalent cation ionophore A23187 is also recognized as a potent agonist for the induction of acrosomal exocytosis. Accordingly, the diagnostic potential of sperm function tests involving A23187 has been demonstrated in the context of in vitro fertilization therapy, using either the acrosome reaction or sperm-oocyte fusion (i.e. hamster egg penetration test) as end-points for such bioassays [28]. Despite this promise, there remains considerable disparity in the literature with respect to the dose and formulation of the A23187 compound that should be used to optimally stimulate spermatozoa, with values as extreme as 100 μM of the Ca^{2+}/Mg^{2+} salt and 2 μM of the free acid being used in different studies. A major problem with this lack of standardization is that high doses of A23187 are cytotoxic, meaning that elevated concentrations may compromise the viability and/or biological responses of the spermatozoa being assessed. If these limitations are addressed, then average levels of acrosome reaction achieved using A23187 (42 percent) are virtually indistinguishable from those obtained in side-by-side comparison with intact zonae pellucidae (43 percent) [29], suggesting similar clinical reference values may be applicable. As a cautionary note however, the processes of acrosomal exocytosis driven by the A23187 chemical agonist proceed differently from those occurring in response to physiological ZP stimuli [19]. This may account for the lack of a direct, linear correlation between acrosome reaction rates and the incidence of downstream sperm-oocyte fusion observed in response to A23187 [24], and also between the results of A23187 and zona pellucida-induced acrosome reaction in the same subjects [29]. Such uncertainties concerning the mechanism of A23187 action inevitably draw into question the biological relevance of diagnostic tests based on this reagent in terms of evaluating the functional competence of human spermatozoa. At present it remains uncertain whether the use of progesterone and/or complex biological fluids such as follicular fluid as the acrosome reaction stimulant are prone to similar limitations. However, the uncontrolled nature of the latter components may well limit their use for the development of defined diagnostic systems.

10.1.2.5 Advantages/Disadvantages of the Test

The histochemical labeling techniques described in this chapter are compatible with the rapid evaluation of human sperm acrosomal status and enable differentiation between physiological acrosome reactions and degenerative acrosomal loss caused by sperm death. Moreover, once mounted with a coverslip, the labeled sperm specimens can be preserved under optimal conditions almost indefinitely with minimal loss of staining intensity; thus permitting future evaluation of the acrosome status and also sperm morphology should the need arise. Importantly, the accuracy and reliability of these techniques in the detection of

89

acrosome reaction frequency has proven comparable to that achieved using fluorophore-conjugated reagents [26, 30]. Setting these techniques apart from fluorescence-based assays is the fact that the chromogenic reagents they employ are readily accessible from multiple commercial sources and are relatively inexpensive. Likewise, the assessment of histochemical labeling profiles does not necessitate specialist infrastructure, highly skilled personnel, or interpretative knowledge; instead relying on conventional light microscopes, which are staple pieces of equipment in virtually all clinical andrology laboratories. Hence, these histochemical protocols represent simple and reliable additions to the armoury of functional tests employed to evaluate sperm fertilizing ability and male fertility.

The major difficulty encountered in the design of sperm acrosome bioassays is not so much the histochemical labeling approaches developed to affirm the acrosomal status of the male gamete, but rather the inability of human spermatozoa to exhibit synchronized capacitation in vitro. Although substantial progress has been made toward this goal, it remains a significant barrier and one that undoubtedly contributes to the variable rates of acrosome reaction recorded among fertile patients (i.e. ranges of 20–98 percent). Indeed, the rate at which human spermatozoa spontaneously acrosome-react in optimal capacitation media does not exceed 10 percent, even after 24 hours of incubation. Instead, capacitation medium must be supplemented with an agonist to actively stimulate acrosomal exocytosis in capacitation-primed spermatozoa and, as discussed above, the selection and optimization of such stimuli presents a number of challenges.

10.1.2.6 Clinical Significance

The acrosome reaction is an irreversible physiological process driven by calcium-dependent molecular events occurring at the level of the acrosomal membrane. Whilst we still have much to learn about the timing, mechanisms, and precise agonists that initiate the in vivo induction of an acrosome reaction, it has been established that the frequency of this event exhibits a significant correlation with human fertility and with fertilization rates in the IVF setting [4]. In addition to prospective evaluation of semen quality and the likelihood of a positive IVF outcome, the acrosome status also has relevance in the context of andrological research for development of male contraception and to detect the cytotoxic effects of

various forms of environmental toxicants. Thus, the precise assessment and quantification of acrosomal loss is of high clinical significance when evaluating sperm fertilizing capacity and damage. Whilst the presence or absence of a human sperm acrosome can be assessed by several methods, the simple and inexpensive histochemical techniques considered in this chapter are permissive of rapid evaluation of whether sperm have completed a physiological acrosome reaction or experienced degenerative acrosomal loss caused by sperm damage and/or death. Moreover, when assessed in parallel, histochemical techniques such as the triple or single stain protocols described, perform with equivalent sensitivity, accuracy, and reliability to that of the most widely used fluorophore-based bioassays of acrosome reaction.

10.1.2.7 When to Order the Test

As we continue to make progress in our understanding of the biochemical and molecular mechanisms that drive the production of functionally competent spermatozoa, we have come to realize that conventional semen profiles that place emphasis on descriptive information (i.e. the numbers of spermatozoa present in the ejaculate, the proportion that display motility and the percentage that are morphologically normal) are relatively blunt instruments for assessing male fertility [31]. To refine the diagnosis, additional functional bioassays tests have been developed to monitor various aspects of sperm function including their potential for movement, cervical mucus penetration, capacitation, zona recognition, the acrosome reaction and sperm–oocyte fusion. Such functional assays provide more information on the fertilizing potential of human spermatozoa rather than just their number or appearance. Determination of the ability of spermatozoa to undergo the acrosome reaction in particular, has been proven to be a useful parameter in the evaluation of sperm fertilizing capacity and hence male fertility. In this context, the difference between spontaneous and inducible acrosome reaction is of prognostic value for identification of men with unexplained infertility who are at risk of zero or very low fertilization rates using standard IVF. Conversely, the acrosome reaction test also identifies men with normal sperm function, and may thus help avoid the need to recourse to ICSI even if IVF is needed for other reasons. In these scenarios, routine screening of patients with the acrosome reaction test may inform rational evidence-based decisions to minimize the risk of unexpected failure of fertilization and the attendant financial and emotional toll on the patient. As an additional dividend, the acrosome reaction test also has diagnostic potential as evidenced by the elevated incidence of DZPIAR in men with relatively low sperm concentration and low proportions of sperm with normal morphology [5, 6]. Such correlations may reflect commonality in the origin of these lesions, possibly attributed to impaired spermatogenesis. We, therefore, support the addition of acrosome reaction monitoring to standard semen analysis as a means by which to improve the diagnosis of male factor infertility and aid in the clinical management of patients in IVF/ICSI programs.

10.2 Conclusion

The sperm acrosome reaction is a unique exocytotic event that leads to the release of the contents of the acrosomal vesicle. Here, we have discussed the physiological significance of the acrosome reaction and described the application of simple histochemical techniques used to study the progression and completion of this event. In accordance with the prevalence of defects in acrosomal exocytosis noted among male infertility patients, we contend that the addition of acrosome reaction monitoring to standard semen analysis may help improve the diagnosis and clinical management of such patients.

References

1. Hermo L, Pelletier RM, Cyr DG, Smith CE. Surfing the wave, cycle, life history, and genes/proteins expressed by testicular germ cells. Part 2: changes in spermatid organelles associated with development of spermatozoa. *Microsc Res Tech* 2010; **73**: 279–319.

2. Aitken RJ, Nixon B, Lin M, Koppers AJ, Lee YH, Baker MA. Proteomic changes in mammalian spermatozoa during epididymal maturation. *Asian J Androl* 2007; **9**: 554–64.

3. Nixon B, Bromfield EG. (2018) Sperm capacitation. In M.K. Skinner, ed., *The Encyclopedia of Reproduction*. Cambridge, MA: Academic Press, Elsevier, pp. 272–8.

4. Baker HW, Liu DY, Garrett C, Martic M. The human acrosome reaction. *Asian J Androl* 2000; **2**: 172–8.

5. Liu DY, Clarke GN, Martic M, Garrett C, Baker HW. Frequency of disordered zona pellucida (ZP)-induced acrosome reaction in infertile men with normal semen analysis and normal spermatozoa-ZP binding. *Hum Reprod* 2001; **16**: 1185–90.

6. Liu DY, Baker HW. Disordered zona pellucida-induced acrosome reaction and failure of in vitro fertilization in patients with unexplained infertility. *Fertil Steril* 2003; **79**: 74–80.

7. Guyonnet B, Egge N, Cornwall GA. Functional amyloids in the mouse sperm acrosome. *Mol Cell Biol* 2014; **34**: 2624–34.

8. Guyonnet B, Zabet-Moghaddam M, SanFrancisco S, Cornwall GA. Isolation and proteomic characterization of the mouse sperm acrosomal matrix. *Mol Cell Proteomics* 2012; **11**: 758–74.

9. Zhou W, Anderson AL, Turner AP, De Iuliis GN, McCluskey A, McLaughlin EA, Nixon B. Characterization of a novel role for the dynamin mechanoenzymes in the regulation of human sperm acrosomal exocytosis. *Mol Hum Reprod* 2017; **23**: 657–73.

10. Buffone MG, Foster JA, Gerton GL. The role of the acrosomal matrix in fertilization. *Int J Dev Biol* 2008; **52**: 511–22.

11. Bourne H, Liu DY, Clarke GN, Baker HW. Normal fertilization and embryo development by intracytoplasmic sperm injection of round-headed acrosomeless sperm. *Fertil Steril* 1995; **63**: 1329–32.

12. Nagy ZP, Liu J, Joris H, Verheyen G, Tournaye H, Camus M, Derde MC, Devroey P, Van Steirteghem AC. The result of intracytoplasmic sperm injection is not related to any of the three basic sperm parameters. *Hum Reprod* 1995; **10**: 1123–9.

13. Stival C, Puga Molina Ldel C, Paudel B, Buffone MG, Visconti PE, Krapf D. Sperm capacitation and acrosome reaction in mammalian sperm. *Adv Anat Embryol Cell Biol* 2016; **220**: 93–106.

14. Nixon B, MacIntyre DA, Mitchell LA, Gibbs GM, O'Bryan M, Aitken RJ. The identification of mouse sperm-surface-associated proteins and characterization of their ability to act as decapacitation factors. *Biol Reprod* 2006; **74**: 275–87.

15. Buffone MG, Hirohashi N, Gerton GL. Unresolved questions concerning mammalian sperm acrosomal exocytosis. *Biol Reprod* 2014; **90**: 112.

16. La Spina FA, Puga Molina LC, Romarowski A, Vitale AM, Falzone TL, Krapf D, Hirohashi N, Buffone MG. Mouse sperm begin to undergo acrosomal exocytosis in the upper isthmus of the oviduct. *Dev Biol* 2016; **411**: 172–82.

17. Hirohashi N, Gerton GL, Buffone MG. Video imaging of the sperm acrosome reaction during in vitro

fertilization. *Commun Integr Biol* 2011; **4**: 471–6.

18. Liu DY, Garrett C, Baker HW. Acrosome-reacted human sperm in insemination medium do not bind to the zona pellucida of human oocytes. *Int J Androl* 2006; **29**: 475–81.

19. Buffone MG, Rodriguez-Miranda E, Storey BT, Gerton GL. Acrosomal exocytosis of mouse sperm progresses in a consistent direction in response to zona pellucida. *J Cell Physiol* 2009; **220**: 611–20.

20. Liu DY, Baker HW. Evaluation and assessment of semen for IVF/ICSI. *Asian J Androl* 2002; **4**: 281–5.

21. Liu DY, Stewart T, Baker HW. Normal range and variation of the zona pellucida-induced acrosome reaction in fertile men. *Fertil Steril* 2003; **80**: 384–9.

22. Talbot P, Chacon RS. A triple-stain technique for evaluating normal acrosome reactions of human sperm. *J Exp Zool* 1981; **215**: 201–8.

23. Mitchell LA, Nixon B, Aitken RJ. Analysis of chaperone proteins associated with human spermatozoa during capacitation. *Mol Hum Reprod* 2007; **13**: 605–13.

24. Aitken RJ, Buckingham DW, Fang HG. Analysis of the responses of human spermatozoa to A23187 employing a novel technique for assessing the acrosome reaction. *J Androl* 1993; **14**: 132–41.

25. Didion BA, Dobrinsky JR, Giles JR, Graves CN. Staining procedure to detect viability and the true acrosome reaction in spermatozoa of various species. *Gamete Res* 1989; **22**: 51–7.

26. Larson JL, Miller DJ. Simple histochemical stain for acrosomes on sperm from several species. *Mol Reprod Dev* 1999; **52**: 445–9.

27. Esterhuizen AD, Franken DR, Lourens JG, van Rooyen LH. Clinical importance of zona pellucida-induced acrosome reaction and its predictive value

for IVF. *Hum Reprod* 2001; **16**: 138–44.

28. Aitken RJ, Thatcher S, Glasier AF, Clarkson JS, Wu FC, Baird DT. Relative ability of modified versions of the hamster oocyte penetration test, incorporating hyperosmotic medium or the ionophore A23187, to predict IVF outcome. *Hum Reprod* 1987; **2**: 227–31.

29. Liu DY, Baker HW. A simple method for assessment of the human acrosome reaction of spermatozoa bound to the zona pellucida: lack of relationship with ionophore A23187-induced acrosome reaction. *Hum Reprod* 1996; **11**: 551–7.

30. Risopatron J, Pena P, Miska W, Sanchez R. Evaluation of the acrosome reaction in human spermatozoa: comparison of cytochemical and fluorescence techniques. *Andrologia* 2001; **33**: 63–7.

31. Aitken RJ. Sperm function tests and fertility. *Int J Androl* 2006; **29**: 69–75.

Chapter

11

Zona Binding: Competitive Sperm-Binding Assay

De Yi Liu, Ying Zhong, Zi-Na Wen

11.1 Introduction/Background

Today, about 10–15 percent of couples at reproductive age worldwide are infertile and they are unable to conceive naturally without medical assistance. Infertility can be caused by male-only factors, female-only factors or a combination of both. However, the cause of infertility is currently unidentifiable in about 20–30 percent of patients, who are classified as "unexplained infertility". Currently, there is a lack of effective medical treatment for most infertile couples to achieve natural pregnancy. Although assisted reproductive technology (ART) such as in vitro fertilization (IVF) and intracytoplasmic sperm injection (ICSI) are popular and effective procedures to treat both female and male factor infertility, they are very expensive and not always successful. Some patients require several attempts of treatment cycles to achieve a pregnancy and bear huge financial and emotional costs in the process.

In clinical ART, the two major treatment procedures – conventional IVF and ICSI – are applied according to the cause of infertility. In general, IVF is effective in treating female factor infertility, whereas ICSI is effective for male factor infertility. Accurate diagnosis of sperm function is therefore critical in determining which treatment option is most suitable, as well as assisting couples to achieve optimal ART outcomes from each oocyte collection cycle. In most ART clinics, assignment of patients to IVF or ICSI treatment is mostly based on routine semen analysis results according to the World Health Organization (WHO) manual [1]. Patients with normal or mildly abnormal results are treated by IVF and those with moderate to severe sperm defects are treated by ICSI. Unfortunately, conventional semen analysis provides limited diagnostic information for the sperm fertilizing ability, and many patients with normal semen analysis but with subtle sperm defects impairing sperm-oocyte interaction go undiagnosed [2, 3].

In conventional IVF, failure of fertilization is highly associated with defective sperm-zona pellucida (ZP) binding and penetration, which is mostly due to sperm and not oocyte abnormalities [4, 5]. Before ICSI became available, patients with failure of fertilization in IVF were commonly associated with abnormal semen such as oligo-, astheno- and teratozoospermia. Now, these patients with abnormal semen analysis are routinely treated by ICSI. However, patients with unexplained infertility and normal semen analysis are usually treated by conventional IVF in the initial cycle. If fertilization is low or completely fails, they are then treated by ICSI in the subsequent cycle. In order to minimize this risk of failure of fertilization in IVF, it is very important to diagnose subtle sperm defects for patients with unexplained infertility before starting ART treatment.

We have developed the bioassays using human oocytes that failed to fertilize in IVF/ICSI to examine the ability of sperm-ZP binding and ZP-induced acrosome reaction (AR) [6, 7]. The ZP-induced AR is a very good marker for the ability of sperm-ZP penetration [8]. The clinical predicative value of these tests for IVF fertilization rate has been extensively studied [9, 10]. Our large set of clinical data shows that defective sperm-ZP interaction is a major cause of male infertility and failure of fertilization in conventional IVF [11–13]. We identified two major defects of sperm-ZP interaction in unexplained infertile men: 1) defective sperm-ZP binding (DSZPB) in which sperm have little to no ability to bind to the ZP [13]; and 2) disordered ZP-induced AR (DZPIAR) in which sperm have normal capacity to bind to the ZP but are unable to undergo the AR induced by the ZP [10, 12]. Both defects severely impair the ability of sperm to penetrate the ZP of human oocytes which then leads to failure of fertilization in conventional IVF. We found that about 25–30 percent of patients with unexplained infertility and normal semen analysis have DSZPB or DZPIAR [11, 13]. These subtle defects are unable to be diagnosed by routine semen analysis and therefore require sperm-ZP binding and ZP-induced AR tests using human oocytes.

11.2 Principle/Mechanism

During the process of human fertilization in vivo or under IVF condition, fertile sperm must be able to bind to the ZP, undergo the AR, penetrate the ZP and finally fuse with the egg plasma membrane [14]. In the literature, the mechanism of human sperm-ZP interaction has been well established. The ZP of the human oocyte consists of four glycoproteins; ZP1, ZP2, ZP3 and ZP4. The ZP3 is regarded as the primary receptor responsible for binding acrosome intact sperm and inducing the AR. If there are defects impairing either sperm-ZP binding or the ZP-induced AR, the sperm will be unable to penetrate the ZP and fertilize oocytes under IVF condition.

In the clinical IVF program, we have observed a large variation in the number of sperm bound to the ZP between individual oocytes in IVF. Due to the variability of ZP quality, the sperm-ZP binding test is designed based on the competitive binding of patient and control (fertile donor) sperm labeled with different fluorochromes (green and red colors) to the same oocyte [6]. Under this experimental condition, if patient sperm have similar ZP binding capacity as fertile control sperm, the number of sperm bound to the same oocyte should be very similar. On the other hand, if patient sperm has DSZPB, the number of sperm bound to the ZP will be significantly lower or may be none.

The ZP-induced AR test is designed to predict the ability of sperm-ZP penetration in infertile men with normal semen analysis and normal sperm-ZP binding [7, 8]. For this test, patient sperm are incubated with a group of four oocytes. If the sperm have normal ZP binding capacity, then all sperm bound to the ZP will be removed from the surface to examine the ZP-induced AR. Our previous study showed that there is a highly significant correlation between the ZP-induced AR and the proportion of ZP penetrated and IVF fertilization rate [8]. Development of the ZP-induced AR test leads us to discover a subtle sperm defect called DZPIAR which causes failure of fertilization in IVF for patients with normal semen analysis and normal sperm-ZP binding [12].

11.3 Brief Methods/Protocol

11.3.1 Sources of Human Oocytes

For clinical tests of sperm-ZP binding and the ZP-induced AR, it is essential to use the ZP of human oocytes as there is currently no artificial human ZP or active recombinant human ZP available. In clinical IVF/ICSI, the average fertilization rate is about 70–80 percent. The remaining 20–30 percent of unfertilized oocytes, as well as immature oocytes (GV and MI) unsuitable for ICSI, can be used for clinical tests of sperm-ZP binding and ZP-induced AR. Our previous study confirmed that the ZP of immature oocytes has similar biological activity to those of mature oocytes for binding sperm and inducing the AR [13]. The oocytes can be used either fresh or after storage in a high concentration of salt solution (1M ammonium sulphate). Salt stored oocytes must be washed with culture medium to remove salt before being used for the test [6, 9].

11.3.2 Competitive Sperm-Zona Pellucida Binding Test

For this test, patient sperm (test) are labeled with the green fluorescence fluorescein isothiocyanate (FITC), and fertile donor (control) sperm are labeled with the red fluorescence tetramethylrhodamine isothiocyanate (TRITC). A mixture of equal numbers (1×10^5/mL) of labeled motile test and control sperm is incubated with a group of four oocytes for two hours. After incubation, the oocytes are washed with a large bore (250–300 μm) pipette to dislodge loosely attached sperm; then the number of green and red sperm tightly bound to the ZP are counted under a fluorescence microscope, and the ratio of test to control sperm is calculated and used as an endpoint [6, 9]. A sample of labeled test and control sperm bound to a salt stored human ZP is shown in Figure 11.1.

11.3.3 Zona Pellucida-Induced Acrosome Reaction Test

The ZP-induced AR test examines the ability of sperm undergoing physiological AR induced by the ZP after binding to the ZP [8]. Defective sperm-ZP induced AR will lead to a failure of sperm-ZP penetration and fertilization in vitro. Thus, the ZP-induced AR is an excellent marker for the ability of sperm-ZP penetration [3, 8]. This test is very simple (see Figure 11.2): a

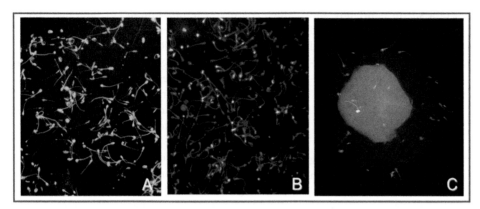

Figure 11.1 These photos are an example of the competitive sperm-ZP binding test using two different colored fluorescent sperm: A shows patient (test) sperm labeled with the green fluorescence (FITC); B is fertile donor (control) sperm labeled with the red fluorescence (TRITC). In image C, there are 14 green sperm and 12 red sperm bound to a salt-stored human ZP.

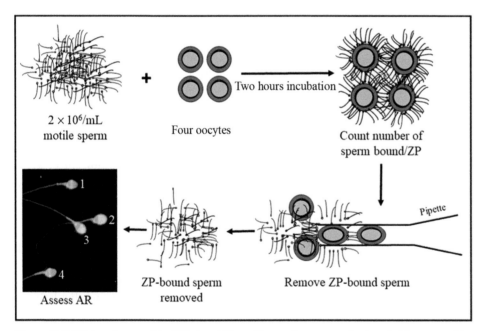

Figure 11.2 This is a diagram of the ZP-induced AR test. First, motile sperm are incubated with a group of four oocytes for two hours. The sperm which bind tightly to the ZP are then assessed after washing the oocytes to dislodge loosely adherent sperm. All sperm which bind to the surface of the ZP are removed by aspiration of the oocyte in and out of a small pipette. The removed ZP-bound sperm are then stained with fluorescein labeled *Pisum sativum* agglutinin for assessment of AR. As illustrated, the two acrosome reacted sperm (1 and 2) show a florescent band in the equatorial region and the two acrosome intact sperm (3 and 4) show uniform florescence of the anterior two-thirds of the head.

group of four oocytes are incubated with motile sperm selected by swim-up or discontinue gradients centrifugation for two hours then transferred to fresh medium to dislodge or remove all sperm loosely bound to the surface of the ZP. The number of tightly bound sperm remaining are counted under an inverted phase contrast microscope with 200× magnification. Then, all the ZP-bound sperm are removed to a glass slide for examination of the AR by staining with *Pisum sativum* agglutinin (PSA-FITC) conjugated with fluorescein isothiocyanate. For each sample, 200 sperm will be scored under fluorescent microscope using excitation wavelengths of 450–490 nm and a magnification of 400×. When more than half the head of a sperm is brightly and uniformly fluorescing, the acrosome is considered intact. Sperm with a fluorescing band at the equatorial segment or without fluorescence are considered acrosome reacted (Figure 11.2) and the percentage of ZP-induced AR is used as an endpoint [3, 11].

11.3.3.1 Reference Values and How to Calculate Cut-Off Values

For the competitive sperm-ZP binding test using patient and fertile donor control sperm labeled with different fluorochromes, a ratio of test and control sperm bound to the same group of four oocytes is used as the endpoint. Our previous study from 106 IVF patients showed that those with sperm-ZP binding ratio <0.3 had significantly low fertilization rate (<30 percent) in IVF [6, 9]. Therefore, the competitive sperm-ZP binding ratio 0.3 is considered as the cut-off for the reference value. If patients with normal semen analysis have a sperm-ZP binding ratio of <0.3, they should be treated using ICSI instead of IVF.

For the sperm-ZP induced AR test, the reference value was considered based on our previous study of 111 fertile men, which showed that an average ZP-induced AR was 48 percent, ranging between 20–98 percent [15]. Another study in IVF patients with unexplained male infertility showed that the fertilization rate was significantly low (<35 percent) if the ZP-induced AR was <25 percent [12]. Furthermore, a group of DZPIAR patients with ZP induced AR <16 percent experienced persistent failure of fertilization in IVF [10]. Therefore, a ZP-induced AR <25 percent is considered as the cut-off for the reference value. Patients with normal semen analysis and normal sperm ZP-binding but ZP-induced AR of <25 percent should be treated by ICSI instead of IVF.

11.3.3.2 Laboratory and Clinical Interpretation

Under IVF conditions, there is a large variation in the number of sperm which bind to the ZP between individual human oocytes, and about 20 percent of oocytes do not bind any sperm [5]. In order to overcome this variability affecting sperm-ZP binding test results, we incubated a group of four oocytes with a mixture of equal numbers of patient (test) and fertile (control) sperm labeled with different fluorescent color [5]. Clinically, if patients are diagnosed with DSZPB (ZP binding ratio of <0.3), they will have a

high risk of low fertilization in IVF, and they should be treated by ICSI instead.

The ZP-induced AR test can predict the subtle sperm defects impairing sperm-ZP penetration. This test is very useful to determine if patients with normal semen analysis and normal sperm-ZP binding have DZPIAR. If patients are diagnosed with DZPIAR, they should be treated by ICSI. Sperm from DZPIAR patients have very little to no chance of penetrating the ZP of oocytes during the fertilization process under IVF conditions. Sperm from these patients generally have very good morphology, motility and normal DNA, but fail to fertilize in IVF due to an inability to penetrate the ZP of the oocyte. DZPIAR patients can be effectively treated by ICSI as a sperm is injected into the cytoplasm of the oocyte. Our previous study showed that patients diagnosed with DZPIAR had high fertilization, implantation and pregnancy rates in ICSI [16]. Therefore, for patients with unexplained infertility and normal semen analysis, the sperm-ZP binding and ZP-induced AR tests will be useful in determining whether patients should undergo IVF or ICSI to achieve optimal ART outcomes in the initial cycle.

11.3.3.3 Advantages/Disadvantages of the Tests

In the initial ART cycle, it is very difficult to determine whether IVF or ICSI is the best procedure to treat couples with unexplained infertility but normal semen analysis. Our study showed that about 25–30 percent of patients with normal semen analysis have DSZPB or DZPIAR [11, 13]. Using the sperm-ZP binding and ZP-induced AR tests, we can identify these subtle sperm defects before a patient commences ART treatment. This results in better fertilization outcomes, as we know that patients diagnosed with either DSZPB or DZPIAR should be treated by ICSI instead of IVF. This will lead to a significant improvement in the clinical management of patients with unexplained infertility.

There is, however, a disadvantage to be considered. The sperm-ZP binding and ZP-induced AR tests require the use of human oocytes, which may be limited in supply for routine diagnostic tests, particularly in small ART clinics with few patients. Currently there is no substitute for the human ZP or active recombinant ZP3 that can be used for clinical tests. This could be overcome in future with the discovery of alternative biological material or development of artificial human ZP, to be used in clinical testing.

11.3.3.4 Clinical Significance

It is known that the ability of sperm binding to the ZP is very important during the process of human fertilization [14]. In fertile men, an average ejaculate contains 100–200 million motile sperm but only about 14 percent are capable of binding to the human ZP and only those sperm bound to the ZP have a chance to penetrate the ZP and fertilize the oocyte [17]. Thus, the majority (over 86 percent) of motile sperm in ejaculate will not bind to the ZP and therefore these sperm may have no fertility potential. During sperm-oocyte interaction, the human ZP selectively binds sperm with normal morphology and normal nuclear chromatin DNA, suggesting that the human ZP plays an important role as a physiological barrier to block abnormal sperm [18, 19] from entering the oocyte.

Before the development of ICSI in 1992, conventional IVF was the only procedure available to treat both male and female factor infertility. A high proportion of those patients (30–50 percent) treated with IVF experienced poor or complete failure of fertilization. Although most patients with poor IVF fertilization were associated with common sperm abnormalities such as severe oligo-, astheno- and terato-zoospermia, about 30 percent of patients had normal semen analysis. To investigate the cause of failed fertilization in the group of patients with normal semen analysis, we identified that a specific sperm defect called DZPIAR caused severe male infertility [10, 11]. Infertile men with DZPIAR have consistently normal semen analysis and normal sperm-ZP binding but the sperm do not undergo the AR induced by the ZP, which is significantly correlated with sperm-ZP penetration. In fertile men, on average 48 percent (range 20–98 percent) of ZP-bound sperm undergo the AR in vitro [15]. In contrast, men with DZPIAR have very low proportions of sperm undergoing the AR on the ZP (mean 6 percent, range 1–16 percent) [10]. Although the pathological mechanisms of DZPIAR are currently not fully understood, our preliminary study suggested that defective protein kinase A and C pathways appear to be a common cause of DZPIAR in men with normozoospermia and normal sperm-ZP binding [20]. ICSI is highly successful in treating those with DZPIAR [16] and thus pre-diagnosis of this defect is critical for the clinical management of patients in IVF/ICSI.

Incidence of DSZPB and DZPIAR occurs in about 25–30 percent of men who have unexplained infertility with normal semen analysis [11, 13]. On the other hand, we have found that the majority (~70 percent) of patients with oligozoospermia and severe teratozoospermia (<5 percent normal sperm morphology), have either DSZPB or DZPIAR [13]. This can be diagnosed by routine semen analysis and most of these patients will be assigned to ICSI treatment in their first cycle and do not require the sperm-ZP binding and ZP-induced AR tests. However, some of these patients may still prefer IVF treatment as they do not like the more interventionist approach of ICSI in which a single sperm is subjectively selected by a scientist. Our previous study found that about 30 percent of patients with oligozoospermia or severe teratozoospermia can have normal sperm-ZP binding and normal ZP-induced AR. For these patients who do not have DSZPB or DZPIAR, IVF treatment is adequate to achieve good fertilization.

11.3.3.5 When to Order the Test

Both sperm-ZP binding and ZP-induced AR tests should be ordered before patients commence ART treatment. Our previous study showed that about 25–30 percent of patients who have unexplained male infertility with normal semen analysis have DSZPB or DZPIAR. As explained above in this chapter, patients with these subtle sperm defects should be treated by ICSI to achieve optimal outcomes in the initial oocyte collection cycle. Without doing these tests, patients are usually treated with conventional IVF first, which may yield low or zero fertilization if they do have these subtle sperm defects. They are then treated by ICSI in the subsequent cycle. The efficiency and effectiveness of ART treatment can be greatly improved by using these tests, which can assist in clinical decision-making, and the overall better fertilization outcomes for patients.

It is worth noting that some patients do not like ICSI treatment, as it involves the manual selection of a single sperm by a scientist. For these patients it can be helpful to undertake the sperm-ZP binding and the ZP-induced AR tests to check whether they have DSZPB or DZPIAR. If both test results are normal, patients can be treated by conventional IVF as their sperm are able to bind and penetrate the ZP of oocytes. In clinical ART, some patients do not have comprehensive sperm tests performed and have persistently low or zero fertilization rates in IVF. These patients should be reviewed by screening sperm-ZP binding and the ZP-induced AR to see if subtle sperm defects are in fact causing failure of fertilization.

11.3.3.6 Clinical Scenario 1

A couple, aged 30 and 34, have been trying to have a child for the last two years. They have regular and frequent intercourse but have never fallen pregnant. So, they seek help from an infertility specialist. After having various tests and examinations performed, the doctor provided a diagnosis of unexplained infertility. The man had consistent normal semen analysis from three separate tests performed, and the woman had a regular period. There were no other factors to indicate the cause of infertility. They were then referred to an Andrology specialist who ordered the sperm-ZP binding and ZP-induced AR tests. The results showed that the sperm-ZP binding ratio was 0.1, which is much lower than the normal range. The doctor suggested the couple undergo ICSI treatment as defective sperm-ZP binding poses a risk of failure in sperm-ZP penetration and fertilization in IVF. The couple agreed to undertake ICSI in the first oocyte collection cycle: 10 oocytes were collected and injected by ICSI, eight of which fertilized with two pronuclei (PN) and six high quality embryos obtained. A single embryo was transferred on day three and the woman became pregnant, and a baby boy was delivered at 39 weeks of gestation. The couple still has five surplus embryos frozen for future use.

11.3.3.7 Clinical Scenario 2

A couple, aged 28 and 32, have been trying to have a baby for the last 18 months. They were having regular and frequent intercourse but did not fall pregnant. So, they sought help from an IVF specialist. After having various tests and examinations performed, the couple was diagnosed as unexplained infertility. The male partner had consistent normal semen analysis according to the WHO manual [1]. The female partner had a regular period and nothing further to indicate the cause of infertility. They were then referred to an Andrology specialist who ordered sperm-ZP binding and ZP-induced AR tests. The results showed that sperm-ZP binding was normal, but the ZP-induced AR was 2 percent, which was diagnosed as DZPIAR. The doctor suggested they needed ICSI treatment rather than conventional IVF as the sperm were unable to penetrate the ZP of the oocyte. The couple agreed and underwent ICSI in the first oocyte collection cycle: 12 mature oocytes were collected and injected by ICSI, all of which fertilized normally with nine high quality embryos obtained. A single embryo was transferred on day three, and the woman fell pregnant, later delivering a baby girl at 37 weeks of gestation. The couple still has eight surplus embryos stored for future use.

11.3.3.8 Clinical Scenario 3

A young couple (man 30 and woman 28) have been trying to have a child for the last two years. The female partner was fit and healthy and had a regular period. The couple have regular and frequent intercourse but have never fallen pregnant. They seek help from an infertility specialist, which involves various tests and examinations. Everything was fine for the female partner, with nothing to indicate a cause of infertility. For the male partner, semen analysis results showed a semen volume of 3.8 mL, sperm concentration of 80 million/mL, total motility of 68 percent, progressive motility of 58 percent and normal sperm morphology of 2 percent according to the WHO manual [1]. The doctor suggested the couple have ICSI treatment, as the normal sperm morphology of 2 percent was too low, which may risk low fertilization rates in IVF. However, the couple insisted on having IVF as they did not like the idea that in ICSI a sperm is subjectively selected by a scientist and force injected into the oocyte. The doctor then ordered the sperm-ZP binding and ZP-induced AR tests to see if the sperm had normal ability to penetrate the ZP under IVF conditions. Test results showed that sperm would bind to the ZP normally, but the ZP-induced AR was only 2 percent, which is much lower than the cut-off reference value of 20 percent. Given these test results, the doctor again advised the couple to consider ICSI treatment. However, the patient insisted on trying IVF treatment for the first oocyte collection cycle. For this treatment, 12 oocytes were collected and inseminated, but none fertilized despite all oocytes being mature and morphologically normal. After the disappointing outcome in IVF cycle, the couple decided to use ICSI for the second cycle. In this treatment, a total of 10 mature oocytes were injected and nine fertilized, with eight good quality embryos obtained. The couple then fell pregnant after the first transfer with a single embryo on day three, and a baby girl was delivered at 38 weeks of gestation. They still have seven surplus embryos frozen for future use.

11.4 Conclusion

Both sperm-ZP binding and ZP-induced AR tests are useful in the clinical management of unexplained male infertility in ART. Patients diagnosed with either defective sperm-ZP binding or DZPIAR should be treated with ICSI to achieve optimal clinical outcomes. The ZP of oocytes which failed to fertilize in clinical IVF and ICSI are valuable biological materials and should be used for clinical sperm-ZP interaction tests. In future, a commercial kit for routine sperm-ZP interaction test could be developed using active recombinant human ZP3 protein or artificial human ZP rather than native human ZP. This means that the current scarcity of human biological materials will no longer limit routine clinical testing.

References

1. World Health Organization. (2010) *WHO Laboratory Manual for the Examination and Processing of Human Semen*, 5th ed. Geneva: The WHO Press.

2. Liu DY, Baker HWG. Tests of human sperm function and fertilization in vitro. *Fertil Steril* 1992; **58**: 465–83.

3. Liu DY, Garrett C, Baker HWG. Clinical application of sperm-oocyte interaction tests in in vitro fertilization-embryo transfer and intracytoplasmic sperm injection programs. *Fertil Steril* 2004; **82**: 1251–63.

4. Liu DY, Baker HWG. A new test for the assessment of sperm-zona pellucida penetration: relationship with results of other sperm tests and fertilization in vitro. *Hum Reprod* 1994; **9**: 489–96.

5. Liu DY, Baker HWG. Defective sperm-zona pellucida interaction: a major cause of failure of fertilization in clinical in-vitro fertilization. *Hum Reprod* 2000; **15**: 702–8.

6. Liu DY, Lopata A, Johnston WIH, Baker HWG. A human sperm-zona pellucida binding test using oocytes that failed to fertilize in vitro. *Fertil Steril* 1988; **50**: 782–8.

7. Liu DY, Baker HWG. A simple method for assessment of the human acrosome reaction of spermatozoa bound to the zona pellucida: lack of relationship with ionophore A23187-induced acrosome reaction. *Hum Reprod* 1996; **11**: 551–5.

8. Liu DY, Baker HWG. Relationship between the zona pellucida (ZP) and ionophore A23187 induced acrosome reaction and the ability of sperm to penetrate the ZP in men with normal sperm-ZP binding. *Fertil Steril* 1996; **66**: 312–15.

9. Liu DY, Clarke GN, Lopata A, Johnston WIH, Baker HWG. A sperm-zona pellucida binding test and in vitro fertilization. *Fertil Steril* 1989; **52**: 281–7.

10. Liu DY, Baker HWG. Disordered acrosome reaction of sperm bound to the zona pellucida (ZP): a newly discovered sperm defect causing infertility with reduced sperm-ZP penetration and reduced fertilization in vitro. *Hum Reprod* 1994; **9**: 1694–770.

11. Liu DY, Clarke GN, Martic M, Garrett C, Baker HWG. Frequency of disordered zona pellucida (ZP)-induced acrosome reaction in infertile men with normal semen analysis and normal sperm-ZP binding. *Hum Reprod* 2001; **16**: 1185–90.

12. Liu DY, Baker HWG. Disordered zona pellucida induced acrosome reaction and failure of in vitro fertilization in patients with unexplained infertility. *Fertil Steril* 2003; 79: 74–80.

13. Liu DY, Liu ML, Garrett C, Baker HWG. Comparison of the frequency of defective sperm-zona pellucida (ZP) binding and the ZP-induced acrosome reaction between subfertile men with normal and abnormal semen. *Hum Reprod* 2007; **22**: 1878–84.

14. Yanagimachi R. Mammalian fertilisation. (1994) In Knobil E, Neill J, eds., *The Physiology of Reproduction*, 2nd ed. New York: Raven Press, pp. 189–317.

15. Liu DY, Stewart T, Baker HWG. Normal range and variation of the zona pellucida-induced acrosome reaction in fertile men. *Fertil Steril* 2003; **80**: 384–9.

16. Liu DY, Bourne H, Baker HWG. Fertilization and pregnancy with acrosome intact sperm by intracytoplasmic sperm injection in patients with disordered zona pellucida induced acrosome reaction. *Fertil Steril* 1995; **64**: 116–21.

17. Liu DY, Garrett C, Baker HWG. Low proportions of spermatozoa can bind to the zona pellucida of human oocytes. *Hum Reprod* 2003; **18**: 2382–9.

18. Liu DY, Baker HWG. Acrosome status and morphology of human sperm bound to the zona pellucida and oolemma determined using oocytes that failed to fertilize in vitro. *Hum Reprod* 1994; **9**: 673–9.

19. Liu DY, Baker HWG. Human sperm bound to the zona pellucida have normal nuclear chromatin assessed by Acridine Orange fluorescence. *Hum Reprod* 2007; **22**: 1597–1602.

20. Liu DY, Liu ML, Baker HWG. Defective protein kinase A and C pathways are common causes of disordered zona pellucida-induced (ZP) acrosome reaction in normozoospermic infertile men with normal sperm-ZP binding. *Fertil Steril* 2013; **99**: 86–91.

Zona Binding: Hemizona Assay

Shubhadeep Roychoudhury, Daniel Franken

12.1 Introduction

The incidence of infertility is up to 20–25 percent in men with poor semen quality with a contribution of the male factor in 30–50 percent of couples undergoing assisted reproduction, including in vitro fertilization (IVF) and intracytoplasmic sperm injection (ICSI). In 17 studies sampling 6410 women, the proportion of couples seeking such medical care was, on average, 56.1 percent (range 42–76.3 percent) in more developed countries and 51.2 percent (range 27–74.1 percent) in less developed countries [1]. Investigation of male infertility or sub-fertility basically comprises of semen analysis [2]. However, a standard semen analysis cannot always assess the multifunctional events and biological properties that spermatozoa express following capacitation. In many cases, it is only when couples fail to achieve conception, the male factor is suspected and advanced laboratory tests are recommended to establish this reliably.

The predictive value of semen analysis has been found to be limited, particularly in cases of oligoasthenoteratozoospermia, idiopathic or unexplained infertility. While considering the conditions of the partner, it is also imperative for the clinician to incorporate an effective and quick test of sperm function into the workup algorithm of such patients who may benefit from a variety of therapeutic options including assisted reproductive technology (ART) [3–5].These functional tests include zona binding, acrosome integrity, reactive oxygen species, chromatin decondensation and DNA integrity, among others.

As a clinically important test in the diagnosis and treatment of infertility [6], sperm-zona binding is one of the most powerful indicators of sperm fertilizing ability of oocytes in vitro [7, 8]. Since defective sperm-zona pellucida binding has been recognized to be a very common cause of fertilization failure in assisted reproduction [9, 10], this test is recommended in cases of poor fertilization, unexpected fertilization failure [5] and failed conventional IVF [11].

As of today, it is well known that fertilization starts when the male gamete binds to the antigenically/biochemically complex translucent extracellular glycoproteinaceous matrix coating of the oocyte, called the zona pellucida (ZP). The ZP is formed during the early stages of folliculogenesis and surrounds the embryo until the time of implantation [12]. The inner surface of the ZP is particulated and granular, whereas the outer surface resembles a fenestrated mesh or lattice [13]. In the human, the zona consists of four major component glycoproteins (ZP1, ZP2, ZP3 and ZP4), of which ZP3 acts as the primary sperm receptor and acrosome reaction inducer, whereas ZP2 is a secondary receptor [14]. During binding, any sperm first attach loosely to the ZP, which is closely followed by tight attachment to specific receptors. This ability of the sperm to bind tightly to the ZP is a critical and mandatory step in fertilization [15] and subsequent embryonic development [16]. Binding capacity depends heavily on the stage of maturity of the oocytes, the presence of complementary binding sites/receptors on the surface of the sperm as well as the surface structure of the ZP [17]. The structural and biochemical changes of the ZP that accompany the oocyte maturation process facilitate the highest binding when oocytes mature to the stage best for fertilization [18, 19].

For the first time, human sperm-oocyte interaction was described in an assay to record zona penetration. The methodology of this assay formed the basis of zona binding assays that developed subsequently [20]. Two tests have been designed to assess sperm capacity to bind to the ZP, namely the hemizona assay (HZA) [21] and the sperm-ZP binding ratio test [22].

12.2 Hemizona Assay

12.2.1 Clinical Utility

In andrology, the identification of specific gamete dysfunction is one of most significant steps prior to assisted reproduction [23]. The clinician usually opts for ART if at least one of the following conditions are fulfiled – i) failure of andrology treatment, ii) diagnosis of idiopathic infertility, iii) moderate to high level of sperm abnormalities revealed by standard semen analysis, and iv) functional abnormalities of sperm detected by advanced tests [24]. The HZA is a highly significant, internally controlled, homologous bioassay providing functional aspects of the sperm, which may assist the clinician in determining the management of men for whom conventional IUI and IVF therapy is likely to be unsuccessful and should rather be referred to ICSI [25, 26]. It has been highly predictive of IVF [27] and IUI fertilization and pregnancy outcomes [18]. Results of this test have also been useful in counseling couples before allocating them into controlled ovarian hyperstimulation (COH/IUI therapy) [26].

The percentage of normal spermatozoa bound to the ZP under HZA conditions reported for both normo- and teratozoospermic men also showed significant improvement when compared to the percentage of normal spermatozoa found after the swim-up procedure (Figure 12.1) [28]. Multiple regression analyses have demonstrated that sperm morphology is the most significant predictor of sperm-zona binding in the HZA, when compared to other sperm variables from the original semen sample (r=0.83, p=0.0001). However, curvilinear velocity (VCL) and hyperactivated motility (HA) have been the most significant predictors of successful zona binding, after separation of the motile sperm fraction (r=0.47 and r=0.46, respectively p=0.001) [28–30]. Sperm morphology and HZA data correlated with fertilization rates in a prospective study of a large number of infertile patients before IVF therapy [11].

The diagnostic utility of HZA has been confirmed based on a set of criteria such as the ability to produce few false-negative and false-positive values, as well as good positive (PPV) and negative (NPV) predictive values [31]. In terms of fertility and fertilization rates, a compilation of studies predicted high HZA sensitivity (75–100 percent), good specificity (57–100 percent), and high PPV (79–100 percent) and NPV (68–100 percent) [32].

12.2.2 Procedure and Evaluation

As shown in Figure 12.2, the ZP of freshly isolated or stored oocytes are divided into half either microsurgically (using a micromanipulator) or manually [25] followed by incubation of one half (called a

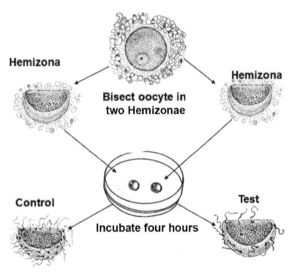

Figure 12.2 The Hemizona Assay [37]. An oocyte is removed from the working droplet and placed in the middle of the microscopic field. The micromanipulation blade is lowered to touch the top surface of the oocyte and the oocyte is flattened by further lowering. The oocyte is bisected into two identical hemizonae using side-to-side excursions. Hemizona pairs are kept together in fresh drops of culture medium after removing the residual cytoplasm. Hemizona pairs are placed in the incubator overnight before transferring into sperm droplets. When sperm are ready for incubation with the hemizonae, one hemizona is transferred into the drop containing control (donor) sperm and the corresponding hemizona is transferred into the drop containing patient's sperm.

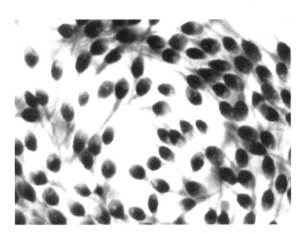

Figure 12.1 Morphologically normal sperm bound to the zona pellucida [28].

101

hemizona) with fertile donor sperm (positive control) and the other half with patient sperm [33]. The 100 µL semen suspension drop containing 500,000 motile sperm/mL are kept under light white mineral oil and are co-incubated with each hemizona in a 35 × 10 mm Petri dish for four hours at 37°C with 5 percent CO_2 in air. Both hemizonae, the control and the test one, are rinsed in a cold medium drop five times with a large drawn glass pipette to dislodge loosely attached sperm and then transferred to a fresh medium drop and positioned with the outer surface upward [21, 23, 34]. The numbers of tightly bound sperm to the respective hemizonae are counted with a 400× phase contrast microscopy [35, 36]. Binding capacity is expressed as the hemizona index (HZI) and calculated by expressing the number of tightly bound patient sperm as a percentage of the number of tightly bound control sperm [23, 35]. The peak number of control sperm bound to the hemizona ranges from 42–215 whereas that of the patient ranges from 27–142, respectively. Based on these findings, a cut-off binding value of 34 sperm was ascertained to be indicative of inferior ZP or subnormal control [23, 35].

12.2.3 Bisecting of Oocytes

Post-mortem oocytes obtained from donated ovarian tissue were used during the developing stages of the assay. A complete micromanipulation system is required for bisecting the oocytes. The assay is performed by separately incubating matching bisected halves of a ZP with sperm from a patient and proven fertile control, respectively. Oocytes are placed in

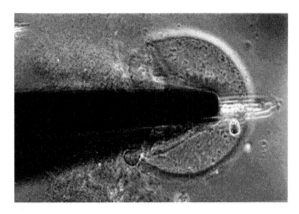

Figure 12.3 Bisecting an oocyte by side by side excursions of the micromanipulation blade [37]. The oocyte is held by a holding pipette and flattened by touching its surface by the micromanipulation blade.

100 mm Petri dish, culture medium is poured into the dish to a depth of 3–4 mm. A holding pipette is used to stabilize the oocyte during cutting [5]. Using total magnification of 200× the cutting blade is lowered flattening the oocyte to initiate a midline cut and, with side-to-side excursions, two identical HZ are subsequently produced (Figure 12.3).

Alternatively, a cost-effective manual hand-cutting method of oocytes recorded comparable recovery rate, diameter size of the hemizonae, sperm binding and HZI thereby advocating the possible elimination of an expensive micromanipulator making the assay more affordable to many fertility clinics across the globe [25, 38].

12.2.4 Oocyte Sources

During experimental studies, hemizonae were obtained from prophase I oocytes from post mortem ovarian tissue from different age groups namely, 7 months, 5 years, 7 years, 12 years and 30 years in the first experiment (Table 12.1) [39]. The age group studies indicated that ovarian age does not have any influence on the ZP's capacity to bind spermatozoa.

Hemizonae can also be recycled for at least a second binding experiment as metaphase II oocytes with previous exposure to sperm were found to retain their binding capacity. Zonae that had been exposed to sperm and that were subsequently stripped from bound sperm, revealed a mean number of bound sperm after re-insemination that were significantly higher than the prophase I oocytes; 115.0±2.8 versus 35.6±12 (P<0.0001) [2]. These results indicate that the upper limit for sperm binding in the presence of sperm populations with known zona binding defects and possibly poor zonae is 34 sperm per hemizona.

Table 12.1 The Mean Number of Bound Sperm among the Different Age Groups [39]

Age	Number sperm bound
7 months	38.9±17
5 years	31.0±27
7 years	49.3±21
12 years	32.8±18
30 years	39.5±17
Pooled data	37.7±7
Donated prophase oocytes	33.0±20.

The lower cut-off value of 34 bound sperm was used for sperm populations with normal (>14 percent normal forms) morphologic features and zona binding potential. Proven fertile sperm samples unavoidably include results with ZP showing inferior sperm binding capacity [40].

The problems of the availability of ZP from oocytes by surgical removal of ovarian tissue or by ovarian follicular aspiration has been largely overcome by utilizing surplus oocytes from IVF programs after gonadotropin stimulation, oocytes derived from post mortem tissue and various storage methods as alternatives of fresh oocytes [25, 39]. Under oocyte storage conditions, the ZP has been able to exhibit good sperm binding [23]. Fresh, long-term DMSO stored [41, 42] and short-term salt-stored oocytes [23, 43] have been used successfully during the initial stages of the assay. Even though the long-term technique of ultralow temperature liquid nitrogen storage could preserve oocytes for up to 12 months, the short-term method of up to seven days storage at 4°C gained gradual widespread use in the HZA [39].

12.3 Perspective

The difficulty in obtaining the precious human ZP for the HZA has largely been overcome by the use of oocytes that fail to fertilize during ICSI or IVF [44]. Furthermore, an easy to perform bioluminescence-enhanced detection system employing a pool of solubilized ZP has been developed for easier routine use in the diagnosis of male infertility. This highly sensitive assay labels the ZP proteins with a luminescent probe and measures the light emission by the luciferin-luciferase system after almost every D-luciferin molecule is oxidized by the enzyme luciferase [45]. Yet, these approaches are still rather laborious and only very specialized laboratories are able to perform the test.

Recently, a 3D system has been developed to facilitate the ART investigations that recreated the spherical shape oocytes and the biochemical characteristics of the ZP [46]. As human sperm bind to the N-terminus of ZP2, thereby acting as a ligand for sperm binding [40, 47], the N-terminus of ZP2 attached agarose beads have been modeled to decoy sperm and prevent fertilization in vitro and in vivo [48]. Another in vitro model based on magnetic sepharose beads coated with single recombinant ZP glycoproteins that mimic the 3D oocyte's shape has been proposed as a diagnostic predictor of sperm function in male infertility patients. The secreted recombinant ZP glycoproteins are capable of conjugating to beads thereby forming a 3D oocyte-like shape that supports sperm binding and reflects the event of capacitation successfully [49]. However, the problem of glycosylation remains to be addressed as the correct amino acid sequence alone is not sufficient as ZP binding with sperm is rather mediated by the glycosidic residues [50].

In conclusion, the HZA may be incorporated into the workup algorithm of patients as an effective test of sperm function, who may benefit from a variety of therapeutic options including ART. As a diagnostic test the HZA may be particularly beneficial in oligoasthenoteratozoospermic males as well as in men with idiopathic or unexplained infertility.

References

1. Boivin J, Bunting L, Collins JA, Nygren KG. International estimates of infertility prevalence and treatment-seeking: potential need and demand for infertility medical care. *Hum Reprod* 2007; **22**: 1506–12.

2. World Health Organization. (2010) *WHO Laboratory Manual for the Examination and Processing of Human Semen*, 5th ed. Geneva: The WHO Press.

3. Franken DR, Kruger TF, Oehninger S, Coddington CC, Lombard C, Smith K. The ability of the hemizona assay to predict human fertilization in different and consecutive in-vitro fertilization cycles. *Hum Reprod* 1993; **8**: 1240–4.

4. Garrett C, Liu DY, Gordon Baker HWG. Selectivity of the human sperm-zona pellucida binding process to sperm head morphometry. *Fertil Steril* 1997; **67**: 362–71.

5. Oehninger S, Toner JP, Muasher SJ, Coddington C, Acosta AA, Hodgen GD. Prediction of fertilization in vitro with human gametes: is there a litmus test? *Am J Obstet Gynecol* 1992; **167**: 1760–7.

6. Paul M, Sumpter JP, Lindsay KS. The paradoxical effects of pentoxifylline on the binding of spermatozoa to the human zona pellucida. *Hum Reprod* 1996; **11**: 814–19.

7. Liu DY, Baker HW. Evaluation and assessment of semen for IVF/ICSI. *Asian J Androl* 2002; **4**: 281–5.

8. Liu DY, Lopata A, Johnston WI, Baker HW. Human sperm zona pellucida binding, sperm characteristics and in-vitro

fertilization. *Hum Reprod* 1989; **4**: 696–701.

9. Liu DY, Baker HW. Defective sperm-zona pellucida interaction: a major cause of failure of fertilization in clinical in-vitro fertilization. *Hum Reprod* 2000; **15**: 702–8.

10. Liu DY, Baker HW. Frequency of defective sperm-zona pellucida interaction in severely teratozoospermic infertile men. *Hum Reprod* 2003; **18**: 802–7.

11. Oehninger S, Coddington CC, Scott R, Franken DR, Burkman J, Acosta AA, Hodgen GD. Hemizon assay: assessment of sperm dysfunction and prediction of in vitro fertilization outcome. *Fertil Steril* 1989; **1**: 665–70.

12. Dunbar BS, Wolgemuth DJ. Structure and function of the mammalian zona pellucida, a unique extracellular matrix. *Mod Cell Biol* 1984; **3**: 77–111.

13. Nikas G, Paraschos T, Psychoyos A, Handyside AH. The zona reaction in human oocytes as seen with scanning electron microscopy. *Hum Reprod* 1994; **9**: 2135–8.

14. Lefievre L, Conner SJ, Salpekar A, Olufowobi O, Ashton P, Pavlovic B. Four zona pellucida glycoproteins are expressed in the human. *Hum Reprod* 2004; **19**: 1580–6.

15. Huszar G, Vique L, Oehninger SC. Creatine kinase immunocytochemistry of human sperm-hemizona complexes: selective binding of sperm with mature creatine kinase staining pattern. *Fertil Steril* 1994; **61**: 129–35.

16. Kruger TF, Oehninger S, Franken DR, Hodgen GD. Hemizona assay: use of fresh versus salt-stored human oocytes to evaluate sperm binding potential to the zona pellucida. *J In Vitro Fert Embry Trans* 1991; **8**: 154–6.

17. Huang TT, Ohzu E, Yanagimachi R. Evidence suggesting that L-Fucose is part of a recognition signal for sperm zona pellucida attachment in mammals. *Gamete Res* 1982; **5**: 355–61.

18. Familiari G, Nottola SA, Micara G, Aragona C, Motta PM. Is the sperm-binding capability of the zona pellucida limited to its surface structure? A scanning electron microscopic study of human IVF. *J In Vitro Fert Embry Trans* 1988; **5**: 134–8.

19. Tesarik J, Kopecny V. Late preovulatory synthesis of proteoglycans by the human oocyte and cumulus cells and their secretion into the oocyte-cumulus-complex extracellular matrices. *Histochem J* 1986; **85**: 523–8.

20. Overstreet JW, Hembree WC. Penetration of zona pellucida of non-living human oocytes by human spermatozoa in vitro. *Fertil Steril* 1976; **27**: 815–31.

21. Burkman LJ, Coddington CC, Franken DR. The hemizona assay (HZA): development of a diagnostic test for the binding of human spermatozoa to the human hemizona pellucida to predict fertilization potential. *Fertil Steril* 1988; **49**: 688–97.

22. Liu DY, Lopata A, Baker HWG. Use of oocytes that failed to be fertilized in vitro to study human sperm-oocyte interactions: comparison of sperm-oolemma and sperm-zona pellucida binding, and relationship with results of IVF. *Reprod Fertil Dev* 1990; **2**: 641–50.

23. Franken DR, Burkman LJ, Oehninger SC, Veeck L, Kruger TF, Coddington CC, Hodgen GD. The hemizona assay using salt stored human oocytes: evaluation of zona pellucida capacity for binding human spermatozoa. *Gam Res* 1989; **22**: 15–26.

24. Sigman M, Baazeem A, Zini A. Semen analysis and sperm

function assays: what do they mean? *Semin Reprod Med* 2009; **27**: 115–23.

25. Janssen M, Ombelet W, Cox A, Pollet H, Franken DR, Bosmans S. The hemizona assay: a simplified technique. *Arc of Andro* 1997; **38**: 127–31.

26. Vasan SS. Semen analysis and sperm function tests: how much to test? *Indian J Urol* 2011; **27**: 41–8.

27. Franken DR, Kruger TF, Oehninger SC, Kaskar K, Hodgen GD. Sperm binding capacity of human zona pellucida derived from oocytes obtained from different sources. *Andrologia* 1994; **26**: 277–81.

28. Oehninger SC, Franken DR, Elyed S, Barosso G, Kolm P. Sperm function and their predictive value for fertilization in IVF therapy: a meta analysis. *Hum Reprod Update* 2000; **6**: 160–8.

29. Aitken RJ. Sperm function tests and fertility. *Int J Aandrol* 2006; **29**: 69–75.

30. Arslan M, Morshedi M, Arslan EO, Taylor S, Kanik A, Duran HF, Oehninger S. Predictive value of the hemizona assay for pregnancy outcome in patients undergoing controlled ovarian hyperstimulation with intrauterine insemination. *Fertil Steril* 2006; **85**: 1697–707.

31. Crosignani PG, Rubin BL. Optimal use of infertility diagnostic tests and treatments. *Hum Reprod* 2000; **15**: 723–32.

32. Vogiatzi P, Chrelias C, Cahill DJ, Creatsa M, Vrachnis N, Iliodromiti Z, Kassanos D, Siristatidis C. Hemizona assay and sperm penetration assay in the prediction of IVF outcome: a systematic review. *Biomed Res Int* 2013: 945825.

33. Samplaski MK, Agarwal A, Sharma S, Sabanegh E. New generation of diagnostic tests for infertility: review of specialized

semen tests. *Int J Urol* 2010; **7**: 839–47.

34. Hodgen GD, Burkman LJ, Coddington CC, Franken DR, Oehninger S, Kruger TF, Rosenwaks Z. The hemizona assay (HZA): finding sperm that have the "right stuff". *J In Vitro Fert Embryo Transf* 1988; **5**: 311–13.

35. Franken DR, Kruger TF, Lombard CJ, Oehninger SC, Acosta AA, Hodgen GD. The ability of the hemizona assay to predict human fertilisation in different and consecutive in-vitro fertilization cycles. *Hum Reprod* 1993; **8**: 1240–4.

36. Windt ML, Franken DR, Kruger TF, Oehninger SC. In vitro fertilization failure: identification of gamete defects by investigation of sperm-zona pellucida binding capacity of unfertilized oocytes. *Andrologia* 1996; **28**: 211–15.

37. Oehninger S, Morshedi M, Franken D. The Hemizona Assay for assessment of sperm function. *Methods Mol Biol* 2013; **927**: 91–102.

38. Sanchez R, Finkenzeller C, Schill WB, Miska W. Comparison of two methods to obtain hemizonae pellucidae for sperm function tests. *Hum Reprod* 1995; **10**: 2945–7.

39. Franken DR, Oehninger S. The clinical significance of sperm-zona pellucida binding: 17 years later. *Front Biosci* 2006; **11**: 1227–33.

40. Bleil JD, Wasserman PM. Structure and function of the zona pellucida: identification and characterization of the proteins of the mouse oocyte's zona pellucida. *Dev Biol* 1980; **76**: 185–8.

41. Hammit DG, Syrop CH, Walker DL, Bennet MR. Conditions of oocyte storage and use of non-inseminated as compared with inseminated, non-fertilized oocytes for the hemizona assay. *Fertil Steril* 1993; **60**: 131–6.

42. Morroll DR, Lieberman BA, Matson PL. Use of human zonae from cryopreserved oocytes in a test to assess the binding capacity of human spermatozoa. *Int J Androl* 1993; **16**: 97–103.

43. Yoshimatsu NR, Yanagimachi R, Lopata A. Zona pellucidae of salt-stored hamster and human eggs: their penetrability by homologous and heterologous spermatozoa. *Gamete Res* 1988; **21**: 115–26.

44. Henkel R, Muller C, Stalf T, Schill W-B, Franken DR. Use of failed-fertilized oocyte for diagnostic zona binding purposes after sperm binding improvement with a modified medium. *J Assist Reprod Genet* 1999; **16**: 24–9.

45. Henkel R, Finkenzeller C, Monsees T, Franken DR, Schill W-B, Miska W. Development of a new, highly sensitive zona pellucid binding assay using a bioluminescence-enhanced detection system. *Andrologia* 2001; **33**: 215–21.

46. Romar R, Funahashi H, Coy P. In vitro fertilization in pigs: new molecules and protocols to consider in the forthcoming years. *Theriogenology* 2016; **85**: 125–34.

47. Avella MA, Baibakov B, Dean J. A single domain of the ZP2 zona pellucida protein mediates gamete recognition in mice and humans. *J Cell Biol* 2014; **205**: 801–9.

48. Baibakov B, Boggs NA, Yauger B, Baibakov G, Dean J. Human sperm bind to the N-terminal domain of ZP2 in humanized zonae pellucidae in transgenic mice. *J Cell Biol* 2012; **197**: 897–905.

49. Hamze JG, Canha-Gouveia A, Algarra B, Gomez-Torres MJ, Olivares MC, Romar R, Jimenez-Movilla M. Mammalian spermatozoa and cumulus cells bind to a 3D model generated by recombinant zona pellucida protein-coated beads. *Sci Rep* 2019; **9**: 179–89.

50. Miranda PV, Gonzalez-Echeverria F, Marin-Briggiler CI, Brandelli A, Blaquier JA, Tezon JG. Glycosidic residues involved in human sperm–zona pellucida binding in vitro. *Mol Human Reprod* 1997; **3**: 399–404.

Chapter 13

Oolemma Binding: Sperm Penetration Assay

Anup Shah, Kathleen Hwang

13.1 Introduction

Infertility is a difficult and stressful condition that impacts about 15 percent of couples attempting to conceive for the first time [1]. In about half of these cases a male factor is causative and, in general, constitutes a major health issue. While the cornerstone of the evaluation of male infertility remains the basic semen analysis, the sperm penetration assay (SPA) is a useful laboratory test for predicting the capacity of an individual male's spermatozoa to fertilize a female oocyte. This assay supplements standard semen parameters and aids clinicians in identifying couples who will have a high chance of success with in vitro fertilization. The test was first developed in the 1970s and gained momentum when, in 1976, Yanagimachi and colleagues noted that enzymatic removal of the zona pellucida of hamster ova allowed penetration by human spermatozoa [2]. The goal of the SPA is to measure the spermatozoa's ability to undergo capacitation, acrosome reaction, fusion and penetration through the oolemma (egg plasma membrane), and decondensation within the cytoplasm of hamster oocytes resulting in the formation of the male pronucleus [3].

13.2 Principle/Mechanism

Hamster oocytes have become widely used in this assay because of one unique feature – their promiscuity. First described in 1956 by Braden et al., hamster oocytes do not possess the same barriers to fertilization by sperm of other mammalian species and have thus become the oocytes of choice for testing fertilization potential [4]. During traditional fertilization, the male spermatozoa bind to the zona pellucida, a prohibitive glycoprotein layer surrounding the mammalian oocyte plasma membrane and ensure that fertilization remains species-specific. In traditional fertilization, the acrosome reaction that occurs with spermatozoa binding to the zona pellucida involves the release of acrosin (a serine protease) and

N-acetylglucoaminindase. These enzymes aid in breakdown of the zona pellucida to allow human spermatozoa fusion with the hamster oolemma – ultimately allowing fertilization and a measurable outcome. The SPA methodology requires analogous enzymes to remove the zona pellucida of hamster oocytes [5].

Currently, no standardized SPA protocol exists. However, the World Health Organization (WHO) has described a protocol for the SPA that involves five detailed steps – 1) sperm preparation, 2) ova preparation, 3) sperm and ova incubation, 4) mounting ova and 5) scoring the final slides [3].

13.2.1 Protocol

The protocol described below is the protocol described in the *WHO Laboratory Manual for the Examination and Processing of Human Sperm* [6].

All equipment and reagents should be stored at room temperature (unless otherwise indicated). All procedures should be carried out at room temperature (unless otherwise indicated).

Reagents needed:

I. **BWW stock solution**

1. Hyaluronidase (300–500 IU/mg)
2. Trypsin Type I (10,000 BAEE U/mg)
3. Wax (melting point 48–66°C)
4. Petroleum jelly
5. Mineral oil
6. Zona-free hamster oocytes: these can be purchased commercially or obtained by superovulation of hamsters
7. Dimethyl sulfoxide (DMSO).

II. **Standard protocol**

1. Mix the semen sample well.
2. Prepare the semen samples by density-gradient centrifugation or swim-up.
3. Remove most of the supernatant from the pellet.

4. Dislodge the pellet by gentle pipetting and establish the concentration of spermatozoa in the pellet.

5. Dilute the pellet to approximately 10×10^6 spermatozoa per mL in approximately 0.5 mL of medium.

6. Incline the tube at an angle of 45 degrees to the horizontal to increase the surface area.

7. Incubate the sperm suspensions for 18–24 hours at 37°C in an atmosphere of 5 percent (v/v) CO_2 in air to induce capacitation (loosen the cap of the tube to allow gas exchange). If a CO_2 incubator is not available, use a Hepes-buffered medium, cap the tubes tightly and incubate at 37°C.

8. Return the tubes to the vertical position for 20 minutes to allow settling of any immotile cells after capacitation.

9. Aspirate motile spermatozoa from the top third of the supernatant, being careful not to disturb the dead spermatozoa at the interface, and transfer them to a new tube.

10. Adjust the concentration to 3.5×10^6 motile spermatozoa per mL of medium.

11. With a positive-displacement pipette, aspirate known volumes (50–150 μL) of a sperm suspension and slowly dispense them into a small Petri dish. With a plastic disposable pipette, cover the droplet with prewarmed mineral oil equilibrated in CO_2, being careful not to disturb the sperm suspension. Add enough oil to surround and just cover each droplet of spermatozoa.

III. **Collecting the ovaries**

1. Recover the oocytes within 18 hours after the injection of hCG by sacrificing the animals according to methods approved by the relevant animal care and use committee.

2. Place the hamsters on their back and dampen the abdominal fur with 95 percent (v/v) ethanol.

3. Grasp the skin with toothed forceps and cut through the skin and muscle with scissors to expose the uterus and ovaries.

4. Wipe the forceps and scissors free of fur with 95 percent (v/v) ethanol.

5. Push the intestines out of the abdominal cavity to expose the uterine horns.

6. Grasp one uterine horn with the forceps and lift it out of the abdominal cavity to expose the oviduct, ovary and ovarian ligament.

7. The oviducts are excised and placed in the first of three ice-cold saline washes after which the oviducts are singularly transferred to a 35×10 mm culture dish containing iced saline on a dissecting microscope.

IV. **Collecting the cumulus masses**

1. Examine the ovaries by transillumination in a dissecting microscope to locate the cumulus cells containing the oocytes in the swollen portion of the oviduct.

2. Hold the oviduct with the forceps and puncture the swollen area with a 21-gauge needle. The cumulus mass will pour out of the puncture hole.

3. Tease out the cumulus mass with the needle. Squeeze the oviduct with the forceps to remove all of the cumulus mass.

V. **Recovering and treating the oocytes**

1. Gather the cumulus cells with the needle and forceps and place the cells in a watch glass dish, spot plate or other shallow container containing 0.1 percent (1g/L) hyaluronidase (300–500 IU/mL) in warm, CO_2-equilibrated BWW.

2. Incubate the container, covered with aluminum foil to protect the cells from light, for 10 minutes at room temperature. Observe the separation of the cumulus cells in a dissecting microscope.

3. Use a flame-drawn glass pipette to transfer freed oocytes from the hyaluronidase to the warm equilibrated BWW.

4. Rinse the recovered oocytes twice in BWW by transferring them into fresh drops of warm, equilibrated BWW. This can be done in a glass multi-well dish or spot plate. Rinse the pipette with BWW between each oocyte transfer.

5. Treat the oocytes with 0.1 percent (1g/L) trypsin (10,000 IU/mL) for approximately one minute at room temperature to remove the zonae pellucidae. Observe the digestion of the zona in a dissecting microscope and remove the oocytes as soon as the zona has dissolved.

6. Wash the oocytes three more times with BWW.

7. Warm the isolated oocytes to 37°C and introduce them into the sperm suspensions. Alternatively, they may be stored at 4°C for up to 24 hours before use.

VI. Co-incubation of gametes

1. Dispense the zona-free hamster oocytes into several droplets, with about five oocytes per drop (i.e. for 20 oocytes per semen sample prepare four aliquots of five oocytes per drop).
2. Load groups of about five oocytes into the glass pipette with little medium so as not to dilute the sperm suspensions too much.
3. Insert the pipette tip directly into the center of one droplet of sperm suspension and slowly dispense the oocytes. Maintain positive pressure to prevent the mineral oil from entering the pipette and take care not to introduce air bubbles into the sperm suspension.
4. Wipe any excess oil from the pipette tip after removal from the sperm suspension.
5. Repeat step 3 until all oocytes have been transferred to the sperm suspensions.
6. Rinse the pipette thoroughly in BWW after each egg transfer to prevent cross contamination of spermatozoa.
7. Incubate the gametes for three hours at 37°C in an atmosphere of 5 percent (v/v) CO_2 in air.
8. Recover the oocytes from the oil droplets. Take care to wipe any oil from the tip of the pipette before transferring the oocytes to BWW.
9. Wash the oocytes free of loosely adherent spermatozoa with the flame-drawn Pasteur pipette, by rinsing in BWW.

VII. Analyzing the oocytes

1. Place four pillars of wax-petroleum jelly mixture in a rectangular pattern to support the coverslip (22 mm × 22 mm, thickness number 1.5, 0.17 mm) at its corners.
2. Place a small droplet of oocyte-containing BWW in the center of the four pillars.
3. Lower the coverslip over the wax pillars and gently press it down, to begin to flatten the oocytes. A well-flattened oocyte is required for optimal observation of decondensed sperm heads.
4. If necessary, add more BWW to flood the slide to prevent squashing of the oocytes.

5. Examine the preparation by phase-contrast microscopy at 200× magnification.
6. Count the number of decondensed sperm heads with an attached or closely associated tail.
7. Record the percentage of eggs penetrated by at least one spermatozoon and the number of spermatozoa per penetrated egg.
8. Record the presence of any spermatozoa that remain bound to the surface of the oocytes after the initial washing procedure, since this may give some indication of the proportion of the sperm population that has undergone the acrosome reaction.

For additional information or further details of the protocol, please see the *WHO Laboratory Manual for the Examination and Processing of Human Sperm*.

13.3 Reference Values with Clinical Interpretation

Clinical interpretation of the SPA is based upon microscopic examination. Once the sperm and ova incubation is complete and the ova have been mounted as described previously, it is the responsibility of the investigator to identify the number of spermatozoa penetrations per ovum. A penetrated sperm is indicated by the presence of a swollen head and must be associated with a tail (Figure 13.1). Occasionally, due to heads merging, it becomes

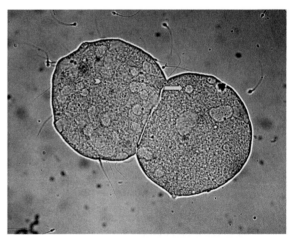

Figure 13.1 Photomicrograph demonstrating two zona-free hamster oocytes with multiple sperm penetrations depicted by the circular, lighter colored areas within the ooplasm [3].

necessary to count the sperm tails without the heads to obtain an accurate representation of sperm penetrations.

Sperm Capacitation Index (SCI) is the metric used to measure the spermatozoon's ability to fertilize an ovum and is calculated by adding up the total number of penetrations divided by the number of ova counted [3]. According to the *WHO Laboratory Manual for the Examination and Processing of Human Sperm*, more than 50 percent of ova in a SPA should demonstrate penetration in the control sperm sample [6].

13.4 Advantages and Disadvantages of Sperm Penetration Assay

The advantages of the SPA lie in its clinical implications for providers trying to direct couples to the appropriate assisted reproductive technology. Clinicians have used a positive SPA to direct couples into in-vitro fertilization (IVF) and the test has been shown in the past to be highly predictive of a positive outcome in IVF [7, 8]. For SPA with a low or absent SCI, couples have been directed to intra-cytoplasmic sperm injection therapy (ICSI).

There are several disadvantages of the SPA to consider prior to offering it to patients considering IVF. First, the SPA is a labor-intensive assay and these time and resource constraints allow it to be offered to only a few patients. Second, there are many costs to consider including, but not limited to an approved animal facility, storage units and freezers for specimens, highly trained staff as well as expensive instruments utilized in the assay. The estimated cost of performing a SPA is approximately $500 to the patient. Finally, there are disadvantages to the assay itself. Despite the enhanced precision and accuracy of the SPA since the original assay was developed in the 1970s, the reliability of the SPA has been called into question. In 2013, Vogiatzi et al. performed a systematic review of 14 SPA studies with outcome parameters and found a considerable variability in the diagnostic accuracy values of SPA with wide sensitivity (52–100 percent), specificity (0–100 percent), positive predictive value (18–100 percent) and negative predictive value (0–100 percent) [9]. Additionally, there was significant fluctuation in methodology and cut-off values employed by each group which likely contributes to the inconsistencies between the groups performing the tests. There have been modified SPA methodologies proposed over the years, but no

individual technique has proven to be superior in its diagnostic accuracy over others [10, 11]. Currently, the presumed standard technique is the one offered through the *WHO Laboratory Manual for the Examination and Processing of Human Sperm*.

13.5 Clinical Significance

The ultimate goal and the clinical value of the SPA lies in its ability to predict success rates with IVF. A meta-analysis of various sperm functional assays by Oehninger et al. included measurement of 842 sperm penetration assays as a predictor of fertilization [12]. One major issue noted is the variability in what constitutes a positive assay. Different studies used varying cut-offs of sperm penetration (10–20 percent) and fertilization rate (either 0 or 50 percent). Overall, as a predictor of IVF success, the SPA showed a high sensitivity but was also accompanied by a high false positive rate. Another similar meta-analysis collected data on 647 patients in 24 studies who had undergone a SPA and showed that SPA alone as a predictor of IVF outcomes was unreliable [13].

Given that the SPA is meant to predict success rates with IVF, many clinicians will continue to offer it to couples with plans to already undergo IVF. The clinical question lies in whether the provider feels that it would be beneficial to perform ICSI with IVF to increase the couple's chances at achieving pregnancy.

13.6 Ordering the Test

Traditionally, the SPA is ordered for couples with unexplained infertility and normal semen parameters and sperm morphology.

13.7 Clinical Case Scenario

A couple with unexplained infertility has been attempting to conceive for 36 months. The male is 31 years of age, the female is 30. Neither partner has had any prior pregnancies. All testing in the female has resulted unremarkable. The male has undergone prior semen analyses that showed morphologically normal sperm, normal semen volume and appropriate sperm density. The couple is interested in pursuing IVF.

13.8 Conclusion

The decision to perform a sperm penetration assay for a couple hoping to undergo IVF goes beyond whether or not a couple wants the test. It becomes a matter of reliability in predicting IVF outcomes and cost effectiveness for both the patient as well as the institution performing the test and analyzing the results. At its core, the test is performed with the well-meaning intent of providing critical information to a couple prior to initiating an expensive IVF cycle. However, a SPA should never be pursued without aggressively counseling the patient about the test's predictive reliability as well as its financial implications.

References

1. Sharlip ID, Jarow JP, Belker AM, Lipshultz LI, Sigman M, Thomas AJ, et al. Best practice policies for male infertility. *Fertil Steril* 2002; **77**(5): 873–82.

2. Yanagimachi R, Yanagimachi H, Rogers BJ. The use of zona-free animal ova as a test-system for the assessment of the fertilizing capacity of human spermatozoa. *Biol Reprod* 1976; **15**(4): 471–6.

3. Hwang K, Lamb DJ. The sperm penetration assay for the assessment of fertilization capacity. *Methods Mol Biol* 2013; **927**: 103–11.

4. Braden AWH, Austin CR. Early reactions of the rodent egg to spermatozoon penetration. *J Exp Biol* 1956; **33**: 358–65.

5. Schoenwolf GC, Bleyl SB, Brauer PR, Francis-West PH, Larsen WJ. (2015) *Larsen's Human Embryology*. Philadelphia, PA: Elsevier/Churchill Livingstone.

6. World Health Organization. (2010) *WHO Laboratory Manual for the Examination and Processing of Human Semen*, 5th ed. Geneva: The WHO Press, p. 271.

7. Freeman MR, Archibong AE, Mrotek JJ, Whitworth CM, Weitzman GA, Hill GA. Male partner screening before in vitro fertilization: preselecting patients who require intracytoplasmic sperm injection with the sperm penetration assay. *Fertil Steril* 2001; **76**(6): 1113–18.

8. Soffer Y, Golan A, Herman A, Pansky M, Caspi E, Ron-El R. Prediction of in vitro fertilization outcome by sperm penetration assay with TEST-yolk buffer preincubation. *Fertil Steril* 1992; **58**(3): 556–62.

9. Vogiatzi P, Chrelias C, Cahill DJ, Creatsa M, Vrachnis N, Iliodromiti Z, et al. Hemizona assay and sperm penetration assay in the prediction of IVF outcome: a systematic review. *Biomed Res Int* 2013; **2013**: 945825.

10. Johnson A, Smith RG, Bassham B, Lipshultz LI, Lamb DJ. The microsperm penetration assay: development of a sperm penetration assay suitable for oligospermic males. *Fertil Steril* 1991; **56**(3): 528–34.

11. Aitken RJ, Thatcher S, Glasier AF, Clarkson JS, Wu FC, Baird DT. Relative ability of modified versions of the hamster oocyte penetration test, incorporating hyperosmotic medium or the ionophore A23187, to predict IVF outcome. *Hum Reprod* 1987; **2**(3): 227–31.

12. Oehninger S, Franken DR, Sayed E, Barroso G, Kolm P. Sperm function assays and their predictive value for fertilization outcome in IVF therapy: a meta-analysis. *Hum Reprod Update* 2000; **6**(2): 160–8.

13. Mol BW, Meijer S, Yuppa S, Tan E, de Vries J, Bossuyt PM, et al. Sperm penetration assay in predicting successful in vitro fertilization. A meta-analysis. *J Reprod Med* 1998; **43**(6): 503–8.

Oxidative Stress Testing: Direct Tests

Renata Finelli, Manesh Kumar Panner Selvam, Ashok Agarwal

14.1 Seminal Oxidative Stress

Seminal oxidative stress (OS) is a condition where the levels of oxidants overwhelm those of the antioxidants (reductants) present in the semen [1]. The most important oxidants are reactive oxygen species (ROS), a group of oxygen-based molecules including radicals (e.g. superoxide anion – $O_2^{\cdot-}$; hydroxyl radical – $OH^{\cdot}$; peroxyl radicals – $ROO^{\cdot}$; alkoxyl radicals – $RO^{\cdot}$; organic hydroperoxides – $ROOH$) and non-radical species (hydrogen peroxide – H_2O_2). Free radicals are molecules with one or more unpaired electrons in the outer orbit, which are highly reactive towards any kind of cellular components (lipids, proteins and DNA). H_2O_2 is not a "radical", but it is classified as ROS because of its strong oxidizing characteristic and reactivity with ferrous ions in the Fenton reaction, leading to the production of hydroxyl radical:

$$H_2O_2 + Fe^{2+} \rightarrow Fe^{3+} + OH^- + OH^{\cdot}$$

Other important oxidants are derived from nitrogen (reactive nitrogen species – RNS), such as peroxynitrite ($ONOO^-$), hypochlorous acid ($HOCl$), nitric oxide ($^{\cdot}NO$) [1].

Reactions between the oxidant and a recipient molecule results in the generation of a radical, triggering a chain reaction that perpetuates the cellular damage. ROS are considered primary mediators of OS, and their presence at physiological levels in semen are essential for important sperm functions including capacitation, hyperactivation, acrosome reaction and sperm-oocyte membrane fusion [1]. When the seminal ROS levels increase beyond a threshold for redox regulation, it disturbs the endogenous antioxidant system to counterbalance the redox potential. This redox imbalance results in OS that is harmful for the spermatozoa and negatively affects the reproductive male potential.

14.2 Sources of Oxidative Stress in Semen

The production of ROS can be classified as endogenous and exogenous (Figure 14.1) [2]. In the human semen, the majority of ROS are produced endogenously by leukocytes, and mitochondria of immature sperm. Mitochondria generate energy by means of oxidative phosphorylation. In this chemical pathway, four protein complexes are involved in the transfer of electrons from donors to acceptors, finally resulting in the reduction of molecular oxygen to H_2O. These redox reactions are coupled with the transfer of protons (H^+) across the mitochondrial membrane in order to produce ATP [2]. Besides water as a final product of oxidative phosphorylation, around 1–2 percent of the oxygen is used by the enzymatic Complex I and III of the electron transport chain to synthetize $O_2^{\cdot-}$ following a single electron addition to the oxygen [3]. At the level of sperm plasma membrane, the enzyme nicotinamide adenine dinucleotide phosphate (NADPH) oxidase catalyzes the synthesis of superoxide by transferring one electron to oxygen from NADPH [3].

Exogenous causes including social behaviors (high intake of alcohol/caffeine, smoking, increased BMI), exposure to pollutants, toxins or radiation, the misuse of drugs and/or medications as well as stress or aging also contribute to increase the levels of seminal ROS. Other sources of ROS include several pathologies such as varicocele, cancer or infections of male reproductive organs [2].

14.3 Role of Oxidative Stress in Male Infertility

The oxidant species are highly reactive molecules which can interact with every cellular component. Sperm membranes are rich in polyunsaturated fatty

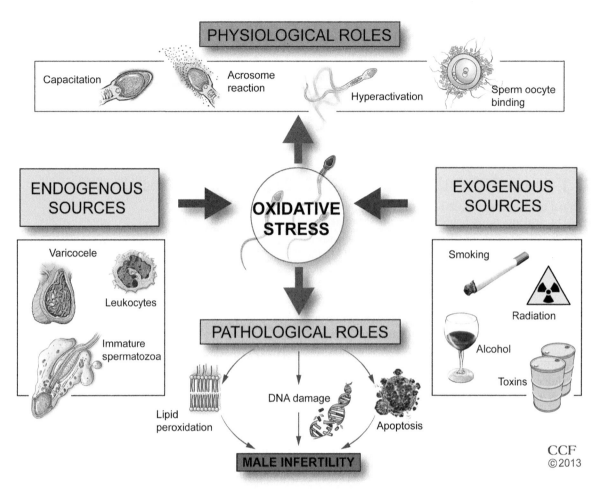

Figure 14.1 Endogenous and exogenous sources of seminal reactive oxygen species [38].

acids and are highly susceptible sites to ROS-mediated damage [1]. The "snatching" of an electron by ROS from the lipids affects the membrane integrity and leads to the production of lipid peroxidation products, such as malondialdehyde, a biochemical marker of OS. Malondialdehyde is a powerful electrophile that further oxidizes other cellular components, such as proteins, resulting in protein degradation, formation of protein-protein cross linkages and loss of function [2]. The damage to the sperm membrane can propagate into the cell from one molecule to the other in a self-perpetuating cycle. The inhibition of the enzyme glucose-6-phosphate dehydrogenase, for example, results in a reduced availability of NADPH and cellular capability to regenerate the antioxidant systems [4].

Due to a very high amount of polyunsaturated fatty acids in the plasma membrane, spermatozoa are highly susceptible to OS, which is a well-established cause of male infertility. Excess levels of ROS impairs sperm production and motility [1]. Genomic and mitochondrial sperm DNA integrity are also affected by OS. Oxidation of nitrogen bases, such as guanosine, leads to the synthesis of 8-hydroxy-2'-deoxyguanosine (8OHdG), and cause single- or double-strand breaks in sperm DNA [2]. Strong correlation exists between the extent of sperm DNA fragmentation (SDF) and different OS markers, such as intracellular ROS, malondialdehyde or 8-OHdG [5–7]. High rates of sperm DNA damage not only lead to a higher mutation rate but can also have negative impact on the fertility potential and embryo development in spontaneous pregnancies and in cycles of artificial reproductive techniques [8, 9]. Idiopathic infertile men show altered semen quality without any apparent cause of infertility, and recently, it has been reported that in 80 percent of cases, the cause could be referred to increasing levels of OS [11]. On the other hand, the percentage of men affected by unexplained male infertility is more uncertain and it could be between 10–30 percent [12]. Varicocele patients show higher ROS and decreased antioxidants levels, as well as increased SDF [10].

14.4 Tests Used to Measure Oxidative Stress

Seminal OS can be measured by both direct and indirect tests (Table 14.1) [13]. Direct tests measure the concentration of oxidant molecules, while indirect tests measure the concentration of antioxidants or analyzes the ROS-induced damage on cellular components, such as DNA, proteins and lipids. Currently, there is no "gold standard" test for the evaluation of seminal OS. Each test has its own advantages and disadvantages (Table 14.2). In this chapter, we focus on direct tests used for the measurement of OS. Direct laboratory tests include measurement of ROS by chemiluminescence method, nitro blue tetrazolium (NBT) assay, cytochrome C reduction test, electron spin resonance technique and oxidation-reduction potential (ORP).

Table 14.1 Direct and Indirect Tests for the Evaluation of Oxidative Stress

Direct tests	Indirect tests
Chemiluminescence	Myeloperoxidase or Endtz test
Nitroblue tetrazolium (NBT)	Lipid peroxidation levels
Cytochrome c reduction test	Chemokines and Interleukins
Electron spin resonance	Antioxidants, micronutrients, vitamins (vitamin E, vitamin C)
Oxidation-Reduction Potential (ORP)	Total antioxidant capacity – TAC
	DNA damage

14.5 Reactive Oxygen Species Measurement by Chemiluminescence Method

14.5.1 Principle

Chemiluminescence is the most widely used direct test for quantification of ROS in semen. The chemiluminescence is a phenomenon characterized by emission of light as a result of a chemical reaction [14, 15]. In this assay, fluorescent probes are used to investigate different ROS (including $O_2^{.-}$, H_2O_2, $OH^.$) at the same time. Luminol (5-amino-2,3-dihydro-1,4-phthalazinedione) is a yellow-colored, membrane-permeable cyclic diacylhydrazide used to detect both, intra- and extracellular ROS. It cannot be used to differentiate between different types of oxidants and cannot be used in association with strong acids/bases or reductive agents. On the other hand, lucigenin (10,10'-dimethyl-9,9'-biacridinium-dinitrate) is membrane-impermeable, used to measure the extracellular $O_2^{.-}$. Both luminol and lucigenin form an unstable endoperoxide and dioxetane after being oxidized and reduced, respectively, followed by a rapid decomposition and emission of photons [14, 15].

14.5.2 Protocol

Reagent – Luminol: 100 mM stock solution in dimethyl sulfoxide (DMSO). A 5 mM working solution should be prepared fresh and stored at room temperature. Since luminol is light-sensitive, tubes need to be covered with aluminum foil.

Sample preparation – Blank (400 µL PBS), a negative (400 µL PBS + 10 µL Luminol) and a positive (400 µL PBS + 10 µL Luminol + 50 µL H_2O_2) controls are included. The liquefied semen samples (400 µL) are mixed with luminol (10 µL) (Figure 14.2A).

ROS determination – The analysis is conducted using a luminometer (Figure 14.2B). The instrument measures sample light output and it consists of: a) a sample chamber, which holds a test tube, microplate, or other type of sample container; b) detection device, which can be photodiodes and photomultiplier tubes; c) signal processing method; d) signal output display. The test is run in triplicate.

113

Table 14.2 Direct Tests Used to Evaluate Seminal Oxidative Stress: Principle, Advantages and Disadvantages.

Tests	Principle	Advantages	Disadvantages
Chemiluminescence	Use of fluorescent probes (luminol and lucigenin)	• High sensitivity and specificity	• Time consuming • Large volume of sample required (800 µL) • Probes are highly sensitive to light • Frozen, azoospermic and hyperviscous samples cannot be analyzed
Nitroblue tetrazolium (NBT)	NBT reaction by superoxide and NADPH oxidase to formazan	• Whole ejaculates, washed sperm or leukocytes can be tested • User friendly, fast and inexpensive • Able to detect neutrophil concentration $\geq 0.5 \times 10^6$/mL	• Non-specific signal due to unspecific NBT reduction • Interpretation of result is subjective
Cytochrome c reduction test	Colorimetric assay based on the reduction of cyt c by NADPH-Cytochrome c reductase	• Suitable test to quantify extracellular O_2^- • Good for high level of ROS production	• Cannot detect NADPH oxidase activity • Cannot detect low concentrations or intracellular O_2^-
Electron spin resonance	Magnetic resonance spectroscopy	• Good for high level of ROS production	• Inference factors leading to possible neutralization of the spin-trap
Flow Cytometry detection of intracellular ROS	Use of fluorescent probes (DCFDA and DHE)	• Fast, accurate and the assay is reproducible • Applicable to oligozoospermic samples	• Expensive instrument is required
Oxidation reduction potential (ORP)	Measurement of redox potential by galvanostat-based instrument	• User friendly device • Fast and results are reliable • Less quantity of sample (30 µL) required • Assay can be performed on both fresh and frozen samples	• Not suitable for azoospermic patients or high viscosity/poorly liquefied samples

14.5.3 Interpretation of Results

The chemiluminescent signals measured by a luminometer are expressed in relative light units (RLU). The average RLU is calculated for both the analyzed tests and controls tubes. The results for ROS samples are obtained by subtracting the average RLU of negative control, and after normalization for sperm concentration/mL (Figure 14.3).

14.5.3.1 Reference Value

Reference values are obtained from the analysis of a large cohort of patient samples. Agarwal et al. analyzed 258 infertile men and 92 controls and suggested a cut-off of <102.2 RLU/s/10^6 sperm/mL to discriminate between fertile and infertile men [16].

14.5.4 Advantages/Disadvantages of the Test

Chemiluminescence methods for the ROS detection present many advantages. Some luminometers calculate the results in the integrated mode, with high sensitivity (76.4 percent) and specificity (53.3 percent). Modern luminometers are equipped with a user-friendly software, to help in the analysis and interpretation of results [16]. On the other hand,

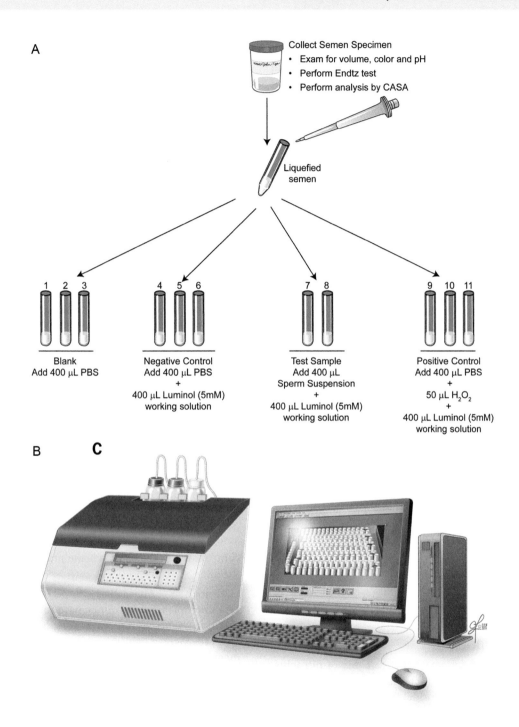

Figure 14.2 A) Processing of sample for ROS analysis by chemiluminescence assay; B) external view of the luminometer connected to the monitor for real-time display of ROS production on the monitor screen [13].

frozen, azoospermic, hyperviscous or poor liquefied semen samples cannot be analyzed with this technique and this represents a limitation of the technique. Moreover, the instrument is expensive, the assay is time-consuming and a minimum of 800 μL of semen is required to carry it out in duplicates. In addition, probes are light-sensitive, and many other factors such as variation in pH, centrifugation of the

115

Sample	Sample ID	Status	RLU Mean	Read Date	Read Time
1	Blank	Done	6269	11/17/2010	1:35:54 PM
2	Blank	Done	6713	11/17/2010	1:35:56 PM
3	Blank	Done	6189	11/17/2010	1:35:57 PM
4	Negative Control	Done	8454	11/17/2010	1:35:59 PM
5	Negative Control	Done	8104	11/17/2010	1:36:00 PM
6	Negative Control	Done	9993	11/17/2010	1:36:02 PM
7	Test Sample	Done	12954	11/17/2010	1:36:03 PM
8	Test Sample	Done	11368	11/17/2010	1:36:05 PM
9	Positive Control	Done	1261225	11/17/2010	1:36:06 PM
10	Positive Control	Done	1207794	11/17/2010	1:36:08 PM
11	Positive Control	Done	1458674	11/17/2010	1:36:10 PM

Example

Patient average (P_{av}) = 12161 RLU / sec   Sperm count = 12.6 x 10^6 /mL

Negative Control average (NC_{av}) = 8850.3 RLU / sec

Corrected value = P_{av} - NC_{av}

12161 - 8850.3 RLU / sec = 3310.7 RLU / sec

Corrected ROS = $\dfrac{3310.7}{12.6}$ = 262.7 RLU / sec / x 10^6 sperms

Result = ROS positive

Figure 14.3 ROS calculation. RLU, relative light units; ROS, reactive oxygen species.

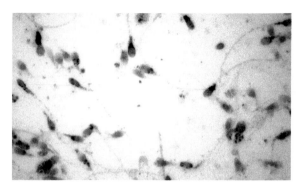

Figure 14.4 Microscopic evaluation of formazan precipitates in sperm [20].

samples and the presence of other molecules (e.g. NADPH, cysteine, ascorbic acid or uric acid) can enhance or decrease chemiluminescent signals even in the absence of spermatozoa [13–15].

14.5.5 Clinical Significance

High concentration of ROS is produced by morphologically abnormal sperm with residual cytoplasm. OS has been associated with lipid peroxidation and sperm DNA damage [17, 18]. Therefore, ROS analysis by chemiluminescence assay can provide information about the quality of spermatogenetic process and the sperm fertilizing potential [15].

14.6 Nitroblue Tetrazolium

14.6.1 Principle

Nitroblue Tetrazolium (NBT) (2,2'-bis (4-nitrophenyl)-5,5'-diphenyl-3,3'-(3,3'-dimethoxy-4,4'-diphenylene) ditetrazolium chloride) is a yellow water-soluble molecule which is reduced by superoxide and NADPH oxidase to water-insoluble formazan crystals [19] and allows the determination of cytoplasmic ROS. In the sperm cytoplasm, the hexose monophosphate pathway is responsible for the synthesis of NADPH by means of glucose-6-phosphate dehydrogenase. The NADPH contributes to the synthesis of superoxide anions by NADPH oxidase. The same enzyme in turn catalyzes

the reduction of NBT into formazan and indirectly provides the measure of ROS generation in cytoplasm. The reduced formazan is bright purple-blue colored, and it is easily detected microscopically or spectrophotometrically (Figure 14.4) [20].

14.6.2 Protocol

Reagents – NBT is usually provided as a powder, dissolved in PBS at concentration of 0.01–0.1 percent.

NBT assay – There are several assay kits in commerce for performing NBT assay. The current protocol is based on the instructions provided by Oxisperm® kit (Halotech® DNA, Madrid, Spain). Semen samples are incubated in equal volume of NBT solution and the suspension allowed to gel at 37°C for 45 minutes. The color of solution is then compared with the color scheme provided by the kit.

NBT analysis – Alternatively, a spectrophotometer or a microplate reader can be used to quantify the resulting color reaction at wavelengths of 530–630 nm. Moreover, a light microscope (100× magnification) can be used to analyze the formazan staining in leukocytes and sperm on air-dried smears as reported in Esfandiari et al [21].

14.6.3 Interpretation of Results

Results of the test sample are expressed as μg of formazan per 10^7 cells and compared with a standard curve of absorbance value derived using known concentration of formazan substrate. Tunc et al. proposed a cut-off of 24 μg formazan/10^7 sperm to discriminate between fertile and infertile men. While

Amarasekara et al. reported a cut-off equal to 40.57 and 42.02 µg formazan/10^7 sperm had high sensitivity and specificity to discriminate asthenozoospermic and unexplained infertile men from fertile men, respectively [19, 22].

14.6.4 Advantages/Disadvantagesof the Test

Since it detects intracellular ROS, NBT test can be used to discriminate the cellular source of ROS in a heterogeneous cell population. The whole ejaculate, washed spermatozoa or leukocytes are tested by NBT assay [20, 21]. The assay can also detect a minimum concentration of neutrophils (0.5×10^6/mL), lower than the WHO (2010) cut-off for leukocytospermia (1.0×10^6/mL) [23]. The test is easy-to perform, fast and inexpensive. However, its specificity in the detection of ROS is quite questionable because the assay is based on the reduction of NBT. Consequently, the reduction of NBT by means of electron donors different from ROS may generate a non-specific signal.

14.6.5 Clinical Significance

Nitroblue Tetrazolium assay is not routinely performed in the andrology laboratories because its chemistry does not detect specifically ROS concentration. In addition, the test still lacks a reference value. The values can be represented qualitatively in spermatozoa and seminal leukocytes [21] as well as quantitatively [19]. Seminal quality, sperm DNA damage and OS was measured by NBT assay in 21 fertile men and 36 infertile patients [19]. A reported cut-off value of 24 µg formazan/10^7 sperm has been suggested clinically appropriate to determine the fertility status of an individual. However, larger multicenter trials are needed to better explore the application of NBT assay for testing OS.

14.7 Cytochrome C Reduction Test

14.7.1 Principle

Cytochrome c reduction test is a colorimetric assay performed to detect extracellular $O_2^{\bullet-}$. It measures the reduction of cytochrome c by NADPH-Cytochrome c reductase in the presence of NADPH and the analysis is conducted spectrophotometrically, evaluating the absorbance at 550 nm [24].

14.7.2 Protocol

Reagents – Different kits are commercially available and the preparation of reagents follows the instructions provided by the manufacturer.

Analysis – The colorimetric analysis can be conducted in cuvette or in microplate by means of a spectrophotometer.

Spectrophotometric detection – The spectrophotometer is set to 550 nm and the kinetic program run at 25°C. A Positive Control (NADPH + Cytochrome c Reductase enzyme) and a Blank (NADPH + Buffer) are included in the analysis.

14.7.3 Interpretation of Results

The test is based on the reduction of cytochrome c. As mentioned earlier for NBT assay, its reduction by means of other electron donors different from $O_2^{\bullet-}$ produces a change in absorbance that is not specific for OS. To selectively analyze the rate of $O_2^{\bullet-}$ -mediated reduction, the test is performed by adding super-oxide dismutase (SOD) [24]. SOD catalyzes the dismutation of $O_2^{\bullet-}$ into hydrogen peroxide and the determination of SOD-inhabitable signal are used to normalize the results. Results are expressed as NADPH-Cytochrome c Reductase (NCR) unit: one unit of NCR activity is the enzyme that generates 1 nmol of the reduction of cytochrome c per minute.

14.7.4 Advantages/Disadvantages of the Test

This test is suitable to quantify $O_2^{\bullet-}$ released during the respiratory burst of neutrophils or by isolated enzyme. However, small quantities of $O_2^{\bullet-}$ cannot be detected. In addition, the enzyme cannot access the intracellular space. So, only the extracellular ROS fraction can be detected [13].

14.8 Electron Spin Resonance

14.8.1 Principle

The Electron Spin Resonance (ESR) or Electron Paramagnetic Resonance (EPR) is a technique used to measure oxygen radicals based on the magnetic resonance spectroscopy [25–27]. EPR spectroscopy can also be used to investigate the sperm membrane fluidity, using lipophilic probes [28]. Electrons are characterized by a spin quantum number (m_s), describing the angular momentum of an electron, which can assume values of ±½. According to Maxwell–Boltzmann distribution, there are typically more electrons in the lower state, described by the angular momentum equal to − ½ [29].

When a fixed frequency of microwave irradiation is used, electrons are excited from the lower energy level to the higher energy level (a phenomenon called "resonance"), with consequent absorption of energy. The absorbed energy is monitored and converted into a spectrum [25].

Reactive oxygen species are molecules characterized by a very short half-life, so some strategies, such as the "spin-trap" or the using of Hydroxylamine Spin probes were developed to detect them [26, 27]. The spin-trap approach is based on diamagnetic compounds (e.g. 5,5-dimethyl-1-pyrroline-N-oxide), which "trap" a radical molecule, generating radical adducts detectable by ESR. According to the type of trapped radical, these adducts show a specific "signature" electron paramagnetic resonance spectrum. Differently from spin-trap compounds, Hydroxylamine Spin probes do not bind the radicals, but they are oxidized to stable nitroxide, which accumulates and is detected by ESR.

14.8.2 Protocol

Sperm preparation – Samples are washed twice with sperm wash medium (700 × g, 10 minutes) and then incubated with the chosen probe (10 minutes, under rotation). Subsequently, the samples are washed again (sperm wash medium, 1 mL, 1000 × g, 60 seconds) and the supernatant loaded into 50 μL glass-capillaries for ESR analysis.

ESR analysis – The analysis is performed by an ESR spectrometer. It is composed by a computer, a microwave unit, a magnet used to apply a strong magnetic field to the unpaired electrons, and finally a spectrometer which amplifies and records the microwave absorption produced by the unpaired electrons. A microwave radiation frequency of about 9–10 GHz is usually applied to excite the electrons. A multi-frequency approach is also performed to improve the resolution of a given ESR spectrum.

14.8.3 Interpretation of Results

Electron Spin Resonance measurements provide information about the quantities, type, nature, surrounding environment, and behavior of unpaired electrons. Specifically, the instrument provides the following parameters:

- The Landé g-factor: which reflects the orbit level occupied by the electron
- Number of unpaired electrons
- Hyperfine structure: which represents the interactions between electrons and nuclei
- Fine structure: which represents the interactions between electron and electron
- Exchange interactions reflecting the exchanges between electrons

14.8.4 Advantages/Disadvantages of the Test

The "ideal" spin-trap molecule is characterized by high solubility, stability of the spin-adduct, insensitivity to inadvertent photolysis and specificity for radicals. The use of spin-trap allows the discrimination between different kinds of oxidative molecules that generate an ESR spectrum specific for the spin adduct produced. However, this technique has certain limitations. The spin-trap can be chemically modified by several enzymes with the result that it can form unspecific adducts independently by the concentration of oxidative molecules. Furthermore, the adduct formation is hampered by the scavenging action of antioxidants, such as SOD and ascorbate present in the sample [25].

14.9 Flow Cytometry Detection of Intracellular Reactive Oxygen Species

14.9.1 Principle

Flow cytometry is an instrument which utilizes laser-based technology to count, sort, and profile cells in a heterogeneous fluid mixture [35]. The interaction between the laser and the cells are measured by an electronic detection apparatus as light scatter and fluorescence intensity that are derived from dyes or monoclonal antibodies targeting either extracellular or intracellular molecules.

The signal's detection allows simultaneous multiparametric analysis of the physical and chemical characteristics of up to thousands of particles per second.

The detection of intracellular ROS by flow cytometry is based on the use of cell permeable reagents. Two specific dyes are available to measure intracellular ROS: a) 2',7'–dichlorofluorescein diacetate

(DCFDA), a fluorogenic dye that measures peroxyl, alkoxyl, $NO_2^{\cdot}$, carbonate ($CO_3^{\cdot}-$) and $OH^{\cdot}$ radicals as well as peroxynitrite within the cell; and b) dihydroethidium (DHE) which detects intracellular $O_2^{-\cdot}$. After diffusion into the cell, DCFDA is de-acetylated by cellular esterases to a non-fluorescent compound, which is later oxidized by ROS into the highly fluorescent compound 2',7'–dichlorofluorescein (DCF) that binds to DNA and emits green fluorescence between 500 and 530 nm. DHE is oxidized by the free intracellular O_2^{-} into ethidium bromide that binds to the DNA and emits red fluorescence between 590 and 700 nm [35].

14.9.2 Protocol

Reagents – DCFDA 25 mM and DHE 1.25 mM are prepared in the dark, to avoid the decay of fluorescent signal.

Sample preparation – Samples are incubated with DCFDA or DHE at 37°C for 40 minutesin the dark. A positive control treated with an organic peroxide, 500 µM tert-butyl hydrogen peroxide (TBHP), is included in the analysis. Samples are incubated in propidium iodide (PI – 1.25 µg/mL), a red-fluorescent nuclear and chromosome counterstain, to identify simultaneously dead cells.

Flow Cytometer analysis – A minimum of 10,000 spermatozoa are examined for each assay.

14.9.3 Interpretation of Results

Reactive oxygen species levels in analyzed sperm cells are expressed as the percentage of fluorescence intensity.

14.9.4 Advantages/Disadvantages of the Test

Flow cytometry is a fast, accurate and reproducible technique, extremely sensitive to changes in the redox state of a cell, and it can be used to follow changes in ROS over time. The incubation with both DCFDA and DHE probes allows the measurement of generalized radicals, even in semen samples with very low sperm counts (oligozoospermia) [35].

14.9.5 Clinical Significance

Flow cytometry has been widely applied in clinical practice for the investigation of male infertility.

Agarwal et al. analyzed three groups of patients with absence of leukocytospermia as well as low and high ($>1.0 \times 10^6$ WBC/mL) levels of leukocytes, based on the reference value provided by WHO guidelines, 2010 [36]. OS was demonstrated in samples with low leukocytospermia using flow cytometer [36]. Ghaleno et al. analyzed the intracellular ROS concentration by flow cytometry in semen selected by density gradient centrifugation, and direct and conventional swim-up [37]. Increase of H_2O_2 associated with the application of conventional swim-up, suggesting the washing and removal of semen plasma as a cause of reduced antioxidant activity. A negative correlation was observed between seminal H_2O_2 and pronuclear formation [37].

14.10 Oxidation Reduction Potential

14.10.1 Principle

The Oxidation Reduction Potential (ORP, or redox potential) is a measure of electron transfer between two chemical species [38], according to the Nernst equation, which determines the cell potential under not standard conditions:

$$E(ORP) = E^0 + RT/nF \ln([Red]/[Ox])$$

E^0, standard reduction potential; R, universal gas constant; T, absolute temperature; n, number of moles of exchanged electrons; F, Faraday's constant; [Red], concentration of reduced species; [Ox], concentration of oxidized species.

The molecule which donates electrons is oxidized while the one that accepts electrons is reduced. In semen, ORP is measured using MiOXSYS (Aytu BioScience, Inc.), a galvanostat-based technology, able to measure the electron transfers between antioxidants and oxidant species, providing a picture of the current redox balance. The sample is loaded into a specific sensor which is inserted into the device, so that the test can automatically begin.

14.10.2 Protocol

Processing of the sample – The entire ejaculate, seminal plasma, fresh and frozen samples can be analyzed, and no sample pre-treatment is required.

Seminal ORP measurement – The sample is loaded onto the sample application port of the sensor, it fills the reference electrode, thereby completing the electrochemical circuit (Figure 14.5).

119

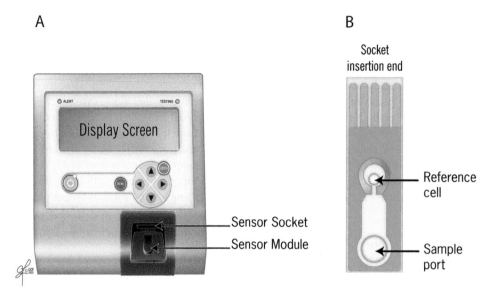

A

B

Socket
insertion end

Reference
cell

Sample
port

Display Screen

ALERT   TESTING

Sensor Socket
Sensor Module

Figure 14.5 MiOXSYS A) analyzer and B) sensor. Fully insert sensor into the analyzer for appropriate sample analysis (A–C) [38].

14.10.3 Interpretation of Results

Initially, the MiOXSYS displays the results in millivolt (mV). The obtained values are normalized with sperm concentration and the final readings are expressed as $mV/10^6$ sperm/mL. ORP is influenced by the concentration of viable cells present in the ejaculate, so the results vary in accordance to the sperm concentration [39]. In addition, the presence of morphologically immature or abnormal sperm with poor motility influences the ROS synthesis and the availability of the antioxidants, reflecting in a change of ORP. Therefore, two samples with an equal number of spermatozoa at different physiological states and OS will have a different ORP [38].

14.10.4 Advantages/Disadvantages of the Test

The MiOXSYS is a cost-effective, small and very easy to use analyzer. It is simple to operate and does not involve special training. It can analyze fresh or frozen samples without any kind of pre-treatment and the analysis is conducted on a very small quantity of sample (30 μL) in a short period of time (<5 minutes). Results are stable up to 120 minutes.

Since ORP readings are normalized to the sperm concentration, it is not possible to analyze azoospermic samples. The loading of the semen sample is difficult in cases of high viscosity or poor liquefied

samples, which can affect the reading. Moreover, the measurement is sensitive to centrifugation. This process generates shear stress which induce spermatozoa to produce more ROS [38].

14.10.5 Clinical Significance

A limited number of studies investigated the use of MiOXSYS in clinics for measurement of ORP. In a multicenter study conducted by Agarwal et al. in 2019, a cut-off of $1.34~mV/10^6$ sperm/mL has been proposed to discriminate between normal and abnormal semen samples with 98.1 percent sensitivity and 40.6 percent specificity. In varicocele patients, a negative association between semen quality and ORP have been reported [11].

14.11 Limitations of Direct Tests for Measuring Oxidative Stress

The direct tests for the detection of OS present different kinds of limitations. In general, they are laborious, time consuming, and can measure only a single marker of OS. According to the technique that is used, a variable amount of sample is required (i.e. 800 μL for chemiluminescence assay) and the use of fluorescent probes has the limitation of fluorescence decay during time. In addition, some techniques such as chemiluminescence assay cannot analyze the OS in frozen or viscous samples and several conditions related to variations in light, pH, centrifugation speed and time can interfere with the analysis, reducing the accuracy of the results.

In addition, the half-life of ROS is very short, rendering their detections extremely challenging. Currently, research is primarily focused to overcome these limitations and, in this context, ORP represents a promising marker for the global detection of oxidant and reductive species in semen [13].

14.12 Conclusion

Currently, there is no "gold standard" test for the evaluation of OS. The direct tests for the detection of OS present different strengths and weaknesses, which limit their use in clinic as diagnostic tools. The ORP represents a promising marker to be used in the andrology laboratory for the evaluation of OS.

References

1. Aitken RRJ. Reactive oxygen species as mediators of sperm capacitation and pathological damage. *Mol Reprod Dev* 2017; **84**(10): 1039–52.

2. Dada R, Bisht S. (2017) Oxidative stress and male infertility. In Singh R, Singh K., eds., *Male Infertility: Understanding, Causes and Treatment.* Singapore: Springer. https://doi.org/10.1007/978-981-10-4017-7_10

3. Sinha K, Das J, Pal P, Sil P. Oxidative stress: the mitochondria-dependent and mitochondria-independent pathways of apoptosis. *Arch Toxicol* 2013; **87**(7): 1157–80.

4. Aitken RJ, Fisher HM, Fulton N, Gomez E, Knox W, Lewis B, et al. Reactive oxygen species generation by human spermatozoa is induced by exogenous NADPH and inhibited by the flavoprotein inhibitors diphenylene iodonium and quinacrine. *Mol Reprod Dev* 1997; **47**(4): 468–82.

5. Aitken RJ, De Iuliis GGN, Finnie JJM, Hedges A, McLachlan RRI. Analysis of the relationships between oxidative stress, DNA damage and sperm vitality in a patient population: development of diagnostic criteria. *Hum Reprod* 2010; **25**(10): 2415–26.

6. Aktan G, Doğru-Abbasoğlu S, Küçükgergin C, Kadioğlu A, Özdemirler-Erata G, Koçak-Toker N, et al. Mystery of idiopathic male infertility: is oxidative stress

an actual risk? *Fertil Steril* 2013; **99**(5): 1211–15.

7. Homa ST, Vassiliou AM, Stone J, Killeen AP, Dawkins A, Xie J, et al. A comparison between two assays for measuring seminal oxidative stress and their relationship with sperm DNA fragmentation and semen parameters. *Genes* 2019; **10**(3): 236.

8. Dhawan V, Kumar M, Deka D, Malhotra N, Singh N, Dadhwal V, et al. Paternal factors and embryonic development: role in recurrent pregnancy loss. *Andrologia* 2019; **51**(1): e13171.

9. Venkatesh S, Thilagavathi J, Kumar K, Deka D, Talwar P, Dada R. Cytogenetic, Y chromosome microdeletion, sperm chromatin and oxidative stress analysis in male partners of couples experiencing recurrent spontaneous abortions. *Arch Gynecol Obstet* 2011; **284**(6): 1577–84.

10. Agarwal A, Sharma RK, Desai NR, Prabakaran S, Tavares A, Sabanegh E. Role of oxidative stress in pathogenesis of varicocele and infertility. *Urology* 2009; **73**(3): 461–9.

11. Agarwal A, Parekh N, Panner Selvam MK, Henkel R, Shah R, Homa ST, et al. Male oxidative stress infertility (MOSI): proposed terminology and clinical practice guidelines for management of idiopathic male infertility. *World J Mens Health* 2019; **37**(3): 296–312.

12. Gunn DD, Bates GW. Evidence-based approach to unexplained infertility: a systematic review. *Fertil Steril* 2016; **105**(6): 1566–74.e1.

13. Agarwal A, Qiu E, Sharma R. Laboratory assessment of oxidative stress in semen. *Arab J Urol* 2018; **16**(1): 77–86.

14. Aitken RJ, Baker MA, O'Bryan M. Shedding light on chemiluminescence: the application of chemiluminescence in diagnostic andrology. *J Androl* 2004; **25**(4): 455–65.

15. Khan P, Idrees D, Moxley MMA, Corbett JAJ, Ahmad F, Von Figura G, et al. Luminol-based chemiluminescent signals clinical and non-clinical application and future uses. *Appl Biotechnol Biochem* 2014; **173**(2): 333–55.

16. Agarwal A, Ahmad G, Sharma R. Reference values of reactive oxygen species in seminal ejaculates using chemiluminescence assay. *J Assist Reprod Genet* 2015; **32**(12): 1721–9.

17. Gomez E, Irvine D, Aitken R. Evaluation of a spectrophotometric assay for the measurement of malondialdehyde and 4-hydroxyalkenals in human spermatozoa: relationships with semen quality and sperm function. *Int J Androl* 1998; **21**(2): 81–94.

18. Oumaima A, Tesnim A, Zohra H, Amira S, Ines Z, Sana C, et al. Investigation on the origin of sperm morphological defects: oxidative attacks, chromatin immaturity, and DNA

fragmentation. *Environ Sci Pollut Res.* 2018; **25**(14): 13775–86.

19. Tunc O, Thompson J, Tremellen K. Development of the NBT assay as a marker of sperm oxidative stress. *Int J Androl* 2010; **33**(1): 13–21.

20. Gosalvez J, Tvrda E, Agarwal A. Free radical and superoxide reactivity detection in semen quality assessment: past, present, and future. *J Assist Reprod Gen* 2017; **34**(6): 697–707.

21. Esfandiari N, Sharma RK, Saleh RA, Thomas Jr AJ, Agarwal A. Utility of the nitroblue tetrazolium reduction test for seminal leukocytes and spermatozoa. *J Androl* 2003; **24**(6): 862–70.

22. Amarasekara DS, Wijerathna S, Fernando C, Udagama PV. Cost-effective diagnosis of male oxidative stress using the nitroblue tetrazolium test: useful application for the developing world. *Andrologia* 2014; **46**(2): 73–9.

23. Kovalski N, de Lamirande E, Gagnon C. Determination of neutrophil concentration in semen by measurement of superoxide radical formation. *Fertil Steril* 1991; **56**(5): 946–53.

24. Dikalov SI, Harrison DG. Methods for detection of mitochondrial and cellular reactive oxygen species. *Antioxid Redox Signal* 2014; **20**(2): 372–82.

25. Kopáni M, Celec P, Danišovič L, Michalka P, Biró C. Oxidative stress and electron spin resonance. *Clin Chim Acta* 2006; **364**(1–2): 61–6.

26. Dikalov SI, Polienko YF, Kirilyuk I. Electron paramagnetic resonance measurements of reactive oxygen species by cyclic hydroxylamine spin probes. *Antioxid Redox Signal* 2018; **28**(15): 1433–43.

27. Kohno M. Applications of electron spin resonance spectrometry for reactive oxygen species and reactive nitrogen species research. *J Clin Biochem Nutr* 2010; **47**(1): 1–11.

28. Ochsendorf FR, Rinne D, Fuchs J, Such P, Zimmer G. Electron paramagnetic resonance spectroscopy for the investigation of the fluidity of human spermatozoa plasma membranes: a feasibility study. *Andrologia* 2000; **32**(3): 169–77.

29. Rowlinson JS. The Maxwell-Boltzmann distribution. *Mol Phys* 2005; **103**(21–23): 2821–8.

30. Hossain MS, Johannisson A, Wallgren M, Nagy S, Siqueira AP, Rodriguez-Martinez H. Flow cytometry for the assessment of animal sperm integrity and functionality: state of the art. *Asian J Androl* 2011; **13**(3); 406–19.

31. Lybaert P, Danguy A, Leleux F, Meuris S, Lebrun P. Improved methodology for the detection and quantification of the acrosome reaction in mouse spermatozoa. *Histol Histopathol* 2009; **24**(8): 999–1007.

32. Du Plessis SS, Agarwal A, Halabi J, Tvrda E. Contemporary evidence on the physiological role of reactive oxygen species in human sperm function. *J Assist Reprod Gen* 2015; **32**(4): 509–20.

33. El-Taieb MA, Ali MA, Nada EA. Oxidative stress and acrosomal morphology: a cause of infertility in patients with normal semen parameters. *Middle East Fertil Soc J.* 2015; **20**(2): 79–85.

34. Ichikawa T, Oeda T, Ohmori H, Schill WB. Reactive oxygen species influence the acrosome reaction but not acrosin activity in human spermatozoa. *Int J Androl* 1999; **22**(1): 37–42.

35. Mahfouz R, Sharma R, Lackner J, Aziz N, Agarwal A. Evaluation of chemiluminescence and flow cytometry as tools in assessing production of hydrogen peroxide and superoxide anion in human spermatozoa. *Fertil Steril* 2009; **92**(2): 819–27.

36. Agarwal A, Alshahrani S, Assidi M, Abuzenadah AMA, Sharma R, Sabanegh E, et al. Reactive oxygen species and sperm DNA damage in infertile men presenting with low level leukocytospermia. *Reproduct Biol Endocrinol* 2014; **12**(1): 1–8.

37. Ghaleno LR, Valojerdi MR, Hassani F, Chehrazi M, Janzamin E. High level of intracellular sperm oxidative stress negatively influences embryo pronuclear formation after intracytoplasmic sperm injection treatment. *Andrologia* 2014; **46**(10): 1118–27.

38. Agarwal A, Bui AD. Oxidation-reduction potential as a new marker for oxidative stress: correlation to male infertility. *Investig Clin Urol* 2017; **58**(6): 385.

39. Pluschkell SB, Flickinger MC. Improved methods for investigating the external redox potential in hybridoma cell culture. *Cytotechnology* 1995; **19**(1): 11–26.

Chapter

15

Oxidative Stress Testing: Indirect Tests

Rakesh Sharma, Kathy Robert, Ashok Agarwal

15.1 Introduction

Oxidative stress (OS) is the consequence of an imbalance between reactive oxygen species (ROS) and the failure of antioxidants to neutralize excessive ROS production. Although many sperm functions require physiological levels of ROS, excessive levels of ROS are detrimental to the sperm [1]. OS is one of the most common etiologies of male infertility affecting 30–80 percent of infertile men [2, 3]. The role of OS in men with unexplained infertility has been clearly established [4]. OS affects sperm quality as a result of alterations in proteins, lipid peroxidation, DNA damage and apoptosis [1]. Damage to sperm DNA can compromise the contribution of paternal genome to the embryo [4]. Hence the advent of numerous tests to diagnose OS in the semen. There are several laboratory tests available to measure OS – both direct and indirect. Direct tests measure OS or free radicals such as ROS and reactive nitrogen species. These include chemiluminescence, nitroblue tetrazolium, cytochrome C reduction test, electron spin resonance, fluorescein isothiocynate (DFITC)-labeled lectins, and measurement of oxidation reduction potential. Indirect tests measure oxidized products resulting from ROS sources such as the oxidized form of nicotinamide adenine dinucleotide (NADPH)-oxidase in the sperm, the reduced form of NAD (NADH)-dependent oxidoreductase in mitochondria, or leukocytospermia. These include myeloperoxidase or Endtz test, antioxidants (both enzymatic and non-enzymatic), lipid peroxidation, and DNA damage. In this chapter we will discuss the indirect tests that are available to assess OS and also elaborate on the interpretation and their clinical significance [4, 5].

15.2 Tests to Detect Factors Causing an Oxidation-Reduction Imbalance

15.2.1 Tests to Detect Leukocyte Products

Apart from immature spermatozoa, presence of white blood cells (WBC) or leukocytes is an important source of ROS in semen [5]. Leukocytes, mainly polymorphonuclear neutrophils (PMN) or granulocytes [6], when activated in the presence of a chronic infection or inflammation due to male accessory gland infection due to prostatitis epididymitis or inflammation of the seminal vesicles can release 100-fold higher levels of ROS compared to abnormal spermatozoa [7, 8]. Leukocyte activation results in increased NADPH production via the hexose monophosphate shunt. This increases superoxide anion concentration which results in oxidative stress [9]. Leukocytes when present in concentrations $>1 \times 10^6$ WBC/mL of semen result in leukocytospermia [10].

15.2.1.1 Granulocyte Elastase Enzyme Immunoassay

Elastase is one of the major proteomic enzymes released by the leukocytes (granulocytes) at the site of inflammation [11]. During inflammation, polymorphonuclear granulocytes (PMN) discharges proteases such as elastase in large quantity. The elastase-α1–protease inhibitor complex (Ela/α1–PI) of the elastase enzyme is a sensitive marker of genital tract inflammation [12]. In addition, elastase itself causes the release of ROS which when in excess triggers cell deterioration. Politch et al. described this method as a gold standard for leukocytospermia using monoclonal antibodies [13].

15.2.1.1.1 Principle

This method is based on the quantitative determination of granulocyte elastase with alpha 1-proteinase inhibitor.

15.2.1.1.2 Methodology

The semen sample is centrifuged at $300 \times g$ for 10 minutes and kept at 37°C for 25 minutes. The supernatant is separated and diluted with phosphate buffered saline (PBS) containing 10 g/L bovine serum albumin (BSA) and 20 mM Ethylenediaminetetraacetic acid (EDTA). The solution is incubated with 500 μL of sample diluent for one hour at 37°C and then washed with distilled water containing 0.5 g/L polyoxyethylene sorbitan monolaurate (PESM). The mixture is then incubated with 500 μL reagent with alkaline phosphatase against α-1 proteinase inhibitor complex for one hour at 37°C. This complex is prepared by adding 2 mL of 30 mM tris(hydroxymethyl)aminomethane/HCl buffer containing 85 mM NaCl to a mixture of 0.5 mg elastase and 2.8 mg α-1 proteinase inhibitor incubated for 30 minutes at 37°C. The sample is washed again with distilled water containing 0.5 g/L PESM and incubated with 500 μL of 10 mM of 4-nitrophenyl phosphate in 1molar diethanolamine/HCl-buffer containing 0.5 mM MgCl$_2$. The reaction of the proteinase enzyme reaction is stopped by adding 500 μL of 2 M NaOH and the absorbance is read at 405 nm [14].

15.2.1.1.3 Interpretation

The concentration of elastase in the sample is determined colorimetrically using a standard curve, and expressed in ng/mL. A three-step grading system of PMN-elastase values are described below:

- <250 ng/mL   normal
- 250–1000 ng/mL   intermediate
- >1000 ng/mL   high (pathologic)

Study shows elastase concentrations to be highly correlated with the number of peroxidase-positive cells ($p < 0.01$) and negatively correlated with sperm vitality ($p < 0.01$). Furthermore, significantly negative correlations were seen with sperm motility ($p < 0.05$), progressive motility ($p < 0.05$) and sperm morphology ($p < 0.05$). In addition, a significant negative correlation was observed between elastase concentrations and percentage of spermatozoa with intact DNA [11].

15.2.1.2 Myeloperoxidase Test or Endtz Test

The test is recommended by the World Health Organization (WHO) to detect leukocytospermia and is performed when the number of round cells is $\geq 1.0 \times 10^6$/mL on routine semen analysis for men presenting with infertility [10].

15.2.1.2.1 Principle

The Myeloperoxidase or Endtz test is based on the principle that peroxidase present in the leukocyte granules or polymorphonuclear granulocytes oxidize the substrate benzidine from a colorless form to an insoluble/brown derivative in presence of hydrogen peroxide (H$_2$O$_2$) [6, 15]. Myeloperoxidase presenting granulocytes such as neutrophils, polymorphonuclear leukocytes, and macrophages can thus be differentiated from germinal cells.

15.2.1.2.2 Methodology

The stock solution is prepared by mixing 50 mL of 96 percent ethanol, 0.125 g benzidine and 50 mL of sterile water. Working Endtz solution is prepared by adding 2 mL of stock solution and 25 μL of 3 percent H$_2$O$_2$. A 20 μL aliquot of the liquefied semen is vortexed and mixed with equal volume of PBS (pH 7.0) in a microfuge tube to which 40 μL of the working Endtz solution is added. The mixture is vortexed and incubated for five minutes at 37°C. The Makler counting chamber is loaded with 5 μL of the above suspension and examined for cells that stain dark brown, indicating that they are peroxidase containing granulocytes (Figure 15.1). These granulocytes are

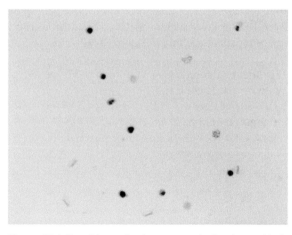

Figure 15.1 Peroxidase-stained semen sample showing positively stained white blood cells.

counted in all 100 squares of the grid in a Makler chamber under 10× bright field objective [16].

15.2.1.2.3 Interpretation
The final value is calculated and recorded as 10^6 WBC/mL of semen [16].

15.2.1.2.4 Clinical Significance
Peroxidase positive leukocytes are proven to be a major source of ROS formation by granulocytes [6]. Leukocytospermia has been shown to have a negative correlation with sperm parameters, ROS [6] as well as DNA integrity [17–20].

15.2.2 Pro-Inflammatory Cytokines and Other Immune Factors
Seminal plasma contains many cytokines and immunological factors such as: interleukins (IL) (IL1α, IL 1β, IL 2, IL6, IL 8, IL10 and IL 12); interferons (IFN-α and γ); macrophage inflammatory protein (MIP-1α and 1β); Regulated on Activation Normal T cell Expressed and Secreted (RANTES) protein also known as chemokine ligand 5; stromal cell-derived factor (SDF-1α); transforming growth factor (TGF-β1) and immunoglobulins (IgA and IgG). These can be measured using Bio-Plex or enzyme-linked immunosorbent assay to determine quantities of immunoglobulin (Ig) isotypes, chemokines, cytokines and growth present in the semen [21]. The concentrations are presented in pg/mL or ng/mL of immunoglobulins.

15.2.2.1 Clinical Significance
Semen of healthy, fertile men contains a broad array of immunologic factors. Many studies demonstrate the significance of elevated pro-inflammatory cytokines in altered sperm function [22]. Pro-inflammatory cytokines increase lipid peroxidation of the sperm membranes [23, 24]. Although they contribute to OS, they are intermediate rather than causative factors of OS [25].

15.2.3 Measurement of Antioxidants
The antioxidant capacity of the seminal fluid can be assessed by measuring individual antioxidants or total antioxidant capacity (TAC) wherein the reducing capacity of various antioxidants against an oxidative reagent is evaluated. The antioxidant capacity of seminal plasma is the sum of enzymatic (superoxide dismutase, catalase, glutathione peroxidase) and non-enzymatic antioxidants (α-tocopherol (Vitamin E), ascorbate (Vitamin C), β-carotene (Vitamin A), folic acid (Vitamin B9), ferritin and carnitines, N-acetyl L-cysteine, coenzyme Q10, ceruloplasmin, selenium, L-arginine, urate and zinc) [26, 27]. A number of assays are available to measure antioxidants. These are described below:

15.2.3.1 Total Antioxidant Capacity Measurement
Total antioxidant capacity (TAC) assay measures the ability of antioxidants in the seminal plasma to scavenge the stable blue-green radical cation ABTS+ (2,2'-azinobis(3-ethylbenzothiazoline-6-sulfonic acid). The ability of the antioxidants to reduce the absorbance at 750 nm by inhibiting the oxidation of ABTS to generate ABTS+ is compared to a water-soluble analogue, Trolox (6-hydroxy-2, 5, 7, 8-tetramethylchroman-2-carboxylic acid) used as a standard [28].

The antioxidant assay buffer concentrate is diluted 10 times in a conical tube. The lyophilized metmyoglobin powder is added to 600 μL of the prepared assay buffer. The working solution is prepared by two serial dilutions, first by adding 10 μL of 8.82 M hydrogen peroxide to 990 μL of ultrapure water and then further diluting 20 μL of this with 3.98 mL of ultrapure water again. Chromogen (containing ABTS) is added to 6 mL of ultrapure water under indirect light as it is light sensitive.

The seminal plasma samples are centrifuged at $300 \times g$ for seven minutes and then diluted with the assay buffer at a ratio of 1:9. Trolox standards and reagents are prepared as per the manufacturer's instructions at the time of the assay. One milliliter of reconstituted lyophilized Trolox is used to prepare the standard curve. Ten microliters of Trolox standard and test samples are loaded into the corresponding wells of a 96-well plate (Cayman Chemical, Ann Arbor, MI). Ten microliters of metmyoglobin along with 150 μL of chromogen are added to all standard and sample wells. The addition of 40 μL of hydrogen peroxide as quickly as possible initiates the reaction. The plate is then covered and incubated for five minutes on a horizontal plate shaker at room temperature (Eppendorf MixMate, Hauppauge, NY). Absorbance is monitored at 750 nm using a microplate reader (BioTek Instruments, Inc., Winooski, VT) [28].

Calculation of assay results: Determination of the reaction rate was done by calculating the average

125

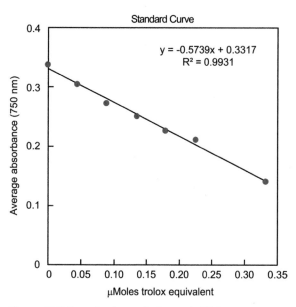

Standard Curve

$$y = -0.5739x + 0.3317$$
$$R^2 = 0.9931$$

Figure 15.2 Example of a standard curve for TAC measurement. Standard Trolox concentrations are represented on the X-axis and the absorbance on the Y-axis.

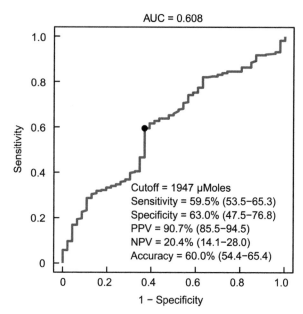

AUC = 0.608

Cutoff = 1947 µMoles
Sensitivity = 59.5% (53.5–65.3)
Specificity = 63.0% (47.5–76.8)
PPV = 90.7% (85.5–94.5)
NPV = 20.4% (14.1–28.0)
Accuracy = 60.0% (54.4–65.4)

Figure 15.3 Receiver Operating Characteristics (ROC) curve showing the Area under Curve (AUC), cut-off, sensitivity, specificity, positive predictive value, negative predictive value and accuracy of the assay.

absorbance of each standard and sample. The average absorbance of the standards as a function of the final Trolox concentration (µM of Trolox equivalent) is plotted for the standard curve in each run, from which the unknown samples are determined.

$$Antioxidant\ (\mu M)$$
$$= [(Unknown\ average\ absorbance - Y - intercept)$$
$$\div Slope] \times dilution \times 1000$$

The total antioxidant concentration of each sample is calculated using the equation obtained from the linear regression of the standard curve by substituting the average absorbance values for each sample into the equation [28] (Figure 15.2). In healthy men, the reference value for TAC levels in seminal plasma is >1900 µM Trolox equivalent. The sensitivity, specificity, positive and negative predictive value and accuracy of the TAC assay is shown in Figure 15.3. Infertile men have lower TAC values compared to healthy men (Figure 15.4).

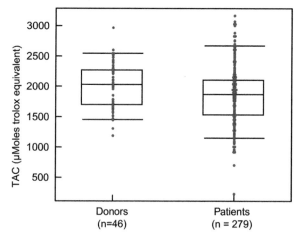

Figure 15.4 Distribution of TAC levels between healthy donors (n = 46) and infertile patients (n = 279).

15.2.3.2 Ferric Reducing Antioxidant Power Assay

Ferric Reducing Antioxidant Power (FRAP) Assay is a spectrophotometric method, that works on the principle of the reducing ability of phenols to convert yellow ferric 2,4,6-tripyridyl-s-triazine (Fe3+-TPTZ) to blue ferrous complex (Fe2+-TPTZ). The change in absorbance is monitored at 593 nm to calculate the antioxidant capacity [29].

The difference in absorbance is translated into a FRAP value expressed in micromoles (µM) by comparing the absorbance at 593 nm of test sample to that of a standard solution of known FRAP value [29].

$$Antioxidant \ (\mu M) = \frac{\text{Change in absorbance at 593 nm of test sample} \times \text{FRAP value of standard}}{\text{Change in absorbance at 593 nm of standard}}$$

The FRAP assay offers a putative index of the antioxidants or reducing agents potential of biological fluids.

15.2.3.3 Oxygen Radical Absorbance Capacity

Oxygen Radical Absorbance capacity (ORAC) is the direct capacity of peroxyl radical-induced oxidation by chain-breaking antioxidants such as α-tocopherol. It measures the hydrogen atom donating ability of antioxidants. In this assay, β-phycoerythrin (β-PE) is used as the fluorescent probe, 2,2′-azobis(2-amidino-propane) dihydrochloride (AAPH) as a peroxyl radical generator and Trolox as a control or standard.

When AAPH is added to the sample, it slows the decrease in the fluorescence intensity. The loss of fluorescence indicates the extent of decomposition, when it reacts with the peroxyl radical. In the presence of antioxidants, this decrease in the intensity is delayed and is proportional to the amount of antioxidants present in the system [30].

The antioxidant capacity is obtained by calculating the difference in the decrease of the fluorescence intensity between sample and Trolox. Results are expressed as ORAC units, where 1 ORAC unit equals the net protection conferred by 1 μM Trolox.

15.2.3.4 Clinical Significance

Proven fertile donors have higher antioxidant values than infertile patients [26, 28, 31], thus suggesting that measuring TAC in semen is an effective and simple test for diagnosing and managing male infertility.

15.2.4 Measurement of Individual Antioxidants, Micronutrients and Vitamins

Individual antioxidants can be identified by assessing the activity of enzymes highly specific to a particular antioxidant, particularly for superoxide dismutase (SOD), catalase, and glutathione peroxidase (GPx) – the three vital ROS scavengers in the semen.

15.2.4.1 Superoxide Dismutase

Superoxide dismutase (SOD) catalyzes dismutation of superoxide and prevents lipid peroxidation. It scavenges both extracellular and intracellular superoxide anion, a major source of ROS, into oxygen and hydrogen peroxide. SOD activity may be quantified according to the method described by Fridovich et al. [32]. In this method, xanthine and xanthine oxidase generates superoxide radicals that react with 2-(4-iodophenyl)-3-(4-nitrophenol)-5- phenyltetrazolium chloride (INT) to produce a red formazan dye. SOD is measured by the inhibition of the reaction indicated by the decrease in red color measured at 505 nm. The assay medium consists of phosphate buffer, a 3-cyclo-hexilamino-1-propanesulfonic acid (CAPS) buffer solution and substrate xanthine, INT and xanthine oxidase. One unit of enzyme activity is defined as the amount of SOD capable of inhibiting 50 percent of nitrite formation at the particular absorbance. SOD activity is expressed as U/mg of protein [32].

15.2.4.2 Catalase

Catalase is the second most abundant enzymatic antioxidant (after superoxide dismutase) responsible to balance the levels of reactive oxygen species. Catalase acts to dissociate hydrogen peroxide (H_2O_2) into oxygen and water. The assay medium consists of EDTA buffer solution, phosphate buffer solution, and H_2O_2. Catalase activity is measured by the spectrophotometric method in which the change of absorbance at 240 nm occurs at high H_2O_2 levels. Hydrogen peroxide inhibits the catalase enzyme and the decrease in concentration of catalase is measured at 240 nm. The calculation is based on the rate of reduction of the absorbance for one minute. The catalase activity is expressed as μmole of H_2O_2 decomposed/min/mg protein [33].

15.2.4.3 Glutathione Peroxidase

Glutathione peroxidase (GPx) is a major enzyme that removes H_2O_2 generated by SOD in cytosol and mitochondria [34]. GPx catalyzes both H_2O_2 and organic peroxide (ROO) decomposition generating glutathione disulphide (GSSG), water and organic alcohol (ROH) with the release of reduced glutathione (GSH). The reaction is initiated by the addition of 25 μL of 0.72 mM cumene hydroperoxide and the change in absorbance is monitored at 340 nm at 30°C for 15 minutes. GPx catalyzes the oxidation of glutathione by cumene hydroperoxide. In the presence of glutathione reductase and NADPH, oxidized glutathione is immediately converted into the reduced form with concomitant oxidation of NADPH to NADP+. Reduced glutathione is used as the control or standard. This oxidation process is associated with a decrease in absorbance at 340 nm, allowing GPx activity to be monitored colorimetrically. GPx activity is expressed as mU/mL seminal plasma. One enzymatic unit is defined as 1 μmole of oxidized NADPH per minute at 30°C by the glutathione reductase-linked kinetic reaction [35].

15.2.4.3.1 Clinical Significance

Although SOD, catalase and GPx levels correlate with routine semen parameters [35], the individual levels required to preserve fertility in men have not yet been established. This is particularly difficult as all the antioxidants combined play a role in scavenging ROS.

15.2.4.4 Ascorbic Acid (Vitamin C)

Ascorbic acid concentration in the seminal fluid (400 μM) is much higher than its concentration in the blood plasma (60 μM), reflecting an important physiological role [36]. The seminal fluid is incubated with 9 vol. of 5 percent metaphosphoric acid (1 mM EDTA and 2 mM cysteine) which reduces ascorbic acid to dehydroascorbate, and is then treated with 2,4-dinitrophenylhydrazine (pH of <2) to form bis-2,4-dinitrophenylhydrazine. Sulfuric acid is mixed with the bis derivative and the red color produced is measured at 520 nm [37].

Fraga et al. demonstrated that a reduction of dietary intake of ascorbic acid from 250 mg/dL to 5 mg/dL reduced the level of ascorbic acid concentration in the seminal plasma [37]. Furthermore, seminal ascorbic acid level was significantly lower in the patients with leukocytospermia compared to patients with normal semen parameters. A significantly greater percentage of men with abnormal DFI were observed in the patients with low levels of seminal ascorbic acid compared with those with normal or high levels of ascorbic acid (59% versus 33%, $p < 0.05$). Men with lower ascorbic acid levels were reported to have sperm DNA damage [37]. However, wide discrepancies in the results have been reported [37, 38]. Assessment of individual antioxidant, micronutrient or vitamin does not provide an overall picture of the seminal antioxidant status.

15.3 Tests to Detect Effect of Oxidative Stress on Sperm

Unlike the somatic cells, the lipid bilayer in the plasma membrane of the human spermatozoa is rich in polyunsaturated fatty acids making them highly susceptible to damage caused by excess ROS [39–41].

The breakdown of polyunsaturated fatty acids to form lipid peroxides is known as lipid peroxidation [42]. Lipid peroxides are unstable and decompose to form complex compounds such as 4-hydroxynonenal (4-HNE), acrolein (ACR) and malondialdehyde (MDA) which freely react and modify lipids, proteins and DNA as they are relatively more stable than free radicals. They act as cytotoxic second messengers of oxidative stress causing alterations in the sperm functions [43, 44]. Measurement of the end products of lipid peroxidation is a widely accepted marker of oxidative stress. Some of the common methods to measure lipid peroxidation and oxidative stress are described below.

15.3.1 Measurement of 4-Hydroxynonenal Histidine (HNE-His) Adduct

15.3.1.1 Principle

Highly reactive aldehyde 4-hydroxynonenal (HNE)-protein adducts can be quantified using ELISA with a monoclonal antibody that rapidly detects the HNE-histidine adducts [45].

15.3.1.2 Methodology

Hydroxynonenal modified BSA (HNE-BSA) standards are prepared. Fatty acid free BSA (without HNE) is diluted in PBS (10 mg/mL). One mM of HNE is added to fatty acid free BSA to give 250 pmol/mg of ELISA with non-commercial antibody or 5000 pmol/mg of ELISA with commercial antibody. These stock solutions are incubated overnight at 4°C to allow binding of HNE to BSA and stored at -20°C.

The samples and standards are diluted in 0.05 M carbonate binding buffer (pH 9.6; 0.015 M sodium carbonate, 0.035 M sodium bicarbonate) and 100 mL of this mixture is placed in ELISA plate wells, kept overnight at 4°C for protein absorption and washed with 300 mL of PBS the following day. Freshly prepared blocking solution consisting of 5 percent fat free dry milk in carbonate is added to these wells and incubated for 2.5 hours at 37°C and washed with 0.1 percent Tween 20 in PBS.

Primary antibody solution (1 percent BSA in PBS; 1:100 for non-commercial; 1:500 for commercial antibody) is incubated for two hours at 37°C and then washed. The plate is then incubated with peroxidase blocking solution containing 3 percent H_2O_2 in PBS for 30 minutes at room temperature and washed again. One hundred mL of the secondary antibody solution (1 percent BSA in PBS) is added to the wells and incubated for one hour at 37°C and washed. The wells are then treated with 0.05 mg/mL of freshly prepared substrate solution for 30 minutes at 37°C followed by 50 mL of stopping solution (2 M sulfuric acid) [45].

15.3.1.3 Clinical Interpretation

Predetermined HNE-BSA standard curves are used to compare the results. The absorbance of each well is read on a microplate reader against a primary wavelength of 450 nm. Results are expressed as pmol/mg.

15.3.1.4 Clinical Significance

4-HNE may impair sperm capacitation by targeting the protein kinase A affecting the tyrosine phosphorylation pathway and thus reducing sperm motility [46].

15.3.2 Measurement of Isoprostanes

F2-isoprostanes (F2-IsoP) is a reliable marker of oxidative stress. Isoprostanes are a series of prostaglandin F2-like compounds formed by peroxidation of arachidonic acid that are bound with phospholipids and are independent of the cyclooxygenase pathway. 8-iso-PGF2α is the most represented isomer for F2-IsoP measurement [47].

15.3.2.1 Methodology

Isoprostanes can be determined by quantification of the amount of F2-IsoP present in the semen which is the sum of free and esterified isoprostanes or 8-iso-PGF2α localization in sperm.

For F2-IsoP determination, samples are incubated in 500 μL/mL of aqueous 1M KOH for 45 minutes at 45°C and 500 μL/mL of 1 M HCl is added to adjust the pH to 3. For an internal standard, 500 pg of derivative of PGF2α (PGF2α-d4) is added to the sample. The sample is then applied to an octadecylsilane (C18) and an aminopropyl (NH2) cartridge to extract the isoprostanes. The carboxylic and hydroxyl groups of F2-IsoP (sum of free and esterified isoprostanes) is derived as pentafluorobenzyl and trimethylsilyl ethers respectively. The F2-IsoP is determined using gas chromatography or negative ion chemical ionization tandem mass spectrometry analysis. The measured ions are derived from precursor ions produced from the 8-iso-PGF2α and PGF2α-d4 [48, 49].

For immunocytochemical staining with polyclonal 8-iso-PGF2α antibody, samples are washed in PBS and air dried on a glass slide and rinsed in PBS again. The sample is treated with methanol for 15 minutes at −20°C to fix the cells. It is further treated with blocking solution containing 1 percent BSA and 5 percent normal goat serum in PBS for 20 minutes at 37°C. The mixture is incubated with monoclonal anti-β-tubulin antibody overnight at 4°C. The following day, the sample is washed thrice and then treated with goat anti mouse IgG antibody. Finally, the samples are mounted on a slide and a cover slip is placed and observed under fluorescence microscope [50].

15.3.2.2 Interpretation

For F2-IsoP determination, 8-isoprostane (IsoP) levels are expressed as ng/mL. For immunocytochemical analysis, a total of 500 sperm are counted in each sample. The signal is absent in normal sperm but shows green fluorescence in sperm with oxidative damage of the lipid membrane.

15.3.2.3 Clinical Significance

Seminal plasma levels free 8-iso-PGF2α are shown to be significantly higher in infertile compared with normozoospermic men [51]. In addition, it has a significant negative correlation with MDA and seminal SOD activity in normozoospermic men [52]. Immunofluorescence analysis shows labeling of mid-piece and tail in as high as 65 percent of sperm in infertile men compared to almost none in fertile men [53].

15.3.3 Thiobarbituric Acid-Reactive Substances Assay

This assay is an indicator of lipid peroxide breakdown products wherein thiobarbituric acid (TBA) reacts with aldehydes mainly derived from peroxides and unsaturated fatty acids. Malondialdehyde (MDA), a reactive and mutagenic end product of lipid peroxidation in semen, is measured using this method [42].

15.3.3.1 Principle

In this assay, MDA (an aldehyde) binds with two molecules of TBA to form the MDA-TBA adduct which is measured colorimetrically or fluorometrically.

15.3.3.2 Methodology

Semen sample is centrifuged and then 100 µL of supernatant containing seminal plasma is diluted with distilled water (1:9) to which 500 µL of TBA reagent containing 0.67 g of TBA in 100 mL of distilled water with 0.5 g NaOH for alkaline denaturation and 100 mL glacial acetic acid is added. This mixture is boiled for one hour at 90–100°C. The samples are quickly cooled in ice and centrifuged for 10 minutes at $4000 \times g$. The supernatant is left for 20 minutes at 37°C [54]. This is loaded onto a microtiter plate and read at wavelength between 530–550 nm [55].

15.3.3.3 Interpretation

The adduct formation is measured either calorimetrically at 530–540 nm or fluorometrically at an excitation and emission wavelength of 530 nm and 550 nm respectively. Lipid peroxidation in sperm is expressed as nmol MDA/10^7 sperm.

15.3.3.4 Clinical Significance

MDA assessed using this assay negatively correlates with semen parameters such as sperm count, motility and morphology [56]. In addition, MDA levels are significantly higher in infertile compared to fertile men [57].

15.3.4 Tests to Detect Abnormal Sperm DNA Integrity

Oxidative stress is one of the major factors responsible for DNA fragmentation [58]. Furthermore, apoptosis as a result of oxidative stress can also explain the generation of DNA fragmentation [59]. Sperm DNA integrity may be compromised due to advanced age, cigarette smoking, chemotherapy, radiation, cancer, varicocele, leukocytospermia and elevated levels of ROS [60, 61]. Studies show that infertile men have high amounts of impaired DNA integrity [62, 63]. Reduced fertility, embryo development, and increased rates of miscarriages have been reported in cases of higher sperm DNA damage [64].

Several tests have been introduced to measure the sperm DNA damage involving different methodological approaches and principles. Currently, several assays are available to assess sperm DNA damage. Some tests measure the maturity and integrity of sperm chromatin (acridine orange, toluidine blue and chromamycin A3 staining), while others measure DNA fragmentation (sperm chromatin structure assay (SCSA); terminal deoxynucleotidyl transferase dUTP nick-end labeling (TUNEL); sperm chromatin dispersion (SCD) or halo sperm test and single-cell gel electrophoresis (Comet) and 8-hydroxy-2-deoxyguanosine (8-OHdG). Of these, SCA, TUNEL, SCD or halo sperm test and Comet are the commonly used tests of sperm DNA fragmentation with well-established and standardized protocols described in the literature. A cross-sectional survey across 19 countries by Majzoub et al. showed that 30.6 percent of SDF measurements are done using TUNEL and SCSA, while 20.4 percent and 6.1 percent are done using sperm chromatin dispersion (SCD) and single-cell gel electrophoresis (Comet), respectively [65]. The details of each of the DNA tests are described in other chapters. A brief description of each test is illustrated in Table 15.1.

15.3.4.1 Clinical Significance of Sperm DNA Fragmentation Tests

The oocyte has the ability to repair sperm DNA damage. Although a sperm with damaged DNA can fertilize an egg, it can result in compromised embryonic growth, miscarriage, or childhood deformities [78–82]. Higher SDF has been shown in men with varicocele compared to fertile men [83]. In a study by Esteves et al. using SCD test, varicocele was identified with 94 percent accuracy based on the rates of degraded sperm determined by the proportion of degraded sperm in the population of spermatozoa with fragmented DNA which was 8-fold higher in men with varicocele than in donors [84]. Following varicocele repair SDF was significantly reduced post-operatively and higher pregnancy rates through natural conception with ART were reported [85]. SDF is also increased in the presence of oxidative stress in these men [86–88]. Other reasons for testing DNA fragmentation are unexplained infertility, failed intrauterine inseminations, recurrent pregnancy loss, in vitro fertilization and intracytoplasmic sperm injection failure, and cancer patients undergoing chemotherapy or

Table 15.1 Common Tests of Sperm DNA Fragmentation

Test	Principle	Method	Result	Cut-off values	Advantage	Disadvantage	Reference
SCSA	Measures the susceptibility of sperm DNA to denaturation.	Acid denaturation, followed by staining by AO. Measurement by flow cytometry.	Normal DNA fluoresces green. Denatured DNA fluoresces orange-red. Result presented as DNA fragmentation index (% DFI) and high DNA stain ability (% HDS).	30% 27%	Reliable estimate of the percentage of DNA damaged sperm. Standardized protocol available. Rapid evaluation of large number of spermatozoa. Correlations with results of other SDF assays. Established clinical thresholds Can be performed on fresh or frozen samples.	Indirect assay involving acid denaturation. Proprietary protocol with no commercial assay. Requires expensive instrument and highly skilled technicians.	[66–68]
TUNEL	Quantifies the enzymatic incorporation of dUTP into DNA breaks as percentage of fluorescent sperm.	Labeled nucleotides are added to the site of DNA fragmentation. Fluorescence is measured by flow cytometry or fluorescence microscopy.	Sperm with fragmented DNA show fluorescence. Result presented as percentage of fluorescent sperm.	36.5% 36% 35% 15%	Direct assay can be performed in fresh or frozen samples. Can be performed on few sperm. Detects both single- and double-strand DNA breaks. Commercial assay available. Reliable estimate of the DNA damaged sperm with minimal interobserver variability	Requires standardization between laboratories. Time-consuming Immature spermatozoa are not evaluated. Variable clinical thresholds reported in the literature.	[69–72]

Table 15.1 (cont.)

Test	Principle	Method	Result	Cut-off values	Advantage	Disadvantage	Reference
SCD or Halo test	Assess dispersion of DNA fragments after denaturation.	Agarose-embedded sperm are subjected to a denaturing solution to remove nuclear proteins. Uses bright field or fluorescent microscopy to observe chromatin dispersion after staining.	Sperm with fragmented DNA do not produce halo. Characteristic halo of dispersed DNA loops are observed in sperm with non-fragmented DNA. Result presented as percentage of sperm with non-dispersed chromatin.	35% 30%	Relatively simple test.	Indirect assay involving acid denaturation. Inter-observer variability. Time-consuming and labor intensive. Inter-observer variability.	[73–75]
Comet	Electrophoretic assessment of DNA fragments of lysed DNA.	Gel electrophoresis performed in alkaline or neutral conditions.	Size of comet tail represents the amount of DNA fragments that stream out of the sperm head. Result presented as mean amount of DNA damage per spermatozoon.	56% 45.6% 44%	Direct assay can be performed on few sperm. Detect multiple types of DNA damage of individual spermatozoon Result correlates well with other SDF assays.	Requires fresh sample. Inter-observer variability. Time consuming. Requires experienced observer.	[76–77]

SCSA: sperm chromatin structure assay; AO: acridine orange; DFI: DNA fragmentation index; HDS: high DNA stainability; SDF: sperm DNA fragmentation; TUNEL: terminal deoxynucleotidyl transferase-mediated deoxyuridine triphosphate-nick end labeling; dUTP: deoxyuridine triphosphate.

radiotherapy [89]. SDF was higher in couples experiencing recurrent pregnancy loss compared to fertile controls (18.8 percent ± 7.0 percent versus 12.8 percent ± 5.3 percent; p<0.9001) [90].

15.3.5 Measurement of Reactive Oxygen Species-Induced Post-Translational Modifications

Post-translational modifications (PTMs) not only confer structural changes in the proteome of the spermatozoa cells, but they also increase the diversity of the proteome and introduce specific modifications that could be translated into functional changes in the affected spermatozoa [91].

A diverse range of PTMs takes place in the developing spermatozoa, of these ROS result in the most common types of PTMs namely, S-glutathionylation (GSS-R), nitrotyrosine modifications (Nitro-Y) and carbonylation [92–94]. Protein modifications by ROS result in altered functions such as activation or inhibition of transcription factors, signal transducers and enzymes [84, 92], thus altering the protein structural and functional integrity.

S-glutathionylation of proteins occurs by the addition of glutathione (GSH) to cysteine residues of certain target proteins under normal conditions as well as under conditions of oxidative stress. The disulfide linkage between the glutathione and the protein is reversible. This modification affects the functions of proteins, enzymes and receptors, thus altering normal cell biology [95].

Nitrotyrosine is formed by the reaction of peroxynitrite or donors of NO• with tyrosine residues [95]. In the sperm cell, the reaction of superoxide and NO• produce nitrotyrosine [96]. The nitrotyrosine protein modification can result in alteration of protein function or structure [97], however low amounts in the spermatozoon are essential for sperm to undergo capacitation [96].

Reactive carbonyls are produced by direct oxidative reaction of specific amino acids namely proline, arginine, lysine and threonine with low- or high-molecular weight dicarbonyls generated during lipid peroxidation and glycoxidation, causing modification of these amino acids to aldehyde or ketone and their eventual cleavage [98, 99].

ELISA is a widely used assay to detect and measure a particular protein using specific antibodies to immobilize proteins in microplate wells. Enzymes are chemically linked with the common antibodies. Such enzyme activities produce a measurable signal when combined with solutions containing appropriate substances [100, 101]. The end-product is a stable color that can be measured colorimetrically or fluorometrically using fluorophore-labeled antibodies particularly in multiplex arrays.

15.3.5.1 Clinical Significance

High amounts of nitrotyrosine were found in patients with impaired motility (asthenozoospermia) or spermatic duct cord blood in varicocele patients [96, 102]. Oxidation products such as protein carbonyls are useful for detection and in estimation of ROS levels in a semen sample [99]. Protein carbonyls are chemically stable, more reliable and frequently used as a marker for protein oxidation [103].

15.3.6 Measurement of Reactive Oxygen Species-Induced Protein Alterations: Proteomic Analysis

Global change occurs in proteomic profile of human spermatozoa and seminal plasma under oxidative stress conditions. Proteomics and bioinformatics tools can be utilized to understand alterations in proteins as a result of exposure of spermatozoa to reactive oxygen species or oxidative stress [104, 105]. Protein alterations present both in the spermatozoa and seminal plasma vary at different levels of ROS or OS which influence fertilization and implantation in infertile men [106–108]. Exposure of seminal proteome to different ranges of ROS (0–<93 RLU/sec/× 10^6 sperm, >93–500 RLU/sec/10^6 sperm and >500 RLU/sec/10^6 representing low, medium and high levels respectively) has shown that proteins involved in biomolecule metabolism, protein folding and protein degradation are differentially modulated in infertile patients compared to fertile controls. In the sperm proteome, differentially expressed proteins (DEPs) with distinct reproductive functions have been demonstrated only in men within these ROS levels [108]. Post-translational modification of proteins, protein folding (heat shock proteins, molecular chaperones) are overexpressed in the seminal plasma

133

proteome with high levels of ROS compared with the fertile control group [107].

The most commonly employed techniques to understand sperm specific proteins include 2D polyacrylamide gel electrophoresis (2D-PAGE), differential in gel electrophoresis (DIGE) and Liquid Chromatography-Mass Spectrometry or LC-MS/MS. Global proteomic analysis involves analysis of pooled or individual test samples (either spermatozoa or seminal plasma from infertile men with OS in semen) [94, 108, 109].

15.3.6.1 Validation of Proteins

Proteins that are modified by ROS and identified by proteomic and bioinformatic analysis can be validated as a potential biomarker of ROS in spermatozoa or seminal plasma. They can be validated by Western blot analysis using protein-specific antibodies or ELISA followed by Immunochemistry [110].

15.3.6.1.1 Western Blot Analysis

Western blot analysis is commonly used in quantification of proteins and in identification of a target protein. In this technique, gel electrophoresis is used to separate proteins on the basis of their 3-D structure or by the length of the polypeptide. The gel produces a band for each protein when transferred onto a PVDF membrane. After washing and blocking, it is incubated with primary antibodies specific to the protein of interest and then with a secondary antibody. The unbound antibodies are rinsed off and the bound antibodies are detected by chemiluminescence. Proteins are quantified by comparing it to a standard protein [109–111].

15.3.6.1.2 Enzyme-Linked Immunosorbent Assay

The protein of interest can also be validated by enzyme-linked immunosorbent assay (ELISA). The protein antigen is immobilized and coated onto the surface of the microplate wells. The unsaturated surface binding sites are then covered by adding blocking antibodies. Antibodies specific to the protein antigens are then added and incubated. The primary or secondary tag present on the specific antibody generates a signal when the antibody binds to the antigen. The quantification of the protein is done by measuring this signal [100, 112].

15.3.6.1.3 Immunochemistry

The antigen expression can be localized using immunocytochemistry. This is based on the principle of interactions between the epitope and the antibody. Using a molecular tag, which can be fluorescent or chromogenic, the positive staining patterns are visualized. Briefly, a concentration of 10×10^6 sperm aliquot is initially centrifuged for five minutes at 500 g. It is then fixed in 2 percent paraformaldehyde for 15 minutes. The fixed cells are then washed in 0.1 M PBS.

The cells are then resuspended in 0.1 M glycine/PBS, and they are then transferred to poly-L-lysine coated coverslips. Triton X-100-PBS (0.2 percent) permeabilization of the sperm at room temperature for 10 minutes, followed by rinsing in PBS. Nonspecific antibodies are blocked by combining 3 percent BSA solution containing 900 mg PBS, 30 mg BSA and 100 μL goat serum for 30 minutes. The cells are rinsed again in PBS and treated with the primary antibody of interest, diluted overnight in a humidified chamber in PBS at 4°C. The cells are washed in PBS and treated with the secondary antibody in PBS for one hour at 37°C. Next the cells are placed on frosted slides and a 530 nm fluorescent microscope captures images and positive staining patterns are identified [111]. The protein(s) are localized in the acrosome, mid-piece, or tail region of the spermatozoa [110, 113]. Similarly, fluorescent images can also be captured by confocal microscopy [110].

Finally, the indirect tests used to measure OS, their advantages, disadvantages and limitations are summarized in Table 15.2.

15.4 Conclusion

Oxidative stress is involved in the pathology of male infertility and results in sperm dysfunction. Effects of OS on sperm function have been extensively studied utilizing various tests to measure OS or OS-mediated sperm damage. However, most assays are complex and cumbersome making the introduction of many of these tests in clinical practice very challenging. There is an urgent need for laboratory tests that are novel, simple, have the ability to measure OS, and provide a comprehensive picture of oxidative status in the infertile male.

Table 15.2 Advantages, Limitations and Reference Value for Infertile Men Using Indirect Tests to Assess Oxidative Stress

Test	Advantages	Limitations	Reference value	References
Granulocyte elastase enzyme immunoassay	Objective, reliable and convenient gold standard	Complex, time consuming and high cost Immunoreactive PMN-elastase content in semen decreases at a constant rate when kept at 37°C.	A PMN-elastase level of > 1000 ng/mL	[11–14]
Myeloperoxidase (Endtz) test	Rapid, easy to perform and inexpensive Recommended by WHO to assess leukocytospermia	Peroxidase-positive leukocytes (PMNs and macrophages) account for 50–60% and 20–30% respectively of all seminal leukocytes. Cannot detect the ROS generation by spermatozoa	$> 1 \times 10^6$ peroxidase positive WBC/mL of semen (leukocytospermia)	[10, 15–20]
Pro-inflammatory cytokines and other immune factors	Commercially available ELISA kits	Costly, requires large sample size, expensive equipment (ELISA plate reader) Discrepant results due to complicated interplay of cytokines that have an inhibitory or synergistic effect on each other	NA	[21–25]
Antioxidants (total antioxidant capacity)	Measures all antioxidants in seminal plasma Automated	Requires expensive assay kit and microplate reader	≥ 1950 µM Trolox equivalents	[28]
FRAP Assay	Sample pretreatment is not required Reproducible and high sensitivity	Does not satisfactorily measure activity of important antioxidants – albumin, ascorbic acid and glutathione		[29]
ORAC assay	Considered biologically relevant as most antioxidants are oxidized by the peroxyl radical	Not sensitive for less reactive ROS		[30]
Individual antioxidants, micronutrients and vitamins	Cofactor of essential enzymatic reactions of ROS Commercially available assay kits	Costly and time consuming Does not provide an overall assessment of the antioxidant activity	NA	[32-38]
Lipid peroxidation				
HNE-His adduct ELISA	Rapid	Cross reactivity	NA	[45, 46]

Table 15.2 (cont.)

Test	Advantages	Limitations	Reference value	References
Measurement of isoprostanes	Isoprostanes – stable compounds, not produced by enzymatic (cyclooxygenase and lipoxygenase) pathways of arachidonic acid	Expensive instrumentation Labor intensive	NA	[47–53]
Thiobarbituric acid assay TBA (TBARS)	Simple Measures lipid peroxidation Detects MDA-TBA adduct by colorimetry or fluoroscopy	Expensive instrumentation Rigorous controls required Non-specific for MDA	NA	[42, 54, 55]
DNA fragmentation	Robust and sensitive method Multiple methods available – TUNEL, SCSA, Comet and SCD	Inter and intra-observervariability Lack of standardized reference value	Multiple cut-offs	[66–77]
Post-translational modifications	Commercially available assay kits	Costly and time consuming Does not provide an overall assessment of the OS	NA	[95–103]
Protein alterations	Highly specific and sensitive	Costly and time consuming	Sperm protein alterations specific to male infertility conditions identified	[104–113]

PMN: polymorphonuclear; WHO: World Health Organization; ELISA: enzyme linked immunosorbent assay; FRAP: ferric reducing antioxidant power assay; ORAC: oxygen radical absorbance assay; HNE-HIS: 4-hydroxynonenal histidine; TBA: thiobarbituric acid; TBARS: thiobarbituric acid reducing substances; TUNEL: terminal deoxynucleotidyl transferase-mediated deoxyuridine triphosphate-nick end labeling; SCSA: sperm chromatin structure assay; SCD: sperm chromatin dispersion; OS: oxidative stress; NA: not available

References

1. Agarwal A, Durairajanayagam D, Halabi J, Peng J, Vazquez-Levin M. Proteomics, oxidative stress and male infertility. *Reprod Biomed Online* 2014; **29**(1): 32–58.

2. Agarwal A, Gupta S, Sikka S. The role of free radicals and antioxidants in reproduction. *Curr Opin Gynecol Obstet* 2006; **18**(3): 325–32.

3. Aitken J, Fisher H. Reactive oxygen species generation and human spermatozoa: the balance of benefit and risk. *Bioessays* 1994; **16**(4): 259–67.

4. Tremellen K. Oxidative stress and male infertility—a clinical perspective. *Hum Reprod Update* 2008; **14**(3): 243–58.

5. Sharma RK, Agarwal A. Role of reactive oxygen species in male infertility. *Urology* 1996; **48**(6): 835–50.

6. Shekarriz M, Sharma R, Thomas A, Agarwal A. Positive myeloperoxidase staining (Endtz test) as an indicator of excessive reactive oxygen species formation in semen. *JAssist Reprod Gen* 1995; **12**(2): 70–4.

7. Plante M, de Lamirande E, Gagnon C. Reactive oxygen species released by activated neutrophils, but not by deficient spermatozoa, are sufficient to affect normal sperm motility. *Fertil Steril* 1994; **62**(2): 387–93.

8. Calogero AE, Duca Y, Condorelli RA, La Vignera S. Male accessory gland inflammation, infertility, and sexual dysfunctions: a practical approach to diagnosis and therapy. *Andrology* 2017; **5**(6): 1064–72.

9. Agarwal A, Saleh RA, Bedaiwy MA. Role of reactive oxygen species in the pathophysiology of human reproduction. *Fertil Steril* 2003; **79**(4): 829–43.

10. World Health Organization (2010). *WHO Laboratory Manual for the Examination and Processing of Human Semen*. Geneva: The WHO Press.

11. Kopa Z, Wenzel J, Papp GK, Haidl G. Role of granulocyte elastase and interleukin-6 in the diagnosis of male genital tract inflammation. *Andrologia* 2005; **37**(5): 188–94.

12. Jochum M, Pabst W, Schill WB. Granulocyte elastase as a sensitive diagnostic parameter of silent male genital tract inflammation. *Andrologia* 1986; **18**(4): 413–19.

13. Politch JA, Wolff H, Hill JA, Anderson DJ. Comparison of methods to enumerate white blood cells in semen. *Fertil Steril* 1993; **60**(2): 372–5.

14. Neumann S, Gunzer G, Hennrich N, Lang H. "PMN-elastase assay": enzyme immunoassay for human polymorphonuclear elastase complexed with α1-proteinase inhibitor. *J Clin Chem Clin Biochem* 1984; **22**(10): 693–8.

15. Endtz A. A rapid staining method for differentiating granulocytes from "germinal cells" in Papanicolaou-stained semen. *Acta Cytol* 1974; **18**(1): 2.

16. Agarwal A, Gupta S, Sharma R. Leukocytospermia quantitation (ENDTZ) test. In A. Agarwal et al., eds., *Andrological Evaluation of Male Infertility*. Geneva: Springer International Publishing, pp. 69–72.

17. Alvarez JG, Sharma RK, Ollero M, Saleh RA, Lopez MC, Thomas Jr AJ, Agarwal A. Increased DNA damage in sperm from leukocytospermic semen samples as determined by the sperm chromatin structure assay. *Fertil Steril* 2002; **78**(2): 319–29.

18. Aziz N, Saleh RA, Sharma RK, Lewis-Jones I, Esfandiari N, Thomas Jr AJ, Agarwal A. Novel association between sperm reactive oxygen species production, sperm morphological defects, and the sperm deformity index. *Fertil Steril* 2004; **81**(2): 349–54.

19. Moskovtsev SI, Willis J, White J, Mullen JBM. Leukocytospermia: relationship to sperm deoxyribonucleic acid integrity in patients evaluated for male factor infertility. *Fertil Steril* 2007; **88**(3): 737–40.

20. Moubasher A, Sayed H, Mosaad E, Mahmoud A, Farag F, Taha EA. Impact of leukocytospermia on sperm dynamic motility parameters, DNA and chromosomal integrity. *Cent European J Urol* 2018; **71**(4): 470–5.

21. Politch JA, Tucker L, Bowman FP, Anderson DJ. Concentrations and significance of cytokines and other immunologic factors in semen of healthy fertile men. *Hum Reprod* 2007; **22**(11): 2928–35.

22. Agarwal A, Virk G, Ong C, Du Plessis SS. Effect of oxidative stress on male reproduction. *World J Mens Health* 2014; **32**(1): 1–17.

23. Camejo M, Segnini A, Proverbio F. Interleukin-6 (IL-6) in seminal plasma of infertile men, and lipid peroxidation of their sperm. *Arch Androl* 2001; **47**(2): 97–101.

24. Martínez P, Proverbio F, Camejo MI. Sperm lipid peroxidation and pro-inflammatory cytokines. *Asian J Androl* 2007; **9**(1): 102–7.

25. Fraczek M, Sanocka D, Kamieniczna M, Kurpisz M. Proinflammatory cytokines as an intermediate factor enhancing lipid sperm membrane peroxidation in in vitro conditions. *J Androl* 2008; **29**(1): 85–92.

26. Mahfouz R, Sharma R, Sharma D, Sabanegh E, Agarwal A. Diagnostic value of the total antioxidant capacity (TAC) in human seminal plasma. *Fertil Steril* 2009; **91**(3): 805–11.

27. Henkel R, Sandhu IS, Agarwal A. The excessive use of antioxidant therapy: a possible cause of male infertility? *Andrologia* 2019; **51**(1): e13162.

28. Roychoudhury S, Sharma R, Sikka S, Agarwal A. Diagnostic application of total antioxidant capacity in seminal plasma to assess oxidative stress in male factor infertility. *J Assist Reprod Gen* 2016; **33**(5): 627–35.

29. Benzie IF, Strain JJ. The ferric reducing ability of plasma (FRAP) as a measure of "antioxidant power": the FRAP assay. *Anal Biochem* 1996; **239**(1): 70–6.

30. Cao G, Alessio HM, Cutler RG. Oxygen-radical absorbance capacity assay for antioxidants. *Free Radic Biol Med* 1993; **14**(3): 303–11.

31. Pasqualotto FF, Sharma RK, Pasqualotto EB, Agarwal A. Poor semen quality and ROS-TAC scores in patients with idiopathic infertility. *Urol Int* 2008; **81**(3): 263–70.

32. Fridovich I. Superoxide radical and superoxide dismutases. *Annu Rev Biochem* 1995; **64**(1): 97–112.

33. Olson KR, Gao Y, DeLeon ER, Arif M, Arif F, Arora N, Straub KD. Catalase as a sulfide-sulfur oxido-reductase: an ancient (and modern?) regulator of reactive sulfur species (RSS). *Redox Biol* 2017; **12**: 325–39.

34. Chance B, Sies H, Boveris A. Hydroperoxide metabolism in mammalian organs. *Physiol Rev* 1979; **59**(3): 527–605.

35. Crisol L, Matorras R, Aspichueta F, Expósito A, Hernández ML, Ruiz-Larrea MB, Ruiz-Larrea MB, Mendoza R. Glutathione peroxidase activity in seminal plasma and its relationship to classical sperm parameters and in vitro fertilization-intracytoplasmic sperm injection outcome. *Fertil Steril* 2012; **97**(4): 852–7.

36. Fraga CG, Motchnik PA, Shigenaga MK, Helbock HJ, Jacob RA, Ames BN. Ascorbic acid protects against endogenous oxidative DNA damage in human sperm. *PNAS* 1991; **88**(24): 11003–6.

37. Song GJ, Norkus EP, Lewis V. Relationship between seminal ascorbic acid and sperm DNA integrity in infertile men. *Int J Androl* 2006; **29**(6): 569–75.

38. Micheli L, Cerretani D, Collodel G, Menchiari A, Moltoni L, Fiaschi A, Moretti E. Evaluation of enzymatic and non-enzymatic antioxidants in seminal plasma of men with genitourinary infections, varicocele and idiopathic infertility. *Andrology* 2016; **4**(3): 456–64.

39. Poulos A, White I. The phospholipid composition of human spermatozoa and seminal plasma. *Reprod* 1973; **35**(2): 265–72.

40. Mack S, Everingham J, Zaneveld L. Isolation and partial characterization of the plasma membrane from human spermatozoa. *J Exp Zool* 1986; **240**(1): 127–36.

41. Alvarez JG, Storey BT. Differential incorporation of fatty acids into and peroxidative loss of fatty acids from phospholipids of human spermatozoa. *Mol Reprod Dev* 1995; **42**(3): 334–46.

42. Halliwell B, Chirico S. Lipid peroxidation: its mechanism, measurement, and significance. *Am J Clin Nutr* 1993; **57**(5): 715S–725S.

43. Zarkovic N. 4-Hydroxynonenal as a bioactive marker of pathophysiological processes. *Mol Aspects Med* 2003; **24**(4–5): 281–91.

44. Spickett CM. The lipid peroxidation product 4-hydroxy-2-nonenal: advances in chemistry and analysis. *Redox Biol* 2013; **1**(1): 145–52.

45. Borovic S, Rabuzin F, Waeg G, Zarkovic N. Enzyme-linked immunosorbent assay for 4-hydroxynonenal–histidine conjugates. *Free Radic Res* 2006; **40**(8): 809–20.

46. Baker MA, Weinberg A, Hetherington L, Villaverde A-I, Velkov T, Baell J, Gordon CP. Defining the mechanisms by which the reactive oxygen species by-product, 4-hydroxynonenal, affects human sperm cell function. *Biol Reprod* 2015; **92**(4): 101–10.

47. Delanty N, Reilly M, Pratico D, FitzGerald D, Lawson J, FitzGerald G. 8-Epi PGF2α: specific analysis of an isoeicosanoid as an index of oxidant stress in vivo. *Br J Clin Pharmacol* 1996; **42**(1): 15–19.

48. Signorini C, Comporti M, Giorgi G. Ion trap tandem mass spectrometric determination of F2-isoprostanes. *J Mass Spectrom* 2003; **38**(10): 1067–74.

49. Signorini C, Perrone S, Sgherri C, Ciccoli L, Buonocore G, Leoncini S, Rossi V, Vecchio D, Comporti M. Plasma esterified F 2-isoprostanes and oxidative stress in newborns: role of nonprotein-bound iron. *Ped Res* 2008; **63**(3): 287–91.

50. Moretti E, Pascarelli NA, Federico MG, Renieri T, Collodel G. Abnormal elongation of midpiece, absence of axoneme and outer dense fibers at principal piece level, supernumerary microtubules: a sperm defect of possible genetic origin? *Fertil Steril* 2008; **90**(4): 1201.e3–8.

51. Khosrowbeygi A, Zarghami N. Fatty acid composition of human spermatozoa and seminal plasma levels of oxidative stress biomarkers in subfertile males. *Prostaglandins Leukot Essent Fatty Acids* 2007; **77**(2): 117–21.

52. Tavilani H, Goodarzi MT, Doosti M, Vaisi-Raygani A, Hassanzadeh T, Salimi S, Joshaghani HR. Relationship between seminal antioxidant enzymes and the phospholipid and fatty acid composition of spermatozoa. *Reprod Biomed Online* 2008; **16**(5): 649–56.

53. Collodel G, Moretti E, Longini M, Pascarelli NA, Signorini C. Increased F2-isoprostane levels in semen and immunolocalization of the 8-iso prostaglandin F2α in spermatozoa from infertile patients with varicocele. *Oxid Med Cell Longev* 2018; 7508014.

54. Rao B, Soufir J, Martin M, David G. Lipid peroxidation in human spermatozoa as related to midpiece abnormalities and motility. *Gamete Res* 1989; **24**(2): 127–34.

55. Grotto D, Santa Maria L, Boeira S, Valentini J, Charão M, Moro A, Nascimento PC, Pomblum VJ, Garcia SC. Rapid quantification of malondialdehyde in plasma by high performance liquid chromatography – visible detection. *J Pharm Biomed Anal*, 2007; **43**(2): 619–24.

56. Colagar AH, Karimi F, Jorsaraei SGA. Correlation of sperm parameters with semen lipid peroxidation and total antioxidants levels in astheno-and oligoasheno-teratospermic men. *Iran Red Crescent Med J* 2013; **15**(9): 780–5.

57. Al-Dujaily SS, Hassan NA, Bilal SA, Salman SL. Malondialdehyde measurements in semen after in vitro sperm activation by pentoxifylline and Glycyrrhiza glabra extract. *Int J Biol Sci* 2013; **3**(4): 828–33.

58. Henkel R, Kierspel E, Stalf T, Mehnert C, Menkveld R, Tinneberg HR, Schill WB, Kruger TF. Effect of reactive oxygen species produced by spermatozoa and leukocytes on sperm functions in non-leukocytospermic patients. *Fertil Steril* 2005; **83**(3): 635–42.

59. Sakkas D, Mariethoz E, Manicardi G, Bizzaro D, Bianchi PG, Bianchi U. Origin of DNA damage in ejaculated human spermatozoa. *Rev Reprod* 1999; **4**(1): 31–7.

60. Zini A, Boman JM, Belzile E, Ciampi A. Sperm DNA damage is associated with an increased risk of pregnancy loss after IVF and ICSI: systematic review and meta-analysis. *Hum Reprod* 2008; **23**(12): 2663–8.

61. Agarwal A, Varghese AC, Sharma RK. (2009). Markers of oxidative stress and sperm chromatin integrity. In Park-Sarge OK, Curry T., eds., *Molecular Endocrinology. Methods in Molecular Biology (Methods and Protocols)*, vol. 590. Totowa, NJ: Humana Press, 377–402.

62. Ribas-Maynou J, García-Peiró A, Fernández-Encinas A, Abad C, Amengual M, Prada E, Navarro J, Benet J. Comprehensive analysis of sperm DNA fragmentation by five different assays: TUNEL assay, SCSA, SCD test and alkaline and neutral Comet assay. *Andrology* 2013; **1**(5): 715–22.

63. Garolla A, Cosci I, Bertoldo A, Sartini B, Boudjema E, Foresta C. DNA double strand breaks in human spermatozoa can be predictive for assisted reproductive outcome. *Reprod Biomed Online* 2015; **31**(1): 100–7.

64. Deng C, Li T, Xie Y, Guo Y, Yang QY, Liang X, Deng CH, Liu GH. Sperm DNA fragmentation index influences assisted reproductive technology outcome: a systematic review and meta-analysis combined with a retrospective cohort study. *Andrologia* 2019; **51**(6): e13263.

65. Majzoub A, Agarwal A, Cho CL, Esteves SC. Sperm DNA fragmentation testing: a cross sectional survey on current practices of fertility specialists. *Transl Androl Urol* 2017; 6(4): S710–S719.

66. Evenson DP, Larson KL, Jost LK. Sperm chromatin structure assay: its clinical use for detecting sperm DNA fragmentation in male infertility and comparisons with other techniques. *J Androl* 2002; **23**(1): 25–43.

67. Evenson DP. Sperm chromatin structure assay (SCSA): 30 years' experience with the SCSA. In Agarwal A, Zini A., eds., *Sperm DNA and Male Infertility and ART*. New York: Springer Publishers, pp. 125–49.

68. Evenson DP. The Sperm Chromatin Structure Assay (SCSA®) and other sperm DNA fragmentation tests for evaluation of sperm nuclear DNA integrity as related to fertility. *Anim Reprod Sci* 2016; **169**:56–75.

69. Sharma RK, Sabanegh E, Mahfouz R, Gupta S, Thiyagarajan A, Agarwal A. TUNEL as a test for sperm DNA damage in the evaluation of male infertility. *Urology* 2010; **76**(6): 1380–6.

70. Sharma R, Ahmad G, Esteves SC, Agarwal A. Terminal deoxynucleotidyl transferase dUTP nick end labeling (TUNEL) assay using bench top flow cytometer for evaluation of sperm DNA fragmentation in fertility laboratories: protocol, reference values, and quality control. *J Assist Reprod Genet* 2016; **33**(2): 291–300.

71. Ribeiro S, Sharma R, Gupta S, Cakar Z, De Geyter C, Agarwal A. Inter-and intra-laboratory standardization of TUNEL assay for assessment of sperm DNA fragmentation. *Andrology* 2017; **5**(3): 477–85.

72. Sharma R, Cakar Z, Agarwal A. (2018) TUNEL assay by benchtop flow cytometer in clinical laboratories. In Zini A, Agarwal A., eds., *A Clinician's Guide to Sperm DNA and Chromatin Damage*. New York: Springer, pp. 103–18.

73. Fernández JL, Muriel L, Goyanes V, Segrelles E, Gosálvez J, Enciso M, LaFromboise M, De Jonge C. Halosperm® is an easy, available, and cost-effective alternative for determining sperm DNA fragmentation. *Fertil Steril* 2005; **84**(4): 860.

74. Gosálvez J, Rodríguez-Predreira M, Mosquera A, López-Fernández C, Esteves SC, Agarwal A, Fernández JL. Characterisation of a subpopulation of sperm with massive nuclear damage, as recognised with the sperm chromatin dispersion test. *Andrologia* 2014; **46**(6): 602–9.

75. Feijó CM, Esteves SC. Diagnostic accuracy of sperm chromatin dispersion test to evaluate sperm deoxyribonucleic acid damage in men with unexplained infertility. *Fertil Steril* 2014; **101**(1): 58–63.

76. Cortes-Gutierrez EI, Davila-Rodriguez MI, Cerda-Flores RM, Fernández JL, López-Fernández C, Aragón Tovar AR, Gosálvez J. Localisation and quantification of alkali-labile sites in human spermatozoa by DNA breakage detection-fluorescence in situ hybridisation. *Andrologia* 2015; **47**(2): 221–7.

77. Cortés-Gutiérrez EI, Fernández JL, Dávila-Rodríguez MI, López-Fernández C, Gosálvez J. (2017). Two-tailed comet assay (2T-Comet): simultaneous detection of DNA single and double strand breaks. In Pellicciari C, Biggiogera M, eds., *Histochemistry of Single Molecules: Methods and Protocols*. New York: Springer Science +Business Media, pp. 285–93.

78. Ashwood-Smith M, Edwards R. DNA repair by oocytes. *Mol Hum Reprod* 1996; **2**(1): 46–51.

79. Meseguer M, Santiso R, Garrido N, García-Herrero S, Remohí J, Fernandez JL. Effect of sperm DNA fragmentation on pregnancy outcome depends on oocyte quality. *Fertil Steril* 2011; **95**(1): 124–8.

80. Cozzubbo T, Neri QV, Rosenwaks Z, Palermo GD. To what extent can oocytes repair sperm DNA fragmentation? *Fertil Steril* 2014; **102**(3): e61.

81. Lewis SEM. Should sperm DNA fragmentation testing be included in the male infertility work-up? *Reprod BioMed Online* 2015; **31**(2): 134–7.

82. Agarwal A, Cho C-L, Esteves SC, Majzoub A. Current limitation and future perspective of sperm

DNA fragmentation tests. *Transl Androl Urol* 2017; **6**(4): S549–S552.

83. Wang Y-J, Zhang R-Q, Lin Y-J, Zhang R-G, Zhang W-L. Relationship between varicocele and sperm DNA damage and the effect of varicocele repair: a meta-analysis. *Reprod BioMed Online* 2012; **25**(3): 307–14.

84. Esteves SC, Gosálvez J, López-Fernández C, Núñez-Calonge R, Caballero P, Agarwal A, Fernández JL. Diagnostic accuracy of sperm DNA degradation index (DDSi) as a potential noninvasive biomarker to identify men with varicocele-associated infertility. *Int Urol Nephrol* 2015; **47**(9): 1471–7.

85. Smit M, Romijn JC, Wildhagen MF, Veldhoven JL, Weber RF, Dohle GR. Decreased sperm DNA fragmentation after surgical varicocelectomy is associated with increased pregnancy rate. *J Urol* 2013; **189**(1): S146–S150.

86. Chen S-S, Huang WJ, Chang LS, Wei Y-H. Attenuation of oxidative stress after varicocelectomy in subfertile patients with varicocele. *J Urol* 2008; **179**(2): 639–42.

87. Agarwal A, Hamada A, Esteves SC. Insight into oxidative stress in varicocele-associated male infertility: part 1. *Nat Rev Urol* 2012; **9**: 678.

88. Blumer CG, Restelli AE, Giudice PTD, Soler TB, Fraietta R, Nichi M, Bertolla RP, Cedenho AP. Effect of varicocele on sperm function and semen oxidative stress. *Br J Urol Int* 2012; **109**(2): 259–65.

89. Agarwal A, Majzoub A, Esteves SC, Ko E, Ramasamy R, Zini A. Clinical utility of sperm DNA fragmentation testing: practice recommendations based on clinical scenarios. *Transl Androl Urol* 2016; **5**(6): 935–50.

90. Carlini T, Paoli D, Pelloni M, Faja F, Dal Lago A, Lombardo F, Lenzi A, Gandini L. Sperm DNA fragmentation in Italian couples with recurrent pregnancy loss. *Reprod BioMed Online* 2017; **34**(1): 58–65.

91. Brohi RD, Huo LJ. Posttranslational modifications in spermatozoa and effects on male fertility and sperm viability. *OMICS* 2017; **21**(5): 245–56.

92. Radi R. Nitric oxide, oxidants, and protein tyrosine nitration. *Pro Nat Acad Sci.* 2004; **101**(12): 4003–8.

93. Dalle-Donne I, Rossi R, Colombo R, Giustarini D, Milzani A. Biomarkers of oxidative damage in human disease. *Clin Chem* 2006; **52**(4): 601–23.

94. Samanta L, Swain N, Ayaz A, Venugopal V, Agarwal A. Post-translational modifications in sperm proteome: the chemistry of proteome diversifications in the pathophysiology of male factor infertility. *Biochem Biophys Acta* 2016; **1860**(7): 1450–65.

95. Halliwell B, Gutteridge J. (2007). Cellular responses to oxidative stress: adaptation, damage, repair, senescence and death. In Halliwell B, Gutteridge J, eds., *Free Radicals in Biology and Medicine*. New York: Oxford University Press, pp. 187–267.

96. Herrero MB, de Lamirande E, Gagnon C. Tyrosine nitration in human spermatozoa: a physiological function of peroxynitrite, the reaction product of nitric oxide and superoxide. *Mol Hum Reprod* 2001; **7**(10): 913–21.

97. Vignini A, Nanetti L, Buldreghini E, Moroni C, Ricciardo-Lamonica G, Mantero F, Boscaro M, Mazzanti L, Balercia G. The production of peroxynitrite by human spermatozoa may affect sperm motility through the formation of protein nitrotyrosine. *Fertil Steril* 2006; **85**(4): 947–53.

98. Bollineni RC, Fedorova M, Blüher M, Hoffmann R. Carbonylated plasma proteins as potential biomarkers of obesity induced type 2 diabetes mellitus. *J Proteome Res* 2014; **13**(11): 5081–93.

99. Dalle-Donne I, Giustarini D, Colombo R, Rossi R, Milzani A. Protein carbonylation in human diseases. *Trends Mol Med* 2003; **9**(4): 169–76.

100. Engvall E, Perlmann P. Enzyme-linked immunosorbent assay (ELISA). Quantitative assay of immunoglobulin G. *Immunochemistry* 1971; **8**(9): 871–4.

101. El-Taieb MA, Herwig R, Nada EA, Greilberger J, Marberger M. Oxidative stress and epididymal sperm transport, motility and morphological defects. *Eur J Obstet Gynecol Reprod Biol* 2009; **144**(1): S199–S203.

102. Romeo C, Ientile R, Impellizzeri P, Turiaco N, Teletta M, Antonuccio P, Basile M, Gentile C. Preliminary report on nitric oxide-mediated oxidative damage in adolescent varicocele. *Hum Reprod* 2003; **18**(1): 26–9.

103. Stadtman ER, Berlett BS. Fenton chemistry. *Amino acid oxidation*. *J Biol Chem* 1991; **266**(26): 17201–11.

104. Hamada A, Sharma R, du Plessis SS, Willard B, Yadav SP, Sabanegh E, Agarwal A. Two-dimensional differential in-gel electrophoresis-based proteomics of male gametes in relation to oxidative stress. *Fertil Steril* 2013; **99**(5): 1216–26.

105. Sharma R, Agarwal A, Mohanty G, Du Plessis SS, Gopalan B, Willard B, Yadav SP, Sabanegh E. Proteomic analysis of seminal fluid from men exhibiting oxidative stress. *Reprod Biol Endocrinol* 2013; **3**(11): 85.

106. Sharma R, Agarwal A, Mohanty G, Hamada AJ, Gopalan B, Willard B, Yadav S, du Plessis S. Proteomic analysis of human spermatozoa proteins with

oxidative stress. *Reprod Biol Endocrinol* 2013; **11**: 48.

107. Agarwal A, Ayaz A, Samanta L, Sharma R, Assidi M, Abuzenadah A M, Sabanegh E. Comparative proteomic network signatures in seminal plasma of infertile men as a function of reactive oxygen species. *Clin Proteomics* 2015; **12**(1): 23.

108. Ayaz A, Agarwal A, Sharma R, Arafa M, Elbardisi H, Cui Z. Impact of precise modulation of reactive oxygen species levels on spermatozoa proteins in infertile men. *Clin Proteomics* 2015; **12**(1): 4.

109. Agarwal A, Sharma R, Samanta L, Durairajanayagam D, Sabanegh E. Proteomic signatures of infertile men with clinical varicocele and their validation studies reveal mitochondrial dysfunction leading to infertility. *Asian J Androl* 2016; **18**(2): 282–91.

110. Samanta L, Agarwal A, Swain N, Sharma R, Gopalan B, Esteves SC, Durairajanayagam D, Sabanegh E. Proteomic signatures of sperm mitochondria in varicocele: clinical use as biomarkers of varicocele associated infertility. *J Urol* 2018; **200**(2): 414–22.

111. Mathews ST, Kim T. Imaging systems for westerns: chemiluminescence vs. infrared detection. *Methods Mol Biol* 2009; **536**: 499–513.

112. Nakane PK, Pierce GB Jr. Enzyme-labeled antibodies for the light and electron microscopic localization of tissue antigens. *J Cell Biol* 1967; **33**(2): 307–18.

113. Salvolini E, Buldreghini E, Lucarini G, Vignini A, Lenzi A, Di Primio R, Balercia G. Involvement of sperm plasma membrane and cytoskeletal proteins in human male infertility. *Fertil Steril* 2013; **99**(3): 697–704.

Chromatin Condensation: Aniline Blue *Stain*

Jesse JP, Vidhu Dhawan, Rima Dada

16.1 Introduction

Spermatozoa, one of the two most pivotal cells of biological existence, are responsible for mediating the transfer of genetic information to subsequent generations. Mammalian fertilization and subsequent embryonic development depend in part on the inherent integrity of sperm genome. Different fertility societies around the globe and the World Health Organization (WHO) estimate that infertility is present in between 7 and 15 percent of couples of reproductive age [1].

The current diagnosis of male infertility is based upon semen analysis, which encompasses the traditional semen parameters, semen volume and sperm concentration, motility and morphology as a gold standard. However, it has become apparent that none of these parameters recommended by the World Health Organization (WHO) is sufficient for the prediction of male fertility capacity. As the WHO parameters only address a few aspects of sperm quality and function, the discriminative power in relation to fertility is quite low [2, 3]. Although there is a direct relationship between semen quality and pregnancy rates, both in spontaneous and assisted conceptions, there is still no definite predictive threshold for success for conventional semen parameters. Conventional semen analysis does not assess all aspects of testicular function and sperm quality. New tests for predicting the chance of pregnancy would be clinically useful. Over the past two decades, sperm DNA testing has been hailed as a more promising method for fertility evaluation [4, 5, 6]. There have been attempts to propose sperm DNA fragmentation as such a new test for male reproductive capability [6, 7].

Sperm cells are remarkably complex and highly specialized cells as compared to somatic cells. Their function is to deliver the paternal genomic blueprint and a highly specialized epigenome along with a pool of proteins and coding and non-coding RNAs to the oocyte. Reproductive success, including optimal embryonic development and healthy offspring, greatly depends on the integrity of the sperm chromatin structure, its genome and epigenome. It is now well documented that DNA damage in sperm is linked to reproductive failures both in natural and assisted conception [8, 9] and is a major cause of defective sperm function and couples opting for assisted conception. Sperm DNA damage is also the underlying etiology of idiopathic recurrent pregnancy losses, idiopathic recurrent congenital malformations and even childhood cancers [10, 11]. The association between DNA damage and diminished reproductive outcomes has led to the introduction of sperm DNA integrity testing into the clinical assessment of male infertility.

There is a growing understanding about the importance of sperm DNA integrity on embryo development and the health of the offspring. Therefore, the purpose of this book chapter is to understand the structure of mammalian sperm chromatin and its impact on the rapidly advancing postgenomic era.

This essay will also evaluate the molecular techniques used for study of sperm DNA fragmentation with a detailed overview of the Aniline Blue staining method.

16.2 Sperm Nuclear Chromatin

The function of sperm is to safely transport the haploid paternal genome to the egg containing the maternal genome. Before the sperm can set out on its adventurous journey, remarkable arrangements need to be made during the post-meiotic stages of spermatogenesis [12]. Spermatogenesis, a continuous and highly conserved process, leads to the formation of haploid sperm cells capable of fertilization. It has been characteristically divided into three critical phases: a) mitotic amplification phase causing proliferation of spermatogonia; b) meiotic phase, where spermatogonia develop into primary and secondary spermatocytes; and c) post-meiotic phase which is also known as spermiogenesis where spermatids differentiate into spermatozoa. The developing germ cells in the post-meiotic phase are further subdivided into early spermatids with round nuclei, intermediate spermatids with elongated nuclei, and spermatids with condensed nuclei [13]. The essential hallmark of spermiogenesis is the replacement of nuclear somatic-cell like histones by small basic proteins known as protamines. This facilitates the condensation/compaction of sperm nucleus and consequently the sperm head. This condensation of the paternal genome in the human spermatozoa is specific to the sperm cell in order to protect the DNA during the transit from the male to the oocyte prior to fertilization [14]. The nuclear proteins found in the sperm form a distinct chromatin structure that is unlike any other cell type and is perfectly suited to support the male gamete [14, 15].

Spermatogenesis is also marked by a shutdown of transcriptional machinery at a defined point of germ cell differentiation [10, 11, 15, 16, 17, 18, 19]. Thus, the resulting translational repression, and storage of long-lived mRNAs, for example those which encode protamines necessary for completion of spermiogenesis and others which are necessary for fertilization and early embryonic development. Mammalian sperm chromatin can be divided into three major structural domains: (1) the vast majority of sperm DNA is coiled into toroids by protamines, (2) a much smaller percent remains bound to histones [20], and (3) the DNA is attached to the sperm nuclear matrix at MARs (matrix attachment regions) at medium intervals of roughly 50 kb throughout the genome [14].

16.2.1 Histones to Protamines: An Overview

Haploid spermatids undergo extensive morphological changes, including a striking reorganization and compaction of their chromatin [12]. Thereby, the nucleosomal histone-based structure is nearly completely substituted by a protamine-based structure. Protamines are the most abundant nuclear proteins found in sperm and are unique to sperm cells. These proteins have a strong positive charge due to their high arginine content, which helps facilitate

their function [11, 17, 18, 19]. The high arginine content facilitates strong DNA binding, while the cysteines in protamines promote the formation of inter- and intra-protamine disulphide bonds during the process of compaction [12, 21]. The vast majority of the sperm chromatin is thus compacted into toroids containing roughly 50 kb of DNA [14]. During the process of spermatogenesis, protamines replace 85–95 percent of histones in the sperm, including both canonical histones and testicular histone variants, via a stepwise process. First, transition proteins, comprising both transition proteins 1 and 2 (T1 and T2), replace histone proteins that are DNA bound. Second, T1 and T2 are replaced by protamine proteins; protamine 1 and protamine 2 (P1 and P2). The ratio of P1:P2 is approximately 1:1 in most fertile humans [17].

After the incorporation of protamines into the paternal chromatin, cysteine residues between protamine molecules form intermolecular disulfide bridges as the cell matures. The strong positive charge of P1 and P2 as well as the formation of disulfide bridges produces a tightly condensed chromatin structure [15, 22]. The compaction of the sperm DNA into a nucleoprotamine complex results in approximately 6–20 times denser structure than the nucleosome-bound chromatin seen in somatic cells [15, 17, 20]. This condensation aids in two important roles: a) sperm motility relies chiefly on condensed nuclear structure as a decondensed sperm head may mechanically inhibit or perturb the cell's potential for motility [23], b) prevents the sperm from impending DNA damage resulting from transit through the male and female reproductive tracts and exposure to oxidative stress due to genital tract inflammation, varicocele, and testicular hyperthermia prior to fertilization, as sperm lacks DNA repair mechanisms [17]. The replacement of histones during spermatogenesis is an incomplete process, as approximately 5–15 percent of the genome remain bound by nucleosomes and is not condensed into a nucleoprotamine complex [22]. This retention of nucleosomes in the peripheral compartment of the sperm genome includes telomeres and genes regulating early embryonic development. The nucleohistone compartment is vulnerable to oxidative stress and also facilitates the maintainance of genomic imprints [11, 20]. The replacement of histones is likely facilitated by incorporation of histone variants, post-translational histone modifications, chromatin-remodeling complexes, as well as transient DNA strand breaks.

16.2.2 Resiliences and Vulnerabilities

Sperm DNA damage has been documented as one of the major factors for defective sperm function. DNA damage includes DNA denaturation and sperm DNA fragmentation (SDF) and may be the common underlying etiology of infertility, recurrent pregnancy loss, pre- and post-implantation losses, accelerated aging, and childhood carcinomas [11, 24]. Oxidative stress is one of the leading causes of DNA damage and this can be determined by quantifying the levels of oxidative DNA adducts like 8-OHdG, a base which induces both mutations and epimutations. Sperm nuclear DNA fragmentation has been positively correlated with lower fertilization rates in IVF, impaired implantation rates, an increased incidence of abortion and disease in offspring, including childhood cancer. Abnormalities in chromatin condensation can cause nuclear damage as DNA denaturation or fragmentation are often associated with male infertility [25].

16.3 Sperm Chromatin Assessment

There has been an increase in the use of sperm DNA and chromatin integrity tests in the evaluation of the infertile man with the hypothesis that these tests may better diagnose infertility and predict reproductive outcomes. The evaluation of sperm chromatin and DNA structure was initially undertaken to improve our understanding of spermatogenesis, sperm physiology, sensitivity to reproductive toxicants and reproductive biology.

It has been suggested that protamine deficiency (with consequent aberrant chromatin remodeling), reactive oxygen species and abortive apoptosis may be responsible for sperm DNA damage [26, 27].

16.4 Various Techniques for Sperm Chromatin Assessment

There are two types of assays that have been developed to measure sperm DNA integrity: a) those that can directly measure the extent of DNA fragmentation through the use of probes and dyes and b) those that measure the susceptibility of DNA to denaturation, which occurs more commonly in fragmented DNA. Various methods to assess sperm DNA fragmentation are briefly described below and summarized in Table 16.1. The most commonly used tests are terminal deoxynucleotidyltransferase UTP nick end labeling (TUNEL), the sperm chromatin dispersion test (SCD), and the sperm chromatin structure assay (SCSA®).

16.5 Aniline Blue Staining

Aniline blue (AB) staining is a histochemical technique that depends on the use of dyes. AB is an acidic dye that has a great affinity for lysine-rich histones in the nucleus of immature sperm, which stain blue.

16.5.1 Background

The chromatin of mature spermatozoa possesses a varying binding capacity for nuclear dyes and stains. The sperm nuclear condensation or maturation can be assessed by the AB test. AB, an acidic dye, has a greater permeability/affinity for proteins in the loose chromatin of the sperm nucleus. This is due to the presence of the residual histones and increased accessibility of the basic groups of the nucleoprotein. Increased AB staining of sperm indicates loose chromatin packing.

Abundant lysine is present in the histone-rich nuclei of immature spermatozoa, which takes up the AB stain, whereas arginine and cysteine present in protamine-rich spermatozoa of mature spermatozoa remain unstained [6, 25, 28, 29]. Thus, this test differentiates between the lysine-rich histones from the arginine- and cysteine-rich protamines. Detection of extra lysine-rich histones indicates lower amounts of protamines in the sperm nucleus and immature chromatin condensation [21, 30]. Infertile males with lower protamine levels show lower sperm counts, motility and abnormal morphology and a higher predisposition to DNA damage [6, 21, 24]. The procedure for the acidic AB staining has been summarized in Figure 16.1 and is based on the protocol previously explained [31].

16.5.2 Methodology

Fresh semen sample obtained by masturbation in a clear sterile room close to the laboratory is left at room temperature for liquefaction and processed for the acidic AB staining (Figure 16.1).

Table 16.1 Sperm chromatin assessment methods

S.NO.	TEST	PRINCIPLE	MEASUREMET/ DETECTION	MERITS	DEMERITS
1.	**AO Test**	Detects metachromatic shift in fluorescence of AO, uses fluorescence microscopy	Single-stranded DNA breaks	Biologically stable measure of sperm quality Technique highly reproducible	Expensive instrumentation Observer subjectivity hinders the result if fluorescent microscopy used
2.	**TB Staining**	Increased affinity of TB to sperm DNA phosphate residues, uses optical microscopy	Single- and Double-stranded DNA breaks	Simple and inexpensive Permanent preparations for use under ordinary microscope Morphological assessment of cells done	Limited number of cells can be reasonably scored Limits of repeatabilit
3.	**CMA3 Staining**	Competitively binds to DNA, uses fluorescent microscopy	Indirectly assesses protamine deficient DNA	Reliable Sensitivity 73%, specificity 75% Strong correlation with other assays	Inter-observer variability
4.	**TUNEL Assay**	Direct assay, done by optical microscopy and fluorescent microscopy	Direct quantification of enzymatic incorporation of dUTP into single- and double-stranded DNA breaks	Sensitive, reliable Intraobserver variability <8%, Interobserver variability <7%	Sophisticated and expensive Requires standarization between different laboratories
5.	**Comet Assay**	Direct assay, electrophoretic assessment of DNA fragments. Done by optical or fluorescent microscopy	Double-stranded DNA breaks	Simple to perform, low performance cost. Well standarized assay Low intra assay coefficient of variation	Requires experienced observer to analyse and interpretation of results
6.	**ISNT**	Direct assay, template-dependent DNA polymerase I, Requires fluorescent microscope	Single-stranded DNA breaks, Incorporates biotinylated dUTP with template-dependent DNA polymerase I	Reaction based on direct labelling of terminal DNA breaks Defects identifiable at molecular level	Less sensitive

Table 16.1 *(cont.)*

S.NO.	TEST	PRINCIPLE	MEASUREMET/ DETECTION	MERITS	DEMERITS
7.	SCSA	Indirect assay based on flow cytometry, Intercalation of acridine orange dye	Susceptibility of sperm DNA to acid induced conformational transition in situ.	Accurately assess percentage of sperm DNA damage Also gives the percentage of high density staining sperm indicative of immature chromatin	Requires expensive instrumentation and skilled technicians.
8.	SCD/ Halo test	Indirect assay, based on the characteristic halo produced by the sperm after denaturation (not produced by sperm with fragmented DNA)	Sperm DNA fragmentation (single stranded DNA fragments)	Simple, fast and reproducible Doesn't require the determination of color or fluorescence	Inter-observer variability
9.	Nuclear protein composition	Indirect assay, protein extraction, and immunoblotting with specific antibodies	Protamine-to-histone ratio	Specific, sensitive,	Requires experienced person to conduct and interpret the results
10.	Sperm nuclear maturity test	Indirect assay, slide based quantification	Sperm DNA integrity Protamine composition	Simple and inexpensive	Inter-observer variability

1) Acridine Orange (AO) Test- Green fluorescence (normal DNA), red fluorescence (denatured DNA), 2) Toluidine Blue (TB) staining- Light blue (normal sperm), violet (sperm with DNA fragmentation), 3) Chromomycin A3 (CMA3)- Bright yellow (protamine deficient sperm), yellowish green (normal protamine content), 4) Terminal deoxynucleotidyl transferase dUTP nick end labeling (TUNEL)- fluorescent activated cell sorting histogram, 5) Comet- migration of fragmented DNA appreciate as tail, intact DNA remains as head, 6) In situ nick translation (ISNT)- measures the number of fluorescent sperm which incorporate dUTP, 7) Sperm chromatin structure assay (SCSA)- AO staining assessed by flow cytometry, measures metachromatic shift of AO fluorescence from green to red, 8) Sperm chromatin dispersion (SCD)- assesses sperm with different DNA dispersion, assesses large, medium or small sized halo.

The sperm cells on the slides are evaluated under bright field microscopy. Sperm heads containing immature nuclear chromatin stain blue, and those with mature nuclei do not take up the stain. This is a simple and inexpensive technique requiring a simple bright field microscope for analysis. The results of AB staining have shown good correlation with those of the Acridine Orange test, but the drawback with the AB staining is heterogenous slide staining [32, 33].

Results of acidic AB staining demonstrate a clear association between abnormal sperm chromatin and male infertility [34, 35]. However, the correlation between the percentage of AB-stained spermatozoa and other sperm parameters remains controversial [35, 36]. AB-positive staining indicates the presence of histones while AB staining negativity indicates the presence of normal chromatin maturity [37].

The adoption of sperm function tests to predict the success rate of IUI was assessed by Irez et al. [37]. They established a cut-off of 24 percent for AB negativity with ROC analysis for prediction of pregnancy, with a sensitivity and a specificity value of 82.35 percent and 51.38 percent (AUC) = 0.653; 95 percent confidence interval: 0.571–0.72 (P value (Area = 0.5) = 0.0267) [37]. The cut-off value for good quality sperm chromatin was stated as 87.2 percent for chromatin maturity assessed by AB staining and 80.2

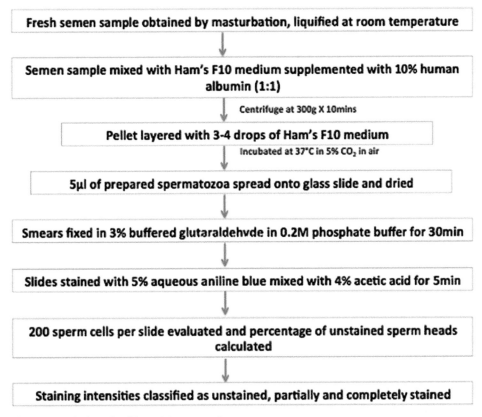

Figure 16.1 Acidic aniline blue staining protocol.

percent for chromatin integrity (toluidine blue staining) in fertile normozoospermic donors [38].

16.6 Implications of Chromatin Condensation: From Benchtop to Clinical Outcomes

The basic semen analysis routinely being done often has left couples with previously failed attempts at fertilization and reproductive outcomes to face daily clinical dilemmas. The limited predictive value for pregnancy in couples trying to achieve natural conception and in couples undergoing advanced assisted reproductive technologies (ART) warrants the adoption of assessment of paternal factors. The assessment of sperm chromatin integrity can be adopted as a reliable indicator of a couple's potential to conceive and is advised in conjunction with routine semen analysis. Though sperm DNA damage does not correlate with fertilization rate, it is associated with

slower cleavage, poor blastocyst morphology and a tendency to develop triploid zygotes [24]. Sperm chromatin and DNA integrity tests have also been studied in the context of ART in order to assess their ability to predict pregnancy outcome because conventional sperm parameters are poor predictors of ART outcomes [7, 39, 40].

Previously studies have been conducted to assess whether AB staining can be employed for male fertility testing and can be included as an indicator to predict pregnancy outcomes. Spermatozoa with increased histone remnants and protamine deficiency results in premature chromatin condensation leading to fertilization failure and impaired embryonic development [25, 41]. Fertilization rate was seen to be significantly higher following intra-cytoplasmic sperm injection (ICSI) in patient groups which were found to have less than 10 percent abnormal chromatin using AB staining [42, 43]. No correlation between AB positive cells and fertilization rate following ICSI was found by [44].

147

Sellami et el. [25] found significant correlation between chromatin maturity assessed by AB staining and sperm head abnormalities but no correlation was found between sperm motility, count and vitality. Increase in sperm head anomalies have also been associated with an increase in AB positive tests [44, 46]. Negative correlation was found between sperm count, progressive motility and morphology by other investigators [35, 47].

This highlights the need for more extended sperm functional testing. Paternal contribution to the fertilization and to the development of healthy offspring is of vital importance.

16.7 Concluding Remarks

The unique chromatin-packing process of the spermatozoon has important implications for both the development of male infertility screening tests and understanding of sperm chromatin characteristics, which may affect ART outcomes. Sperm deoxyribonucleic acid (DNA) integrity tests have been proposed as a means to assess male gamete competence. Although these assays are currently gaining popularity, and are more often used as a supplement to traditional semen analysis, the point at which DNA damage occurs during spermiogenesis, and to what degree, remains to be elucidated [48].

References

1. Louis JF, Thoma ME, Sørensen DN, McLain AC, King RB, Sundaram R, Keiding N, Buck Louis GM. The prevalence of couple infertility in the United States from a male perspective: evidence from a nationally representative sample. *Andrology* 2013; **1**: 741–8.

2. Bungum M. Sperm DNA integrity assessment: a new tool in diagnosis and management of male infertility. *Obstet Gynecol Int* 2012; **2012**: 531042.

3. Cissen M, Wely MV, Scholten I, Mansell S, de Bruin JP, Mol BW, Bratt D, Repping S, Hamer G. Measuring sperm DNA fragmentation and clinical outcomes of medically assisted reproduction: a systematic review and meta-analysis. *PLOS One* 2016; **11**(11): e0165125.

4. Aitken RJ, de Iuliis GN, McLachlan RI. Biological and clinical significance of DNA damage in the male germ line. *Int J Androl* 2008; **32**: 46–56.

5. Barratt CL, Aitken RJ, Bjorndahl L, Carrell DT, de Boer P, Kvist U, Lewis SE, Perreault SD, Perry MJ, Ramos L, Robaire B, Ward S, Zini A. Sperm DNA: organization, protection and vulnerability: from basic science to clinical applications–a position report.

Hum Reprod 2010; **25**: 824–38.

6. Shamsi MB, Inam SN, Dada R. Sperm DNA integrity assays: diagnostic and prognostic challenges and implications in management of infertility. *J Assist Reprod Genet* 2011; **28**: 1073–85.

7. Lewis SE, Agbaje I, Alvarez J. Sperm DNA tests as useful adjuncts to semen analysis. *Syst Biol Reprod Med* 2008; **54**(3): 111–25.

8. Aitken RJ, De Iuliis GN. On the possible origins of DNA damage in human spermatozoa. *Mol Hum Reprod* 2010; **16**: 3–13.

9. Champroux A, Torres-Carreira J, Gharagozloo P, Drevet JR, Kocer A. Mammalian sperm nuclear organization: resiliences and vulnerabilities. *Basic Clin Androl* 2016; **26**: 17.

10. Dhawan V, Kumar M, Dada R. Effect of sperm molecular factors, oxidative damage and transcripts in childhood disorders. *J Child Dev Disord* 2017; **3**(1): 6.

11. Dhawan V, Kumar M, Deka D, Malhotra N, Singh N, Dadhwal V, Dada R. Paternal factors and embryonic development: role in recurrent pregnancy loss. *Andrologia* 2018; **51**(1): e13171.

12. Rathke C, Baarends WM, Awe S, Renkawitz-Pohl R. Chromatin

dynamics during spermiogenesis. *Biochem Biophys Acta* 2014; **1839**: 155–68.

13. Dadoune JP. Expression of mammalian spermatozoal nucleoproteins. *Microsc Res Tech* 2003; **61**: 56–75.

14. Ward WS. Function of sperm chromatin structural elements in fertilization and development. *Mol Hum Reprod* 2010; **16**: 30–6.

15. Miller D, Brinkworth M, Iles D. Paternal DNA packaging in spermatozoa: more than the sum of its parts? DNA, histones, protamines and epigenetics. *Reproduction* 2010; **139**: 287–301.

16. Krawetz SA. Paternal contribution: new insights and future challenges. *Nat Rev Genet* 2005; **6**: 633–42.

17. Jenkins TG, Carrell DT. The sperm epigenome and potential implications for the developing embryo. *Reproduction* 2012; **143**(6): 727–34.

18. Kumar M, Kumar K, Jain S, Hassan T, Dada R. Novel insights into genetic and epigenetic paternal contribution to the human embryo. *Clinics* 2013; **68**(S1): 5–14.

19. Kumar M, Dhawan V, Kranthi V, Dada R. Paternal factors: role in idiopathic recurrent pregnancy

losses. *Int J Reprod Fertil Sex Health S2*; **001**: 1–6.

20. Hammoud SS, Nix DA, Zhang H, Purwar J, Carrell DT, Cairns BR. Distinctive chromatin in human sperm packages genes for embryo development. *Nature* 2009; **460**(7254): 473–8.

21. Carrell DT, Emery BR, Hammoud S. Altered protamine expression and diminished spermatogenesis: what is the link? *Hum Reprod Update* 2007; **13**: 313–27.

22. Wykes SM, Krawetz SA. The structural organization of sperm chromatin. *J Biol Chem* 2003; **278**: 29471–7.

23. Carrell DT, Hammoud S. The human sperm epigenome and its potential role in embryonic development. *Mol Hum Reprod* 2010; **16**(1): 37–47.

24. Dada R. Sperm DNA damage diagnostics: when and why? *Transl Androl Urol* 2017; **6**(Suppl. 4): S691–4

25. Sellami A, Chakroun N, Zarrouk BS, Sellami H, Kebaili S, Rebai T, Keskes L. Assessment of chromatin maturity in human spermatozoa: useful aniline blue assay for routine diagnosis of male infertility. *Adv Urol* 2013; **2013**: 1–8.

26. Sakkas D, Mariethoz E, St. John JC. Abnormal sperm parameters in humans are indicative of an abortive apoptotic mechanism linked to the Fas-mediated pathway. *Exp Cell Res* 1999; **251**: 350–5.

27. Aitken RJ, De Iuliis GN. Origins and consequences of DNA damage in male germ cells. *Reprod Biomed Online* 2007; **14**: 727–33.

28. Hammadeh M, Zeginiadov T, Rosenbaum P. Predictive value of sperm chromatin condensation (aniline blue staining) in the assessment of male fertility. *Arch Androl* 2001; **46**: 99–104.

29. Agarwal A, Said MT. (2004) *Sperm Chromatin Assessment*. Abingdon: Taylor and Francis, pp. 93–103.

30. Aoki VW, Moskovtsev SI, Willis J, Liu L, Mullen JB, Carrell DT. DNA integrity is compromised in protamine-deficient human sperm. *J Androl* 2005; **26**: 741–8.

31. Hammadeh ME, Hasani SA, Stieber M, Rosenbaum P, Kupker D, Diedrich K, Schmidt W. The effect of chromatin condensation (Aniline Blue staining) and morphology (strict criteria) of human spermatozoa on fertilization, cleavage and pregnancy rates in an intracytoplasmic sperm injection programme. *Hum Reprod* 1996; **11**: 2468–71.

32. Erenpreiss J, Bars J, Lipatnikova V, et al. Comparative study of cytochemical tests for sperm chromatin integrity. *J Androl* 2001; **22**: 45–53.

33. Agarwal A, Majzoub A, Esteves SC, Ko E, Ramasamy R, Zini A. Clinical utility of sperm DNA fragmentation testing: practice recommendations based on clinical scenarios. *Trans Androl Urol* 2016; **5**(6): 935–50.

34. Muratori M, Tamburrino L, Marchiani S, Cambi M, Olivito B, Azzari C, et al. Investigation on the origin of sperm DNA fragmentation: role of apoptosis, immaturity and oxidative stress. *Mol Med* 2015; **21**: 109–22.

35. Pourmasumi S, Khoradmehr A, Rahiminia T, Sabeti P, Talebi AR, Ghasemzadeh J. Evaluation of sperm chromatin integrity using Aniline Blue and Toluidine Blue staining in infertile and normozoospermic men. *J Reprod Infertil* 2019; **20**(2): 90–101.

36. Talebi AR, Sarcheshmeh AA, Khalili MA, Tabibnejad N. Effects of ethanol consumption on chromatin condensation and DNA integrity of epididymal spermatozoa in rat. *Alcohol* 2011; **45**(4): 403–9.

37. Irez T, Dayioglu N, Alagoz M, Karatas, Guralp O. The use of aniline blue chromatin condensation test on prediction of pregnancy in mild male factor and unexplained male infertility. *Andrologia* 2018; **50**(10): e13111.

38. Ahmad SA, Umar LA, Lestari SW, Mansyur E, Hestiantoro A, Paradowszka-Dogan A. Sperm chromatin maturity and integrity correlated to zygote development in ICSI program. *Syst Biol Reprod Med.* 2016; **62**(5): 309–16.

39. Simon L, Brunborg G, Stevenson M, Lutton D, McManus J, Lewis SE. Clinical significance of sperm DNA damage in assisted reproduction outcome. *Hum Reprod* 2010; **25**:1594–608.

40. Zini A. Are sperm chromatin and DNA defects relevant in the clinic? *Syst Biol Reprod Med* 2011; **57**: 78–85.

41. Lin MH, Lee RK, Li SH, Lu CH, Sun FJ, Hwu YM. Sperm chromatin structure assay parameters are not related to fertilization rates, embryo quality, and pregnancy rates in in vitro fertilization and intracytoplasmic sperm injection, but might be related to spontaneous abortion rates. *Fertil Steril* 2008; **90**(2): 352–9.

42. Esterhuizen AD, Franken DR, Lourens JGH, van Zyl C, Müller I, Van Rooyen LH. Chromatin packaging as an indicator of human sperm dysfunction. *J Assist Reprod Genet* 2000; **17**(9): 508–14.

43. Sadeghi MR, Hodjat M, Lakpour N et al. Effects of sperm chromatin integrity on fertilization rate and embryo quality following intracytoplasmic sperm injection. *Avicenna J Med Biotechnol* 2009; **1**(3): 173–80.

44. Razavi S, Nasr-Esfahani MH, Mardani M, Mafi A, Moghdam A. Effect of human sperm chromatin anomalies on fertilization outcome post-ICSI. *Andrologia* 2003; **35**(4): 238–43.

45. Abu DA, Franken DR, Hoffman B, Henkel R. Sequential analysis of sperm functional aspects involved in fertilization: a pilot study. *Andrologia* 2012; **44**(Suppl. 1): 175–81.

46. Jayaraman V, Upadhya D, Narayan PK, Adiga SK. Sperm processing by swim-up and density gradient is effective in elimination of sperm with DNA damage. *J Assist Reprod Genet* 2012; **29**(6): 557–63.

47. Kazerooni T, Asadi N, Jadid L, Kazerooni M, Ghanadi A, Ghaffarpasand F, et al. Evaluation of sperm's chromatin quality with acridine orange test, chromomycin A3 and aniline blue staining in couples with unexplained recurrent abortion. *J Assist Reprod Genet* 2009; **26**(11–12): 591–6.

48. Palermo GD, Neri QV, Cozzubbo T, Rosenwaks Z. Perspectives on the assessment of human sperm chromatin integrity. *Fertil Steril* 2014; **102**: 1508–17.

Chromatin Condensation: Chromomycin A3 (CMA3) Stain

Sara Marchiani, Lara Tamburrino, Francesca Benini, Sandra Pellegrini, Elisabetta Baldi

17.1 Introduction

In order to transport an intact and complete paternal genome to the oocyte, spermatozoa are characterized by an extremely compacted nuclear DNA as compared to the nucleus of somatic cells. Such packaging of the chromatin is obtained through a dramatic nuclear reorganization occurring in developing spermatids leading to an almost complete replacement of histones with protamines. During the epididymal transit, spermatozoa complete the process of chromatin packaging by formation of disulphide bridges in nucleoproteins [1]. This process of sperm maturation is critical for male fertility. Indeed, it has been demonstrated that alterations in chromatin structure could impact male fertility potential compromising both in vivo and in vitro fertilization and the subsequent embryo development [2, 3].

For this reason, in recent years, assays to evaluate the sperm chromatin status have gained increased value in order to find a possible marker useful in male infertility work-up. Among the several methods that have been proposed, staining with chromomycin A3 (CMA3, 4) is commonly used. This method gives an indication of the degree of sperm protamination. In a recent paper, it has been demonstrated that in an adjusted model for confounding factors including female age and female factors, the sperm chromatin status evaluated by CMA3 is able to predict the achievement of good quality embryos with 78 percent sensitivity and 65 percent specificity [5]. Although the possible use of CMA3 in clinical practice is still debated, it could represent a simple and promising tool to be added to routine semen analysis for evaluation of male reproductive health before infertility treatment.

17.2 Principle

Chromomycin A3 (CMA3, Figure 17.1) is an antibiotic glycoside produced by the fermentation of a certain strain of Streptomyces griseous. In the presence of bivalent metal ions, CMA3 binds reversibly to DNA, preferentially to contiguous G/C base pairs. As mentioned, the probe is used as a fluorescent DNA stain for detection of protamine deficiency in sperm chromatin, since it competes with protamines for binding to DNA minor grooves.

When bound to DNA, CMA3 has a maximum excitation wavelength of 445 nm and a maximum emission wavelength of 575 nm. Two types of staining patterns are identified with fluorescence microscopy: bright green fluorescence (reflecting abnormal chromatin packaging) and weak green staining (normal chromatin packaging) of the sperm head (Figure 17.2A).

17.3 Protocol

17.3.1 Equipment Needed

- Fluorescence microscope with filters able to match the spectral excitation and emission characteristics of the fluorophore, CMA3, (excitation wavelength of 445 nm and emission wavelength of 575 nm);
- Slides.

Figure 17.1 Chromomycin A3 chemical structure

A **B**

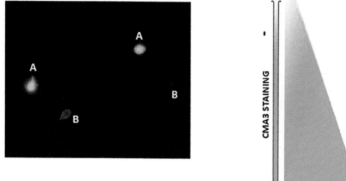

Figure 17.2 (A) Staining with CMA3 of human spermatozoa. Two patterns are identified at fluorescence microscopy: bright green fluorescence of sperm head (A, abnormal chromatin packaging) and weak green staining (B, normal chromatin packaging). (B) CMA3 staining and is an index of protamine content and, consequently a sign of sperm chromatin maturity.

17.3.2 Reagent Needed

- Chromomycin A3 (empirical formula: $C_{57}H_{82}O_{26}$; molecular weight: 1183.25);
- Medium for washing spermatozoa (human tubal fluid, etc.);
- Paraformaldehyde solution 4 percent in phosphate buffer;
- Phosphate buffered saline (PBS);
- Mc Ilvaine Buffer (0.2 M Na_2HPO_4 and 0.1 M citric acid, pH7.00) added with 10 mM $MgCl_2$;
- PBS/glycerol solution (1:1).

17.3.3 Sperm Preparation

The percentage of spermatozoa stained with CMA3 can be evaluated either in whole semen or selected (Swim up or PureSperm) spermatozoa after sperm separation.

Procedure:

- take 1×10^6 spermatozoa;
- in case of whole semen, wash spermatozoa twice in sperm culture medium (centrifuge at 500×g for five minutes, room temperature). In case of selected spermatozoa centrifuge once at 500×g for five minutes;
- remove supernatant and fix the pellet in 50 µL of 4 percent paraformaldehyde for 30 minutes at room temperature;

- take 20 µL of the sample and centrifuge at 300×g for seven minutes, room temperature;
- remove supernatant and wash once in PBS by centrifuging at 300×g for seven minutes, room temperature.

17.3.4 Incubation of Spermatozoa with CMA3 Solution

To prepare stock solution of CMA3 (0.5 mg/mL), 5 mg of CMA3 powder should be dissolved in 10 mL of Mc Ilvaine buffer added with 10 mM $MgCl_2$. Aliquots of CMA3 stock solution can be stored at −20°C.

At the time of use, dilute aliquots 1:1 in Mc Ilvaine buffer added with 10 mM $MgCl_2$ to obtain a final concentration of CMA3 of 0.25 mg/mL. Add 100 µL CMA3 solution (0.25 mg/mL) to sperm pellet (after washing and fixation in paraformaldehyde) and incubate for 20 minutes at room temperature. Then, add 200 µL Mc Ilvaine buffer added with 10 mM $MgCl_2$ and centrifuge at 300×g for seven minutes at room temperature, discard supernatant and re-suspend the pellet in 10 µL Mc Ilvaine buffer added with 10 mM $MgCl_2$.

17.3.5 Mounting of Slides

After staining and washing, make a spot on a slide, dry the slide on air, add a drop of PBS: glycerol and place a coverslip over.

17.3.6 Analysis by Fluorescence Microscopy

Spermatozoa exhibiting a bright green fluorescence in the head are scored as CMA3-positive. At least 200 spermatozoa from each sample should be scored and the percentage of CMA3-positive sperm calculated.

17.4 Reference Values/Laboratory and Clinical Interpretation

The percentage of spermatozoa which exhibits bright green fluorescence of the sperm head is reported as CMA3-positive and represents an index of the sperm protamination status. The higher the percentage of brightly stained spermatozoa, the lower the protamine content (Figure 17.2B).

Since this method has not been standardized yet, a universal reference value for CMA3 staining has not been established, even though this technique is used in numerous research laboratories. In our study [5], a cut-off value of 19.5 percent CMA3-positive sperm was able to predict the attainment of good embryo quality (AUC=0.778, CI 95 percent: 0.616–0.940, p=0.005). Moreover, by applying a logistic regression model including confounding factors such as female age, female factor and number of MII oocytes, we found that the probability of obtaining good quality embryos was higher when the CMA3-positivity was $\leq$19.5 percent (OR=6.6, CI 95 percent: 1.29–33.63, p=0.02).

17.5 Advantages/Disadvantages of the Test

17.5.1 Advantages

This test is simple and easy to perform, inexpensive, and does not require sophisticated instrumentation for its evaluation, enabling its use in virtually all clinical laboratories.

17.5.2 Disadvantages

This test may be affected by inter-observer variability since it is an operator-dependent assay. Moreover, the standardization of the method among laboratories remains a challenge.

17.6 Clinical Significance

Several studies investigating the association between sperm protamine content as determined by CMA3 staining, and both semen quality and assisted reproduction outcomes, have been published. Concerning the relationship with semen quality, all studies agree that poor protamination is associated with worse sperm parameters [6–8]. However, studies investigating assisted reproductive technologies (ART) outcomes and their association with the chromatin status evaluated by CMA3 do not allow us to draw firm conclusions, due to a high heterogeneity in couple selection, male and female factors, male and female age etc. Some studies report no association between CMA3-positivity and ART outcomes (fertilization, embryo quality, pregnancy and rate of miscarriage) [9–10], whereas others show that poor protamination negatively impacts fertilization rate and embryo quality [5, 11]. Overall, such data suggest that CMA3-staining could represent a promising tool to be added to routine semen analysis for the evaluation of male reproductive health before infertility treatment, but further large studies are required.

17.7 Ordering the Test

The test could be useful for couples with unexplained infertility when the male partner has normal semen parameters and the female partner does not present with signs of infertility (see clinical cases below). In addition, all couples undergoing ARTs could take advantage of this test because its value included in a statistical model including female age, female factor and number of oocytes in metaphase II could be predictive of obtaining good quality embryos, considered as a strong predictor of implantation and pregnancy [12].

17.8 Clinical Case Scenarios

Four clinical cases are reported, selected from our database [5]. In cases 1–3, the male partner showed CMA3 levels above and in case 4 below the cut-off value of 19.5 percent, which predicts the attainment of $\geq$50 percent embryos of high quality according to the following criteria: two-cell stage at 40/44 hours or four-cell stage at 44/48 hours or eight-cell stage at 66/72 hours; degree of fragmentation less than 10 percent; absence of any blastomere abnormalities.

17.8.1 Clinical Case 1

A couple with idiopathic infertility have been attempting to conceive for two years. The female partner was 30 years old and did not show detectable female factors. The male partner was 32 years old, normozoospermic (sperm concentration: 70 million/mL, progressive motility: 42 percent, normal morphology: 11 percent) and did not present with other detectable male factors. After ovarian stimulation, 11 oocytes were retrieved, of which five were mature (MII) and inseminated by IVF. Three out of the five oocytes were fertilized, but only one progressed to the embryo stage. Embryo quality was classified as C (embryos showing considerable deviation in the degree of fragmentation, symmetry and division pace). The embryo was transferred on day 5, no clinical pregnancy was obtained. CMA3-positivity, evaluated on selected spermatozoa after sperm separation used for insemination, was 29 percent.

17.8.2 Clinical Case 2

A couple with idiopathic infertility have been attempting to conceive for three years. The female partner was 34 years old and did not show detectable female factors. The male partner was 31 years old, normozoospermic (sperm concentration 22 million/mL, progressive motility: 45 percent, normal morphology: 6 percent) with first grade varicocele on left testis. After ovarian stimulation, 12 oocytes were retrieved, of which nine were mature (MII) and inseminated by ICSI. Seven out of the nine oocytes were fertilized, but only one progressed to embryo. Embryo quality was classified as C (embryos showing considerable deviation in the degree of fragmentation, symmetry and division pace). The embryo was transferred on day 5, no clinical pregnancy was obtained. CMA3-positivity, evaluated on selected spermatozoa used for insemination, was 35 percent.

17.8.3 Clinical Case 3

A couple with idiopathic infertility have been attempting to conceive for two years. The female partner was 32 years old and did not show any detectable female factors. The male partner was 38 years old, normozoospermic (sperm concentration 60 million/mL, progressive motility: 66 percent, normal morphology: 10 percent) with no detectable male

factors. After ovarian stimulation, 12 oocytes were retrieved of which seven were mature (MII) and inseminated by ICSI. Seven of the seven oocytes were fertilized, of which four progressed to embryo. Embryo quality were B, B/C (embryos showing slight deviation in the degree of fragmentation, symmetry and division pace) and C (embryos showing considerable deviation in the degree of fragmentation, symmetry and division pace). The three embryos were transferred on day 5, no clinical pregnancy was obtained. CMA3-positivity, evaluated on selected spermatozoa used for insemination, was 22 percent.

17.8.4 Clinical Case 4

A couple with idiopathic infertility have been attempting to conceive for two years. The female partner was 33 years old and did not show any detectable female factors. The male partner was 37 years old, normozoospermic (sperm concentration: 20 million/mL, progressive motility: 55 percent, normal morphology: 5 percent) and did not present with other detectable male factors. After ovarian stimulation, 14 oocytes were retrieved, of which 12 were mature (MII) and inseminated by IVF. Eleven of the twelve oocytes were fertilized and six progressed to embryo. Four embryos were classified as A quality (embryos showing the best properties) and two embryos as B quality (embryos showing slight deviation in the degree of fragmentation, symmetry and division pace). An embryo of A quality was transferred on day 5 and clinical pregnancy was achieved. CMA3-positivity, evaluated on selected spermatozoa used for insemination, was 9 percent.

The four reported clinical cases suggest that evaluation of CMA3 may be useful in the management of selected cases with infertile couples. Our previous study [5] and the clinical cases presented above, highlight a possible employment of the test in those couples with no identifiable factors. The test may be useful to predict the attainment of good quality embryo. Clearly, further studies are needed to establish the possible role of CMA3 evaluation as a diagnostic test in the work-up of male infertility.

References

1. Ward WS. Function of sperm chromatin structural elements in fertilization and development. *Mol Hum Reprod* 2010; **16**: 30–6.

2. Ni K, Spiess AN, Schuppe HC, Steger K. The impact of sperm protamine deficiency and sperm DNA damage on human male fertility: a systematic review and meta-analysis. *Andrology* 2016; **4**: 789–99.

3. Simon L, Castillo J, Oliva R, Lewis SE. Relationships between human sperm protamines, DNA damage

and assisted reproduction outcomes. *Reprod Biomed Online* 2011; **23**: 724–34.

4. Nijs M, Creemers E, Cox A, Franssen K, Janssen M, Vanheusden E, De Jonge C, Ombelet W. Chromomycin A3 staining, sperm chromatin structure assay and hyaluronic acid binding assay as predictors for assisted reproductive outcome. *Reprod Biomed Online* 2009; **19**: 671–84.

5. Marchiani S, Tamburrino L, Benini F, Fanfani L, Dolce R, Rastrelli G, Maggi M, Pellegrini S, Baldi E. Chromatin protamination and catsper expression in spermatozoa predict clinical outcomes after assisted reproduction programs. *Sci Rep* 2017; **7**: 15122.

6. Dehghanpour F, Fesahat F, Yazdinejad F, Motamedzadeh L, Talebi AR. Is there any relationship between human sperm parameters and protamine deficiency in different groups of infertile men? *Rev Int Androl* 2019; pii: S1698–031X(19)30039-1.

7. Manochantr S, Chiamchanya C, Sobhon P. Relationship between chromatin condensation, DNA integrity and quality of ejaculated spermatozoa from infertile men. *Andrologia* 2012; **44**: 187–99.

8. Kazerooni T, Asadi N, Jadid L, Kazerooni M, Ghanadi A, Ghaffarpasand F, Kazerooni Y, Zolghadr J. Evaluation of sperm's chromatin quality with acridine orange test, chromomycin A3 and aniline blue staining in couples with unexplained recurrent abortion. *J Assist Reprod Genet* 2009; **26**: 591–6.

9. Gill K, Rosiak A, Gaczarzewicz D, Jakubik J, Kurzawa R, Kazienko A, Rymaszewska A, Laszczynska M, Grochans E, Piasecka M. The effect of human sperm chromatin maturity on ICSI outcomes. *Hum Cell* 2018; **31**: 220–31.

10. Sadeghi MR, Lakpour N, Heidari-Vala H, Hodjat M, Amirjannati N, Hossaini Jadda H, Binaafar S, Akhondi MM. Relationship between sperm chromatin status and ICSI outcome in men with obstructive azoospermia and unexplained infertile normozoospermia. *Rom J Morphol Embryol* 2011; **52**: 645–51.

11. Iranpour FG. Impact of sperm chromatin evaluation on fertilization rate in intracytoplasmic sperm injection. *Adv Biomed Res* 2014; **3**: 229.

12. Cai QF, Wan F, Huang R, Zhang HW. Factors predicting the cumulative outcome of IVF/ICSI treatment: a multivariable analysis of 2450 patients. *Hum Reprod* 2011; **26**: 2532–40.

Chapter 18

Sperm Chromatin Structure: Toluidine Blue Staining

Mohammad Nasr-Esfahani, Marziyeh Tavalaee

18.1 Introduction

Gametogenesis is a central biological process for sexual reproduction. In this process, both haploid male and female gametes are needed for successful fertilization. Male gamete or sperm are produced during spermatogenesis; a complex, unique, and tightly regulated process, which includes a series of physiological, biochemical and morphological events. During this process, round diploid spermatogonia are differentiated into haploid spermatozoa with an acrosome, flagellum, and condensed nucleus. Condensation of nucleus or chromatin compaction play a paramount role in formation of morphology, especially the size of sperm. Therefore, during spermiogenesis, nucleo-histones are replaced by protamines. To achieve this aim, histones become hyper-acetylate to reduce their binding affinity to DNA. Subsequently, hyper-acetylated histones are replaced by transition proteins and next by protamines. According to the literature, in the human, 85–95 percent of the histones are replace with protamines while 5–15 percent of histones remain bounded to mature sperm DNA in humans [1, 2]. Therefore, through this process, sperm chromatin becomes six-fold more condensed than chromatin of other cells. This condensation will protect sperm chromatin from chemical and mechanical damages, bacterial infections, detrimental molecules such as oxidants, and also damaging molecules within the female reproductive system [2]. Alterations in the sperm histone/protamine ratio due to reduction of hyper-acetylation of histones or excessive histone retention are associated with abnormal chromatin packaging which can increase susceptibility to DNA damage, and eventually result in male infertility [1]. Therefore, normal chromatin packaging in the spermatogenesis process is essential for maintaining genomic integrity and accomplishment of fertility. In this regard, numerous studies have shown that there is a significant positive

correlation between proper sperm chromatin condensation with clinical outcomes of infertile couples being candidates for assisted reproductive technology (ART) [3]. In addition, a significant positive association has been reported between sperm abnormal chromatin packaging with recurrent pregnancy loss [4]. Therefore, numerous studies suggested that the evaluation of "sperm chromatin condensation" may have a prognostic value in the assessment of male infertility. For this aim, several analytical methods based on cyto-chemical or fluorescent dyes have been proposed for the assessment of sperm nuclear compaction such as acidic aniline blue (for direct detection of excessive presence of histones), toluidine blue staining and chromomycin A3 (for indirect assessment of protamine deficiency), sperm chromatin structure assay (SCSA) or acridin orange test (for indirect assessment of sperm chromatin DNA stability based on chromatin compaction termed "high DNA stability structure"). Toluidine blue (TB) staining is one of the procedures used for evaluation of chromatin structure. Therefore, this chapter, provides detailed practical advice on TB staining, optimization, and interpretation of results in the field of medically assisted reproduction.

18.1.1 Sperm Chromatin Structure

The entire human genome is two meters in length when it is disassociated from histones. In somatic cells, this genome, with aid of nucleo-histones, is packaged into a micrometer-size nucleus. In mature sperm, DNA is compacted in a volume of less than 10 percent of a somatic cell nucleus. This degree of compaction is achieved through replacement of histones with protamines. Protamines are small proteins rich in cysteine and arginine. They induce chromatin compaction by neutralizing the negative charges of the phosphate groups of DNA backbone. Then, the chromatin structure is stabilized by –S-S- bridges formed between and within the protamines during passaging sperm through the epididymis [1, 2]. It is noticeable that sperm chromatin packaging in all species is not similar and the type of protamine (P1 or P2) and their ratio may vary between species. For example, in ram, bull and bear, only P1 plays an important role in chromatin compaction, while in the human and mice both, P1 and P2 are present [5]. In addition, a small percentage of histones, which varies depending on the species, remains in connection with DNA; approximately 5–15 percent in the human, while in other species such as mice, bulls, stallions and hamsters, this value is around 5 percent [5].

Several studies have envisaged important functional roles for the retained histones, including: maintenance of paternally imprinted genes, early embryonic developmental events, regulation of transcription factors (like HOX gene family) and, microRNA clusters. Organization of sperm chromatin is based on three main domains; 1) protamine-bound DNA, the majority of sperm DNA is packaged with protamines in a toroid structure, 2) histone-associated DNA, a small portion of DNA, is bound to histones, and 3) matrix attachment regions, remaining DNA is connected to nuclear matrix regions. Protamine-bound DNA regions not only provide chromatin compaction, but also protect the DNA structure against chemical and mechanical damages, control gene expression through silencing of gene expression during spermatogenesis, and improve the hydrodynamic structure of sperm which can facilitate sperm reaching and penetrating the oocyte [5].

Toluidine blue is a basic nuclear dye that can be used to distinguish quality and the quantity of sperm DNA fragmentation and nuclear chromatin condensation through binding to DNA-phosphate groups. Therefore, in case of high DNA damage, this dye can also bind to free phosphate groups of DNA and to some degree may reveal the integrity of chromatin structure [6–7].

18.1.2 Chemical Properties of Toluidine Blue Dye

Toluidine or tolonium chloride dye is a member of the thiazine group and was discovered by William Henry Perkin in 1856. This metachromatic dye selectively stains acidic components such as sulfates, carboxylates, and phosphate in cells or tissues. Therefore, it has a high affinity for nucleic acids in DNA and RNA content and appears as blue, while upon binding to polysaccharides it appears as purple. Several applications in medicine and industry have been envisaged for toluidine blue and the most important of these applications is vital staining for mucosal lesions, and as a metachromatic dye for assessment of chromatin integrity [6]. This dye is soluble in both water and alcohol.

18.1.3 Principle of Toluidine Blue Dye in Identifying Sperm Chromatin

The toluidine blue staining procedure is performed at pH 4.0. At this condition, cationic dye molecules can bind to negatively charged ionized phosphates, but not to other possible unionized anions binding sites. Based on this feature, if sperm DNA is highly and tightly compacted, toluidine cannot bind to DNA and therefore sperm will appear from green to light blue. Contrary, in sperm with loosely compacted or unpacked DNA, toluidine will bind to phosphate residues of DNA and sperm appear as dark blue to magenta [8].

18.2 Protocol of Toluidine Blue Staining

The below protocol is a modification of the previous protocols [7, 9–11].

1. Allow the ejaculate to liquefy at 37°C for 30 minutes
2. Centrifuge the liquefied sample at $250 \times g$ for 10 minutes
3. Remove the supernatant and re-suspend pellets in sperm washing media containing 5 percent BSA
4. Prepare smears on pre-cleaned defatted slides
5. Allow the smears to dry for 30 minutes, and then fix the slides with freshly prepared 96 percent ethanol: acetone (1:1) at 4°C for 30 minutes. Allow the fixed slides to dry.
6. After 12 hours, hydrolysis the slides with 0.1 M HCl at 4°C for five minutes
7. Wash slides with distilled water, three times for two minutes each time
8. Prepare TB working solution (0.05 percent of TB in 50 percent McIlvain's citrate phosphate buffer at pH=3.5–4)
9. Cover the slides for 5–10 minutes with TB working solution
10. Wash slides in distilled water

157

11. Dehydrate slides in tertiary butanol at 37°C (2×3 minutes) or ethanol (70 percent, 96 percent and 100 percent)
12. Mount slides with xylene at room temperature (two to three minutes)
13. Evaluate the slide for positive- or negative-TB spermatozoa using oil immersion on light microscope
14. Count of 200–500 sperm per sample
15. Report percentage of sperm with dark blue stain of TB as abnormal chromatin packaging (Figure 18.1)

> ➤ Fixed slides can be stored before staining in the dark box for up to one week at room temperature and for up to two weeks in an exicator in the cold room. This duration will not affect the results
> ➤ The TB working solution can be prepared monthly from 1 percent TB with distilled water and stored at 4°C.
> ➤ One percent TB can be stored at 4°C for up to one year.

18.3 Advantages and Disadvantages of Toluidine Blue Staining

Several advantages are mentioned for the assessment of sperm chromatin structure by the TB staining through light microscopy as it is a simple, easy to perform, fast, and inexpensive method. The disadvantages of this test are that only a limited number of sperm can be assessed as compared to flow cytometry where a minimum of 5000–10,000 sperm per sample are assessed. In addition, the technique is labor-intensive.

18.4 Clinical Interpretation of the Results of Toluidine Blue Staining

The sperm chromatin integrity is essential for fertilization, early embryonic development and even development to term. Recently, researchers suggested that besides standard semen parameters, sperm chromatin integrity should be evaluated in parallel with semen analysis [12]. Sperm chromatin integrity is influenced by both external and internal factors such as lifestyle,

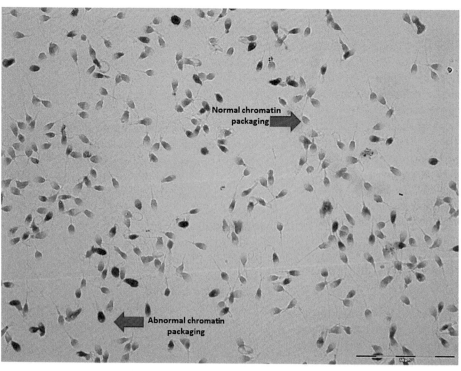

Figure 18.1 Assessment of sperm chromatin packaging by toluidine blue (TB) staining. Sperm with dark blue stain of TB dye were considered as abnormal chromatin packaging while sperm with light blue stain of TB dye were considered as normal chromatin packaging.

age, overproduction of oxidative stress, apoptosis, and protamine deficiency [13]. In this regard, several studies demonstrated the mean values of sperm DNA fragmentation and abnormal chromatin packaging were significantly higher in different groups of infertile men such as men with varicocele, globozoospermia, and abnormal sperm parameters, compared to fertile men or individuals with normal semen parameters (14–16).

Evenson, the pioneer of SCSA, believes that a high level of DNA damage in a semen sample could be considered as a predictive parameter for "subfertility and infertility". On the other hand, since fertility is a complex orchestrated process and is influenced by numerous factors, a high level of DNA integrity in a semen sample could not be considered as a direct predictor of "fertility" [17]. Indeed, during natural fertilization and even in the process of in vitro fertilization (IVF), numerous barriers exist that help to select the most competent sperm and thereby, through these selection barriers, the chance of sperm with damaged DNA or chromatin anomalies to participate in the process of fertilization is reduced. However, in intracytoplasmic sperm injection (ICSI), all these barriers are bypassed and the chance of sperm with reduced chromatin integrity to be inseminated is increased. In this context, Avendaño et al. (2010) believe that in the case of male infertility there is a likelihood of oocytes being inseminated with sperm with normal morphology and reduced chromatin integrity and damaged DNA [18]. Clinical outcomes in the field of infertility treatment revealed significant negative correlations between sperm DNA damage with fertilization, embryo quality and pregnancy rates [18–20] while there are studies that reported no influence of sperm DNA damage on reproductive outcome [21]. When systematic review and meta-analysis studies are checked, it was suggested that sperm DNA damage could have adverse effects on ART outcome, especially as it decreases the likelihood of formation of a good-quality embryo [19, 20].

DNA repair mechanisms in male germ cells are active during mitotic and meiotic stages of spermatogenesis. However, at the time when the excess cytoplasm becomes redundant and the sperm nucleus becomes highly compacted, the ability of DNA repair machinery is nearly completely reduced [22]. Therefore, if sperm are exposed to oxidants, the chance of DNA damage is increased. In this state, fertilization of sperm with highly damaged DNA can result in the formation of embryos with retarded development, which may eventually arrest and result in implantation failure or pregnancy loss [18–20]. Although it has been stated the DNA repair machinery of oocytes could repair sperm DNA damages, this process is highly dependent on the degree of sperm DNA damage and the age of the female [23]. In light of these considerations, assessment of chromatin structure by TB, which has a high affinity to chromatin DNA phosphate residues, could be considered as one of the approaches for assessment of DNA integrity.

Although several direct and indirect methods are introduced for the assessment of DNA integrity and chromatin packaging in sperm, recently, it has been suggested that the TUNEL assay and the SCSA are the most reliable tests for clinical assessment of chromatin integrity and cut-off values of 30–35 percent and 10–20 percent, respectively, have been proposed for SCSA and TUNEL assay [20]. In this regard, Erenpreiss et al. (2004) demonstrated a strong significant correlation between the results of TB with the SCSA and TUNEL assay [r=0.84; r=0.8; p<0.001, respectively] (24). In addition, Tsarev et al. (2009) observed a significant difference in TB-positive spermatozoa or abnormal sperm chromatin structure between fertile and infertile men [7]. They presented a cut-off value of 45 percent for this test and concluded that the results of the TB test can be considered as a predictor for "infertility" and not "fertility" with high specificity (92 percent) and low sensitivity (42 percent).

In addition, Ajina et al. (2016) showed that the mean of abnormal sperm chromatin structure by TB and DNA denaturation by acridine orange were significantly higher in infertile men with astheno-teratozoospermia than in fertile groups. They also observed significant correlations between these two parameters with sperm morphology and viability [10].

In support of these results, Alves et al. (2018) concomitantly assessed the sperm head area, sperm DNA fragmentation with acridine orange and the sperm head area with chromatin compaction by TB in caput, corpus and caudal regions of the cat epididymis. These authors showed that the percentage of sperm DNA fragmentation as well as major and minor defects of sperm morphology were reduced, while the percentage of DNA compaction and DNA integrity were increased as sperm move from caput to cauda. In addition, they showed that the head area of

TB-stained sperm decrease as sperm move from caput toward caudal region. Therefore, the sperm head size and TB stainability could predict the quality of chromatin condensation [25]. From this study we conclude that in addition to semen analysis, TB staining could provide better information regarding chromatin integrity for the assessment of hidden anomalies in the sperm chromatin packaging.

A number of studies suggested that a major contributor of DNA damage in sperm is oxidative stress and that this phenomenon could lead to compromised sperm quality and decreased fertility outcome with advanced age [26]. In this regard, a significant negative correlation was observed between male age and reproductive outcomes in ART [27]. When Kim et al. (2013) used the TB test for assessment of sperm chromatin structure, they did not find any significant correlation between percentage of sperm abnormal chromatin structure with age, while significant correlations were observed between sperm chromatin structure with abnormal sperm chromatin condensation (r=0.594, p=0.000) and strict morphology (r=-0.219, p=0.029) [28]. These controversies could be related to sample size, evaluation method, type of sample, and age range of individuals, but one rational conclusion is that TB staining does not appear to be able to detect oxidative stress-induced DNA damage.

Sperm processing is an inevitable step for separation of normal viable spermatozoa from plasma and also from heterogeneous population, including abnormal sperm and other cells in semen samples in an ART setting. To achieve this goal, swim-up and density gradient centrifugation (DGC) are two commonly used procedures for semen preparation in the andrology laboratory. A number of studies show that these procedures can reduce the number of spermatozoa with abnormal chromatin packaging and DNA fragmentation, while some studies demonstrated centrifugation force could aggravate production of oxygen reactive species and effect DNA integrity of sperm [29, 30]. In this regard, Kim et al. (2015) assessed sperm chromatin integrity by the TB test and observed that this parameter and sperm DNA oxidation significantly increased after swim-up procedure compared to before swim-up. When they divided their participants into smoker and non-smoker groups, mean sperm DNA oxidation significantly increased after swim-up procedure compared to before in the smokers (not the non-smokers), while sperm chromatin integrity assessed by TB test was not different before and after swim-up in smoking and non-smoking men [11].

Talebi et al. (2012) assessed the sperm chromatin packaging status and DNA integrity in couples with a history of recurrent spontaneous abortion (RSA). Except sperm motility, sperm chromatin and DNA status were similar between the control and RSA group. However, the percentages of abnormal spermatozoa higher than the proposed cut-off values for various sperm chromatin tests (aniline blue>35 percent, chromomycin A3>30 percent, TB>45 percent, acridine orange>50 percent and nuclear chromatin stability assay) were significantly higher in RSA compared to the control group. Therefore, they emphasized the importance of the assessment of sperm chromatin status and DNA integrity in couples with unexplained RSA [31]. In addition, the aforementioned sperm chromatin tests were also assessed in infertile men with varicocele, and the results demonstrated that percentages of abnormal spermatozoa for each of the aforementioned tests were significantly higher in infertile men with varicocele compared to fertile men [32]. In this regard it has been shown that microsurgical varicocelectomy reduces these anomalies and significantly improves the quality of sperm chromatin, DNA integrity, and sperm parameters. Therefore, sperm function tests such as TB staining can be used to assess whether a surgical procedure like varicocelectomy has improved the quality of sperm [33].

18.5 Conclusion

Toluidine blue has high affinity to bind to phosphate groups of DNA. In sperm, due to high chromatin compaction, TB cannot access the phosphate groups of DNA. Therefore, normal sperm show light blue while sperm with low chromatin packaging appear as dark blue. Based on this differential staining, researchers have used this test and showed that there is significant correlation between TB stainability and sperm DNA integrity tests like SCSA and TUNEL. The application of TB staining in ART has been very limited in comparison to other tests, despite it being a simple, easy to perform and inexpensive test. Therefore, there is more room for future research to define the diagnostic value of this test in andrology settings.

References

1. Muratori M, De Geyter C. Chromatin condensation, fragmentation of DNA and differences in the epigenetic signature of infertile men. *Best Pract Res Clin Endocrinol Metab* 2019; 33(1): 117–26. doi: 10.1016/j.beem.2018.10.004

2. Hao SL, Ni FD, Yang WX. The dynamics and regulation of chromatin remodeling during spermiogenesis. *Gene* 2019; 706: 201–10. doi: 10.1016/j.gene.2019.05.027

3 Irez T, Sahmay S, Ocal P, Goymen A, Senol H, Erol N, Kaleli S, Guralp O. Investigation of the association between the outcomes of sperm chromatin condensation and decondensation tests, and assisted reproduction techniques. *Andrologia* 2015; 47(4): 438–47. doi: 10.1111/and.12286

4. Zidi-Jrah I, Hajlaoui A, Mougou-Zerelli S, Kammoun M, Meniaoui I, Sallem A, Brahem S, Fekih M, Bibi M, Saad A, Ibala-Romdhane S. Relationship between sperm aneuploidy, sperm DNA integrity, chromatin packaging, traditional semen parameters, and recurrent pregnancy loss. *Fertil Steril* 2016; 105(1): 58–64. doi: 10.1016/j.fertnstert.2015.09.041

5. Ioannou D, Tempest HG. Does genome organization matter in spermatozoa? A refined hypothesis to awaken the silent vessel. *Syst Biol Reprod Med* 2018; 64(6): 518–34. doi: 10.1080/19396368.2017.1421278

6. Sridharan G, Shankar AA. Toluidine blue: a review of its chemistry and clinical utility. *J Oral Maxillofac Pathol* 2012; 16(2): 251–5. doi: 10.4103/0973-029X.99081

7. Tsarev I, Bungum M, Giwercman A, Erenpreisa J, Ebessen T, Ernst E, Erenpriess J. Evaluation of male fertility potential by Toluidine Blue test for sperm chromatin structure assessment. *Hum Reprod* 2009; 24(7): 1569–74. doi: 10.1093/humrep/dep068

8. Beletti ME, Costa LDF, Guardieiro MM. Morphometric features and chromatin condensation abnormalities evaluated by toluidine blue staining in bull spermatozoa. *Braz J Morphol Sci* 2005; 22(2): 85–90.

9. Erenpreisa J, Erenpreiss J, Freivalds T, Slaidina M, Krampe R, Butikova J, Ivanov A, Pjanova D. Toluidine blue test for sperm DNA integrity and elaboration of image cytometry algorithm. *Cytometry A* 2003; 52(1): 19-27.

10. Ajina T, Ammar O, Haouas Z, Sallem A, Ezzi L, Grissa I, Sakly W, Jlali A, Mehdi M. Assessment of human sperm DNA integrity using two cytochemical tests: acridine orange test and toluidine blue assay. *Andrologia* 2017; 49 (10). doi: 10.1111/and.12765

11. Kim SK, Jee BC, Kim SH. Histone methylation and acetylation in ejaculated human sperm: effects of swim-up and smoking. *Fertil Steril* 2015; 103(6): 1425–31. doi: 10.1016/j.fertnstert.2015.03.007

12. Agarwal A, Cho CL, Esteves SC. Should we evaluate and treat sperm DNA fragmentation? *Curr Opin Obstet Gynecol* 2016; 28(3): 164–71. doi: 10.1097/GCO.0000000000000271

13. Durairajanayagam D, Agarwal A, Ong C. Causes, effects and molecular mechanisms of testicular heat stress. *Reprod Biomed Online* 2015; 30(1): 14–27. doi: 10.1016/j.rbmo.2014.09.018

14. Tavalaee M, Kiani-Esfahani A, Nasr-Esfahani MH. Relationship between phospholipase C-zeta, semen parameters, and chromatin status. *Syst Biol Reprod Med* 2017; 63(4): 259–68. doi: 10.1080/19396368.2017.1298006

15. Tavalaee M, Nomikos M, Lai FA, Nasr-Esfahani MH. Expression of sperm PLCζ and clinical outcomes of ICSI-AOA in men affected by globozoospermia due to DPY19L2 deletion. *Reprod Biomed Online* 2018; 36(3): 348–55. doi: 10.1016/j.rbmo.2017.12.013

16. Nasr-Esfahani MH, Abasi H, Razavi S, Ashrafi S, Tavalaee M. Varicocelectomy: semen parameters and protamine deficiency. *Int J Androl* 2009; 32(2): 115–22.

17. Evenson DP, Jost LK, Marshall D, Zinaman MJ, Clegg E, Purvis K, de Angelis P, Claussen OP. Utility of the sperm chromatin structure assay as a diagnostic and prognostic tool in the human fertility clinic. *Hum Reprod* 1999; 14(4): 1039–49.

18. Avendaño C, Franchi A, Duran H, Oehninger S. DNA fragmentation of normal spermatozoa negatively impacts embryo quality and intracytoplasmic sperm injection outcome. *Fertil Steril* 2010; 94: 549–57.

19. Deng C, Li T, Xie Y, Guo Y, Yang QY, Liang X, Deng CH, Liu GH. Sperm DNA fragmentation index influences assisted reproductive technology outcome: a systematic review and meta-analysis combined with a retrospective cohort study. *Andrologia* 2019; 51(6): e13263. doi: 10.1111/and.13263

20. Simon L, Liu L, Murphy K, Ge S, Hotaling J, Aston KI, Emery B, Carrell DT. Comparative analysis of three sperm DNA damage assays and sperm nuclear protein content in couples undergoing assisted reproduction treatment. *Hum Reprod* 2014; 29(5): 904–17. doi: 10.1093/humrep/deu040

21. Lin MH, Kuo-Kuang Lee R, Li SH, Lu CH, Sun FJ, Hwu YM. Sperm chromatin structure assay parameters are not related to fertilization rates, embryo quality, and pregnancy rates in in vitro fertilization and intracytoplasmic sperm injection, but might be related to spontaneous abortion rates. *Fertil Steril* 2008; 90: 352–9.

22. Marchetti F, Bishop J, Gingerich J, Wyrobek AJ. Meiotic interstrand DNA damage escapes paternal repair and causes chromosomal aberrations in the zygote by maternal misrepair. *Sci Rep* 2015; 5: 7689. doi: 10.1038/srep07689

23. Esbert M, Pacheco A, Vidal F, Florensa M, Riqueros M, Ballesteros A, Garrido N, Calderón G. Impact of sperm DNA fragmentation on the outcome of IVF with own or donated oocytes. *Reprod Biomed Online* 2011; 23(6): 704–10. doi: 10.1016/j.rbmo.2011.07.010

24. Erenpreiss J, Jepson K, Giwercman A, Tsarev I, Erenpreisa J, Spano M. Toluidine blue cytometry test for sperm DNA conformation: comparison with the flow cytometric sperm chromatin structure and TUNEL assays. *Hum Reprod* 2004; 19(10): 2277–82.

25. Alves IP, Cancelli CHB, Grassi TLM, Oliveira PRH, Franciscato DA, Carreira JT, Koivisto MB. Evaluation of sperm head dimensions and chromatin integrity of epididymal sperm from domestic cats using the toluidine blue technique. *Anim Reprod Sci* 2018; 197: 33–9. doi: 10.1016/j.anireprosci.2018.08.001

26. Alshahrani S, Agarwal A, Assidi M, Abuzenadah AM, Durairajanayagam D, Ayaz A, Sharma R, Sabanegh E. Infertile men older than 40 years are at higher risk of sperm DNA damage. *Reprod Biol Endocrinol* 2014; 12: 103. doi: 10.1186/1477-7827-12-103

27. Naher ZU, Ali M, Biswas SK, Mollah FH, Fatima P, Hossain MM, Arslan MI. Effect of oxidative stress in male infertility. *Mymensingh Med J* 2013; 22(1): 136–42.

28. Kim HS, Kang MJ, Kim SA, Oh SK, Kim H, Ku SY, Kim SH, Moon SY, Choi YM. The utility of sperm DNA damage assay using toluidine blue and aniline blue staining in routine semen analysis. *Clin Exp Reprod Med* 2013; 40(1): 23–8. doi: 10.5653/cerm.2013.40.1.23. 29.

29. Younglai EV, Holt D, Brown P, Jurisicova A, Casper RF. Sperm swim-up techniques and DNA fragmentation. *Hum Reprod* 2001; 16(9): 1950–3.

30. Taherian SS, Khayamabed R, Tavalaee M, Nasr-Esfahani MH. Alpha-lipoic acid minimises reactive oxygen species-induced damages during sperm processing. *Andrologia* 2019; 51(8): e13314. doi: 10.1111/and.13314

31. Talebi AR, Vahidi S, Aflatoonian A, Ghasemi N, Ghasemzadeh J, Firoozabadi RD, Moein MR. Cytochemical evaluation of sperm chromatin and DNA integrity in couples with unexplained recurrent spontaneous abortions. *Andrologia* 2012; 44: 462–70. doi: 10.1111/j.1439-0272.2011.01206.x

32. Talebi AR, Moein MR, Tabibnejad N, Ghasemzadeh J. Effect of varicocele on chromatin condensation and DNA integrity of ejaculated spermatozoa using cytochemical tests. *Andrologia* 2008; 40(4): 245–51. doi: 10.1111/j.1439-0272.2008.00852.x

33. Vahidi S, Moein M, Nabi A, Narimani N. Effects of microsurgical varicocelectomy on semen analysis and sperm function tests in patients with different grades of varicocele: role of sperm functional tests in evaluation of treatments outcome. *Andrologia* 2018; 50(8): e13069. doi: 10.1111/and.13069

Chapter 19

DNA Damage: TdT-Mediated dUTP Nick-End-Labelling Assay

Rakesh Sharma, Concetta Iovine, Ashok Agarwal

19.1 Introduction

Male infertility affects men worldwide with about 20 percent of couples having male factor infertility [1]. The routine semen analysis is the first step in the assessment of male infertility. However, conventional semen analysis does not provide a complete understanding of fertility potential, especially in patients with idiopathic infertility [2]. In this scenario, DNA integrity is the most important feature to ensure normal fertilization, implantation, pregnancy and embryonic development. Sperm DNA fragmentation (SDF) can be due to several intrinsic factors such as varicocele, oxidative stress, apoptosis, and chromatin packaging defects. Further, SDF can be caused by extrinsic factors such as lifestyle alterations, infections, exposure to xenobiotics, etc. [3–7].

Sperm nuclear DNA is highly compacted because of its protamine content. DNA fragmentation can be attributed to several factors such as oxidative stress [4–6], abortive apoptosis [5], failure to repair DNA strand breaks [6], and environmental exposure of sperm DNA to toxins, defective chromatin packaging and protamine deficiency [7]. Sperm DNA damage results in infertility, miscarriage, and birth defects in offspring [8]. Oxidative stress is the main cause of sperm DNA damage. Oxidative stress is caused by an imbalance between the levels of oxidants or reactive oxygen species (ROS) and the ability of the antioxidants or reductants to scavenge them. A number of factors can lead to oxidative stress, including (viral or bacterial) infections, exposure to xenobiotics, tobacco and alcohol consumption, consumption of fatty diet, drug abuse, radiation, psychological stress, consumption of medications (cyclophosphamide, opioids, etc.), exposure to environmental and air pollutions, chronic diseases, cryptorchidism, and testicular torsion [3, 9–12].

19.2 Mechanisms of Sperm DNA Damage

DNA fragmentation may occur during spermiogenesis where DNA is condensed as a result of replacement of histones with protamines and packaged into the differentiating sperm head as a result of the nuclear exchange of proteins (transition proteins and protamines). This supercoiling of the nucleosomal DNA can result in torsional stress. Endogenous endonucleases (topoisomerases) may induce DNA fragmentation to counter this stress [13, 14]. Although spermatozoa are transcriptionally and translationally inactive and cannot undergo conventional programed cell death or "regulated cell death" called "apoptosis", they exhibit some of the hallmarks of apoptosis. This includes caspase activation and phosphatidylserine exposure on the surface of the sperm. This process is termed "abortive apoptosis" [5, 15]. During spermatogenesis, sperm cells have the ability to repair some DNA damage, however this innate ability is lost once they mature [16, 17]. Therefore, post-testicular sperm are more vulnerable to DNA damage [18–21]. Studies have shown that the accurate assessment of sperm DNA integrity expressed as SDF is a good predictor of semen quality [22–25]. Many tests have been developed to measure SDF, but the most commonly used tests are terminal deoxynucleotidyl transferase deoxyuridine triphosphate (dUTP) nick end labeling (TUNEL) assay, Sperm Chromatin Structure Assay (SCSA®), Comet and Sperm Chromatin Dispersion (SCD) assay [26]. The tests that assess SDF can be classified as direct and indirect tests. Direct tests include TUNEL and Comet assay, and they measure single or double strand damage. SCSA and SCD are the indirect tests that measure the susceptibility of sperm DNA breaks after acid or heat denaturation (Table 19.1).

Table 19.1 Common Direct and Indirect Assays of Sperm DNA Integrity

Assay	Principle	Parameter measured
Direct assays		
TUNEL	Adds labeled nucleotides to free DNA ends Template independent Labels SS and DS breaks	% Cells with labeled DNA
COMET	Electrophoresis of single sperm cells	% Sperm with long tails (tail length, % of DNA in tail)
	DNA fragments form tail Intact DNA stays in head Alkaline COMET Alkaline conditions, denatures all DNA Identifies both DS and SS breaks Neutral COMET Does not denature DNA Identifies DS breaks, maybe some SS breaks	
In situ nick translation	Incorporates biotinylated dUTP at SS DNA breaks with DNA polymerase I Template-dependent Labels SS breaks, not DS breaks	% Cells with incorporated dUTP (fluorescent cells)
Indirect assays		
DNA break detection FISH	Denatures nicked DNA	Amount of fluorescence proportional to number of DNA breaks
	Whole genome probes bind to SS DNA	
SCD	Individual cells immersed in agarose Denatured with acid then lysed Normal sperm produce halo	% Sperm with small or absent halos
Acridine orange flow cytometric assays (example: SCSA)	Mild acid treatment denatures DNA with SS or DS breaks	DFI – the percentage of sperm with a ratio of red to (red + green) fluorescence greater than the main cell population
	Acridine orange binds to DNA DS DNA (nondenatured) fluoresces green SS DNA (denatured) fluoresces red Flow cytometry counts thousands of cells	
Acridine orange test	Same as above, manual counting of green and red cells	% Cells with red fluorescence

DFI = DNA fragmentation index; DS = double-stranded; FISH = fluorescence in situ hybridization; SCD = sperm chromatin dispersion test; SCSA = sperm chromatin structure assay; SS = single-stranded; TUNEL = terminal deoxynucleotidyl transferase-mediated dUTP nick end-labeling.

Each of these tests is related to properties of the DNA damage and provides semi-quantitative estimates only. They do not provide information of the specific DNA sequences that may be affected [27]. High DNA integrity is generally observed in fertile men with normal semen parameters, whereas infertile men with abnormal semen parameters have higher percentage of DNA damage. However, men with normal semen parameters can have poor DNA integrity [28, 29]. There is, however, some evidence to suggest that increased DNA fragmentation is associated with reduced fertility [30]. Yet, this evidence is not conclusive for these tests to be truly predictive of fertility status.

Five percent of women experience two consecutive miscarriages and approximately 1 percent have three or more consecutive miscarriages [31–33]. This is linked with sperm DNA damage [34, 35].

A panel of experts in the reproductive field extensively analyzed the utility of SDF as part of the male fertility evaluation [2]. They recommended SDF analysis for men with high grade varicocele and normal semen parameters as well as low grade varicocele and abnormal semen parameters [2]. Other conditions include unexplained infertility, recurrent pregnancy loss, and recurrent intrauterine insemination (IUI) failures [2]. Nevertheless, many reproductive societies such as the American Society for Reproductive Medicine (ASRM), European Association of Urology (EAU), American Urological Association (AUA) and National Institute of Clinical Excellence (NICE) do not recommend its use as part of the routine assessment of male infertility [25, 26].

In this chapter, we summarize the step-by-step protocols established for the measurement of SDF in human spermatozoa using the bench top flow cytometer. Data acquisition and analysis as well as the necessity for quality control evaluation is further discussed. These steps are required for the standardization of laboratory protocols and the establishment of reference values for TUNEL assay applicable to their patient population.

19.3 Assays for the Evaluation of Sperm DNA Damage

Sperm DNA damage can be assessed by a number of techniques that measure different aspects of DNA damage (Table 19.1). Each assay has its own advantages and disadvantages (Table 19.2). One of the most commonly used assays is the TUNEL assay. TUNEL identifies what is termed as "real" DNA damage – that is, damage that has already occurred – as opposed to "potential" damage caused by exposing sperm to denaturing conditions tested by indirect tests (Table 19.3).

All of the assays shown in Table 19.1 strongly correlate with each other. Unfortunately, none is able to selectively differentiate clinically important from clinically insignificant DNA fragmentation. Moreover, DNA nicks that occur physiologically or pathologically cannot be differentiated with these assays, which cannot evaluate the genes that may be affected by DNA fragmentation. All the assays, including TUNEL, can only determine the amount of SDF that occurs with the assumption that higher level of DNA fragmentation is pathological.

19.4 Measurement of DNA Damage in Spermatozoa by TUNEL Assay

DNA damage can be measured using the TUNEL assay by various protocols such as: fluorescein isothiocynate (FITC) labeled dUTP system (In Situ Cell Detection kit, Roche Diagnostics, Indianapolis, IN); biotin-d(UTP)/avidin system; BrdUTP/anti-Br-dUTP-FITC system and the Apoptosis detection kit (Apo-Direct kit; BD Pharmingen, San Diego, CA)

Here we will briefly describe these protocols and elaborate on the step-by-step measurement of SDF by TUNEL test by a bench top flow cytometer using the Apo-Direct kit. In addition, we will describe the detection of SDF using TUNEL kit and fluorescence microscopy.

19.4.1 Principle of TUNEL Assay

The TUNEL assay was first developed for somatic cells and then later adapted for sperm cells. It shows the percentage of apoptotic cells with damaged DNA. Apoptosis in spermatozoa results in activation of endonucleases, enzymes that induce sperm DNA fragmentation [40]. During apoptosis, endonucleases break down high order sperm chromatin into smaller DNA fragments of ~50kb. These breaks are labeled by FITC-dUTP. This is accomplished with the template independent enzyme called terminal deoxyribonucleotidyl transferase (TdT) that transfers the deoxyribonucleotides to the 3-hydroxyl (3-OH) end of the single- and double-strand breaks [1, 36–38] (Figure 19.1). The intensity of fluorescent labeling examined by fluorescence microscope or flow cytometry is proportional to the number of DNA strand break sites.

19.4.1.1 In Situ Cell Detection Kit to Detect DNA Fragmentation

The (FITC dUTP system or the In Situ Cell Detection kit (Roche Diagnostics) is used to detect SDF. Spermatozoa are centrifuged (at 600 × g for four minutes) before being resuspended in 100 μL of fresh permeabilization solution (10 mg sodium citrate, 10 μL Triton X-100 in 10 mL dH$_2$O) and incubated for two minutes at 4°C. The cells are centrifuged again (600 × g for four minutes) and the pellet is washed with PBS. The positive control samples are treated with 100 μL of DNase I provided by the kit (1 mg/mL) supplemented with 10 μL MgSO$_4$ (100 mM) for one

Table 19.2 Advantages and Disadvantages of Various DNA Integrity Assays

Direct Assays	Advantages	Disadvantages
TUNEL	Can be performed on few sperms Expensive equipment not required Simple and fast High sensitivity Indicative of apoptosis Correlated with semen parameters Associated with fertility Available in commercial kits	Thresholds not standardized Variable assay protocols Not specific to oxidative damage Special equipment required (flow cytometer)
Comet	High sensitivity Simple and inexpensive Correlates with seminal parameters Small number of cells required Can perform on few sperm Alkaline: identifies all breaks Neutral: may identify more clinically relevant breaks	Labor intensive Not specific to oxidative damage Subjectiveness in data acquired No evident correlation in fertility Lack of standard protocols Requires imaging software Variable assay protocols Alkaline: may identify clinically unimportant fragmentation May induce breaks at "alkaline-labile" sites
In situ nick translation	Simple	Unclear thresholds
Indirect assays		Less sensitive
DNA break detection FISH	Can perform on few sperm	Limited clinical data
SCD	Easy, can use bright-field microscopy	Limited clinical data
Acridine orange flow cytometric assays (SCSA)	Many cells rapidly examined Most published studies reproducible	Expensive equipment required Small variations in lab conditions affect results Calculations involve qualitative decisions
Manual acridine orange test	Simple	Difficulty with indistinct colors, rapid fading, heterogeneous staining
8-OHdG analysis	High specificity Quantitative High sensitivity Correlated with sperm function Associated with fertility	Large amount of sample required Introduction of artifacts Special equipment required Lack of standard protocols

FISH = fluorescence in situ hybridization; SCD = sperm chromatin dispersion test; TUNEL = terminal deoxynucleotidyl transferase-mediated dUTP nick end-labeling; SCSA = sperm chromatin structure assay.

hour at 37°C. Cells are washed twice in PBS, diluted to a final volume of 500 μL in PBS and kept in the dark for analysis via flow cytometry.

19.4.1.2 Evaluation by Apo-BrdUTP Apoptosis Detection Kit

Apo-BrdUTP in situ DNA fragmentation kit is also used to measure SDF. The kit includes the positive and the negative controls. The DNA labeling is done with BrdUTP which binds to the 3'-OH terminals of the DNA strand breaks and terminal deoxynucleotidyl transferase (TDT). The antibodies to the BrdUTP molecule are linked to fluorescein molecule. These are detected in FL1 channel [39, 40]. Sample analysis is done with flow cytometer. FL3 channel records the propidium iodide fluorescence.

Table 19.3 TUNEL Test as a Method of Choice for DNA Damage

	TUNEL	SCSA	COMET	SCD
Principal	1. Adds labeled nucleotides to free DNA ends 2. Template independent 3. Labels SS and DS breaks	1. Mild acid treatment denatures DNA with SS or DS breaks 2. Acridine orange binds to DNA 3. Double stranded DNA (nondenatured) fluoresces green. Single stranded DNA (denatured) fluoresces red 4. Flow cytometry counts thousands of cells.	1. Electrophoresis of single sperm cells 2. DNA fragments form tail 3. Intact DNA stays in head Alkaline COMET 1. Alkaline conditions, denatures all DNA. 2. Identifies both DS and SS breaks Neutral COMET 1. Does not denature DNA 2. Identifies DS breaks, maybe some SS breaks.	Individual cells are immersed in agarose. Cells are denatured and lysed A distinct halo is seen in spermatozoa with intact DNA integrity.
What is measured	% Cells with labeled DNA	DFI – the percentage of sperm with a ratio of red to (red + green) fluorescence greater than the main cell population	% Sperm with long tails (tail length, % of DNA in tail)	Percentage of sperm with small or absent halo The distinct halo of deprotenized nuclei (nucleoids) is measured by bright field or fluorescent microscopy.
Type of Assay	Direct	Indirect	Direct	Indirect
	Objective	Objective	Subjective	Subjective
Ease of assay	Many labs run this assay	Samples have to be shipped to reference lab.	Very few labs perform this assay.	Simple, fast and reproducible
Instrumentation	Flow cytometry	Flow cytometry	Microscopy	Microscopy
Nature of assay	TUNEL kit available	Only in reference or designated labs.	Manual, no assay kits available	Manual and Halosperm kit available
Reference values	Ranges from 10–30%	Robust, >30% DFI indicative of decreased pregnancies	Clinically useful reference values not established	Limited clinical data
Type of samples	Fresh or frozen	Fresh or frozen	Fresh	Fresh
Repeatability of assay	Good	Good	Poor	
Cost	Inexpensive	Expensive	Inexpensive	

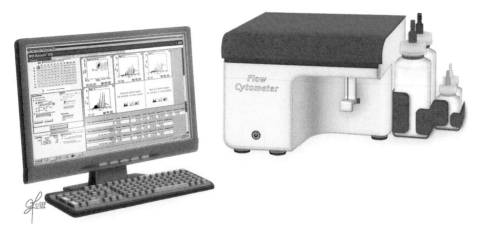

Figure 19.1 Set-up of a benchtop flow cytometer.

19.4.1.3 Measurement of DNA Fragmentation by TUNEL Assay Using a Bench Top Flow Cytometer and Apo-Direct Assay Kit

The TUNEL assay can be evaluated by the Bench top Accuri C6 flow cytometer (BD Pharmingen) (Figure 19.2) [1, 36]. Propidium Iodide (PI) is used as a fluorescent counterstain that allows to count all the other intact cells. The TUNEL kit utilized in the following procedure is the APO-DIRECT™ kit (BD Biosciences Pharmingen, San Diego, CA).

A minimum of 10,000 events are examined for each measurement at a flow rate of about 100 events/second on the flow cytometer. The excitation wavelength is 488 nm supplied by an argon laser at 15 mW. Green fluorescence (480–530 nm) is measured in the FL-1 channel and red fluorescence (580–630 nm) in the FL-2 channel. Spermatozoa obtained in the plots are gated using a forward-angle light scatter (FSC) and a side-angle light scatter (SSC) dot plot to gate out debris, aggregates and other cells different from spermatozoa [1, 36].

19.4.1.3.1 Protocol

19.4.1.3.1.1 Materials – Reagent solutions used, equipment, test specimens

A. Sheath fluid (blue bottle): it comprises of 0.22 μm filtered, deionized water with or without bacteriostatic concentrate solution (PN 653156).

   If bacteriostatic concentrate solution is used (optional), add one bottle per 1 L of water.

B. Cleaning solution (green bottle) (PN 653157): cleaning concentrate solution. To dilute add 3 mL

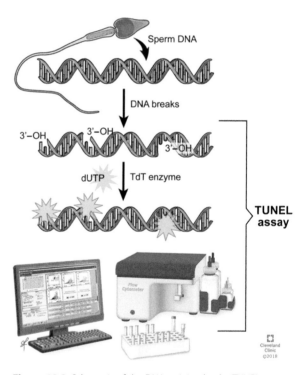

Figure 19.2 Schematic of the DNA staining by the TUNEL assay.

of cleaning concentrate to 197 mL of filtered deionized water. Use the solution within two weeks.

C. Decontamination solution (yellow bottle) (PN653154):

   Add entire bottle to 180 mL of filtered, deionized water.

D. Extended flow cell clean (PN 653159): this solution is provided in working concentrate.

E. APO-DIRECT™ Kit (BD Pharmingen, Catalog #556381)

1. PI/RNase staining buffer
2. Reaction buffer
3. FITC-dUTP
4. TdT Enzyme
5. Rinsing buffer
6. Wash buffer
7. Negative control cells
8. Positive control cells

F. Serological pipettes (2 mL and 5 mL)

G. Eppendorf pipette and tips (20 μL, 100 μL and 1000 μL)

H. Sperm counting chamber

I. Paraformaldehyde (3.7 percent)

19.4.1.3.1.2 Preparation of Paraformaldehyde––Add 90 mL of phosphate buffered saline (PBS, pH 7.4) to 10 mL of formaldehyde (37 percent) and store at 4°C.

J. Microfuge tubes

K. Ethanol (70 percent)

L. Flow cytometer (BD Biosciences, San Jose, CA)

M. 8-Peak Validation Beads (Spherotech, BD)

19.4.1.4 General Set-Up of the Bench Top Cytometer

A. Open the software.

B. Inspect all the reagent bottles to ensure that the fluid levels are fine.

C. Waste bottle should be empty.

D. The sheath, cleaner and the decontamination bottles must be full.

E. Turn on the cytometer.

F. At the beginning, the software light turns yellow. This is an indication that the peristaltic pump has started to run.

G. Allow five minutes for the fluidics line to get flushed with the sheath fluid.

H. Wait for the cytometer software light to turn green, indicating that the C6 Accuri is connected and ready.

I. Flush the tubing to remove any bubbles from the cytometer system.

J. Place a 0.22 μm deionized (DI) water tube on the sheath injection port (SIP).

K. Run a cycle with criteria selected as "Run with limits".

L. Select "Fluidics speed" as "Fast".

M. Click the "Run" button.

N. Leave the SIP tube on the tube holder. Save the file as "Flush".

19.4.1.5 Instrument Quality Control

The quality control is performed with eight-peak beads. The eight-peak beads are 3.2 μm particles excited by the blue laser and emitting light at eight different wavelengths. The validation of the bench top flow cytometer is done by running the eight-peak beads and determining the coefficient of variation (CV) and mean fluorescence intensity (MFI) each time the instrument is used. These can be plotted as CV and MFI in the Levy Jennings chart.

19.4.1.6 Preparation of Eight-Peak Beads

A. Use a 12 × 75 mm tube and label it as "Eight-Peak QC Beads". Also mark the date of preparation.

B. Add 1 mL of deionized DI water to each of the tubes.

C. Vortex each of the bead vials provided by manufacturer.

D. Place four drops of eight-peak beads to the tube and vortex. Cover the tube with the aluminum foil.

19.4.1.6.1 Preparation for the Run of the Eight-Peak QC Beads

A. Double click and open the eight-peak bead template provided with the instrument (Figure 19.3).

B. Turn on the cytometer by pressing the power button.

C. A green light will be displayed under the "Collect tab" indicating that the machine is ready for sample acquisition.

D. Start the acquisition by clicking on the well "A1".

E. Place a tube with 2 mL of 0.22 μm-DI water on the SIP.

F. Check "Run with limits" and set the time limit to "15 minutes".

G. Set "Fluidics" speed to "Fast".

H. Click the "Run" button.

I. The software will prompt to "Save" the file.

J. After completion of the "Run" place the tube with DI on the SIP.

19.4.1.6.2 Acquisition of the Eight-Peak Bead Data

A. Select an empty field from left heading towards the right selecting one well at a time from A1 to H12.

169

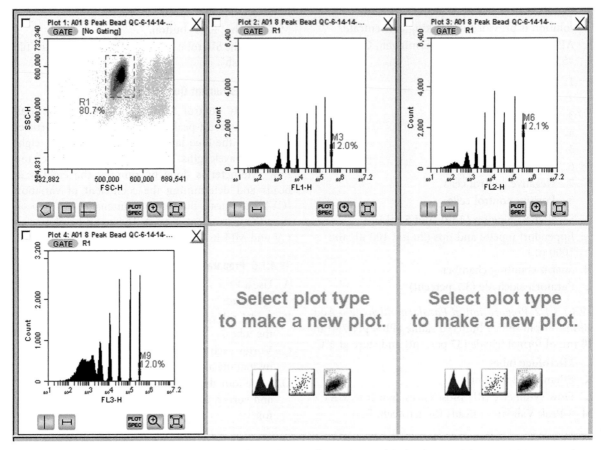

Figure 19.3 Eight-peak quality control beads as seen after analysis in software; the CV of the brightest peak (M3, M6, M9) is measured.

B. Enter in the empty space above the wells the acquisition date for the eight-peak beads as "eight-peak-beads-date-tech initials".

C. The acquisition is performed under the "Collect tab".

D. Unselect the "Time" check-box next to "Min." and "Sec.".

E. Select the "Events" check-box and check the "50,000" option in the "Events" field.

F. From the drop-down menu click on "Ungated sample".

G. Set "Fluidics" speed to "Slow."

H. Mix the eight-peak QC bead suspension by vortexing the tube.

I. Remove tube of deionized water from the SIP.

J. Place the "Eight-Peak QC Bead" tube under the SIP.

K. Click the "RUN" button to start the acquisition.

L. Save the file as "Eight-Peak QC-DATE-TECH INITIALS".

M. After the cytometer has recorded 50,000 events, acquisition will stop.

N. When the run is finished, remove "Eight-Peak QC Bead" tube from SIP and clean the SIP using a lint-free wipe.

O. Place the tube containing 2 mL of DI water on the SIP.

19.4.1.6.3 Ending the Run

A. Place a 2 mL tube of DI water on the SIP and select an empty well in the BD Accuri software.

B. Check "Time" and set the time to "2 min.".

C. Set "Fluidics" speed to "Fast."

D. Click the "Run" button.

E. When the run is finished, place the tube with 2 mL of DI water on the SIP.

F. Before running any other samples click "delete events" to erase the data collection from the water run.

G. At the completion off the run, use a 10 percent solution of bleach for two minutes, followed by a DI water run before shutting down the instrument.

19.4.1.6.4 Analyzing the Eight-Peak Bead Acquisition Data

A. The analysis is done in the "Collect" tab only.

B. Select the well (example: well A1) where the data was acquired for the eight-peak beads run.

C. Adjust the R1 gate to include 75–85 percent of all events.

D. The first plot is labeled "FSC-H" and "SSC-H", click on the border of the "R1" gate. The border will become bold and handles will appear to adjust the gate settings.

E. Include all the "Singlets" or the main bead population making sure to exclude all the doublets which appear as light-gray dots.

F. All the three plots "FL1-H", "FL2-H" and "FL3-H" must be gated on R1.

G. Measure the CV of the brightest peak (right most peak) of the "FL1-H", "FL2-H" and "FL3-H" histograms (Figure 19.3).

19.4.1.6.5 Criteria for Successful Eight-Peak Bead Quality Control

The CV for all three peaks must be less than 5 percent for validation of the three channels of the instrument.

A. To select the brightest peak, use the zoom tool over the histogram and zoom in on the brightest peak in the "FL1-H" histogram.

B. The "M1" marker is adjusted tightly around the brightest peak.

C. The above two steps need to be repeated around the "FL2-H" and "FL3-H" histograms as well.

D. Save this template for future runs of the eight-peak quality control.

19.4.1.6.6 Tracking Performance of the Eight-Peak Bead Quality Control

Open the file for the acquisition data obtained from the eight-peak bead run. Highlight all the statistics that need to be copied and transferred to the excel spread sheet. In the "statistics column selector", check the boxes for the mean and CV of the brightest peak (M3, M6, and M9) for the following parameters: "FL1-H", "FL2-H" and "FL3-H". The Levy-Jennings chart gets populated by the data and the data is saved.

19.4.2 Sample Preparation for TUNEL Assay

A. Semen sample is kept in the incubator for 30–60 minutes at 37°C to undergo liquefaction.

B. After liquefaction, sample is evaluated for volume, sperm concentration, total sperm count, sperm motility and round cell concentration.

C. The sample volume for TUNEL needs to be adjusted to 2.5×10^6/mL.

D. This can be achieved by the following formula:

$$\frac{2.5 \times 1000 \ \mu L}{\text{Sperm Concentration} \ (10^6/\text{mL})} = X \ \mu L$$

E. Save two tubes each for the test sample, negative control and positive control samples.

F. Label tubes with the following information:

   a. TUNEL

   b. Patient name

   c. Medical record number

   d. Date

G. Aliquot the required volume for an adjusted sperm concentration of 2.5×10^6/mL cells to each of the four tubes.

H. Spin the aliquoted sample at $300 \times$ g for seven minutes.

I. Remove the supernatant after the spin.

J. Replace the supernatant with 1 mL PBS.

K. Centrifuge at $300 \times$ g for seven minutes.

L. Remove the supernatant and replace with 1 mL PBS.

19.4.2.1 Preparation of the "Positive Control" Sample

A. Add 100 μL of the stock hydrogen peroxide of 37 percent solution to 1400 μL of PBS 1× to prepare a diluted solution (1:15 dilution) of H_2O_2.

B. Add and suspend the sperm cells in 1 mL of diluted H_2O_2 solution.

C. Place the sperm cell resuspended in H_2O_2 on the heating block at 50°C for 60 minutes.

D. After incubation, centrifuge the tube for seven minutes at $300 \times$ g.

E. Aspirate the supernatant with a transfer pipette, resuspend in 1 mL PBS 1× and centrifuge at $300 \times$ g for seven minutes.

F. Remove the supernatant and replace with 1 mL PBS.

   Along with the "Test" "Negative" sample tubes, repeat centrifugation step for seven minutes at $300 \times$ g.

171

G. Remove the supernatant and replace with 1 mL PBS.

H. Proceed to the next steps of "Fixation" and "Permeabilization."

19.4.2.2 Fixation and Permeabilization

A. Fixation of the sperm cells is done with paraformaldehyde.

B. The supernatant from the "Test", "Negative" and "Positive" control sample is removed after centrifugation at 300 × g for seven minutes, followed by addition of 1 mL of 3.7 percent paraformaldehyde solution.

C. Incubate the samples by resuspending in 3.7 percent paraformaldehyde at room temperature for 15 minutes.

D. Centrifuge the samples at 300 × g for four minutes.

E. Carefully aspirate the paraformaldehyde and replace it with 1 mL of PBS.

F. Centrifuge at 300 × g for four minutes.

G. Aspirate the supernatant and replace with 1 mL of ice-cold ethanol (70 percent). Place the sample at 4°C for 15–30 minutes.

H. Perform a second wash with PBS.

19.4.2.3 Staining Protocol

The negative kit control and positive kit controls are provided as part of kit components.

A. The "Negative" controls, "Positive" controls, and "Test" samples should be mixed well by vortexing them.

B. Aliquot 2 mL suspensions of the well mixed "Kit control" samples into 12 × 75 mm polystyrene tubes.

C. The 2 mL suspension contains approximately $1 × 10^6$ cells/mL.

D. Include "Internal" controls – both positive and negative (two of each) with each run. These controls are sperm samples with known DNA fragmentation.

E. The "Kit control" samples, "Test" samples as well as the "Internal" control samples should be centrifuged for seven minutes at 300 × g.

F. Remove 70 percent ethanol with a transfer pipette by aspirating it, without disturbing the cellular pellet.

G. Add 1.0 mL of the "Wash Buffer" (blue cap) and mix well.

H. Centrifuge at 300 × g for seven minutes.

I. Aspirate and remove the supernatant from the tubes.

J. Repeat the washing step with the "Wash Buffer" and discard the supernatant.

K. Number all the tubes starting from the "Negative controls", "Positive controls", "Test samples" and "Internal controls".

19.4.2.4 Staining for TUNEL Assay

A. Count the total number of tubes or test samples including the kit controls and the internal controls.

B. Prepare stain for an additional five to seven tubes.

C. Remove "Reaction buffer" vial (green cap) from 4°C and the TdT (yellow cap) and FITC-dUTP (orange cap) vials (Figure 19.4) from −20°C and place them at room temperature for 20 minutes (Table 19.4). Give a quick vortex to bring the reagent to the bottom of the vial.

D. Prepare the stain as shown in Table 19.5.

E. Add the reagents in the same sequence as indicated in the table.

F. All the steps for the stain preparation must be carried out in the dark.

G. Omit the "TdT" from the "Negative" controls.

H. Resuspend the pellet in each tube in 50 μL of the "Staining solution".

I. Incubate the sperm suspension for 60 minutes at 37°C.

J. The tubes should be covered by an aluminum foil.

K. After the 60 minute incubation add 1.0 mL of "Rinse buffer" (red cap) to each tube. Centrifuge

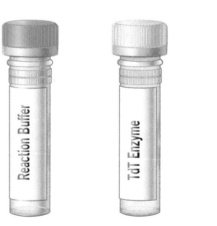

Figure 19.4 Components of the staining reagents: reaction buffer, TdT enzyme and FITC.

Table 19.4 Components of the Apo-Direct Kit
Part A: Reagents Stored at 4°C

Size (mL)	Description	Color code
25	PI/ RNase staining buffer (5 µg/ mL PI, 200 µg/mL RNase)	Amber bottle
0.50	Reaction buffer (contains cacodylate acid (dimethylarsenic))	Green cap
100	Rinsing buffer (contains 0.05% sodium azide)	Red cap
100	Wash buffer (contains 0.05% sodium azide)	Blue cap

Part B: Reagents Stored at −20°C

Size (mL)	Description	Color code
0.40	FITC-dUTP (0.25 nmole/reaction; contains 0.05% sodium azide)	Orange cap
5	Negative control cells (contain 70% vol./ vol.) ethanol)	Clear cap
5	Positive control (contains 70 % vol./ vol. ethanol)	Brown cap
0.038	TdT enzyme (10,000 U/ mg) 20 ug/ mL in 50% vol./ vol. glyceriol solution)	Yellow cap

Table 19.5 Preparation of Staining Solution for the TUNEL Test

Staining solution	Number of assays	
	1 Assay	12 Assays
Reaction buffer (green cap)	10.00 µL	120.00 µL
TdT enzyme (yellow cap)	0.75 µL	9.00 µL
FITC-dUTP (orange cap)	8.00 µL	96.00 µL
Distilled H_2O	32.25 µL	387.00 µL
Total volume	**51.00 µL**	**612.00 µL**

the tubes for seven minutes at 300 × g. Aspirate and remove the supernatant.

L. Repeat the wash with addition of 1 mL of "Rinse buffer".

M. Repeat the centrifugation step for seven minutes at 300 × g.

N. Aspirate and discard the supernatant.

O. Resuspend the pellet in 0.5 mL of PI/RNase buffer.

P. Incubate the suspension mixture for 30 minutes at room temperature.

19.4.3 Running Kit Controls and Acquisition of Data for Kit

Run the kit controls using the "Kit Control template". The settings include "Run with limits" for a total of 10,000 events with a slow fluidics speed and threshold set at 80,000 on FSC-H. Data is recorded on four plots: "FSC-A/SSC-A", "FSC-A/FL2-A", "FL2-A/FL2-H" and "FL1A/FL2-A". Observe the right upper quadrant and record percent positive value for each kit control (Figures 19.5 and 19.6).

19.4.4 Running Patient Samples

Patient samples are run under the "Collect" tab. Use the standardized data acquisition template (Figure 19.7).

The complete acquisition data should be saved in a designated folder for patient results.

A. Double-click on the "TUNEL patient template" saved under folder.

B. Wait till the software loads.

C. Ensure that there is no data in any of the wells in the template file. If there is data in any of the wells, select "Delete all events icon" at the bottom left of the software and remove the data (Figure 19.7).

D. Select well "F1" and import the standard sample file (.fcs).

E. Select the first well "A1." In the space provided above the well, insert "TUNEL patient result, tech initials, date and well number. Hit the save button.

F. Begin with tube #1 (first test sample).

G. Remove DI water tube from the SIP.

H. Vortex the sample and place on the SIP.

I. The run parameters are set as follows for patient samples:

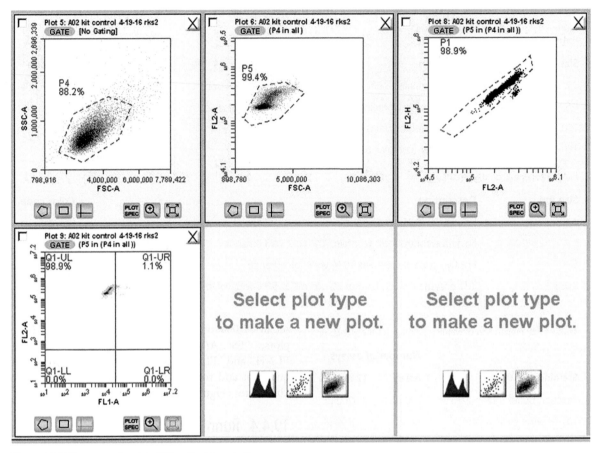

Figure 19.5 Representative plot of "Negative kit control".

1. "Run with limits": check "10,000 events".
2. "Fluidics" speed: select "Slow".
3. Select gate "P3 in P1".
4. Threshold: set at 80,000 on "FSC-H".

J. The acquisition of data is begun by clicking on the "Run" button.

K. After 10,000 events the run will be completed.

L. Remove the tube from the SIP.

M. Use a lint-free wipe to clean the SIP.

N. Vortex and place the second sample on the SIP.

O. Select the next well (A2, and so on) for the next samples.

P. The above steps are repeated for each sample to allow processing of all samples.

Q. The data acquisition workspace is saved under a subfolder e.g. "TUNEL Patient Results" "date", "tech" initials.C6. Save the workspace and close the file.

R. Remove the tube from the SIP and replace with "bleach tube" on the SIP.

S. A "bleach cycle" is run at the end with the following parameters:

1. "Run with limits": two minutes.
2. "Fluidics" speed: Fast.
3. Threshold: 80,000 on FSC-H.

T. Wipe the SIP at the end of the run.

U. Remove the tube and replace it with DI water tube.

V. Repeat steps (1–3) in S with DI water.

W. Follow the shutdown steps at the end of the run.

19.4.4.1 Data Analysis

The dual strategy outlined below is used for data analysis

1. Alignment strategy is performed under the "Collect tab": A standard sample file is used for alignment of all the samples.

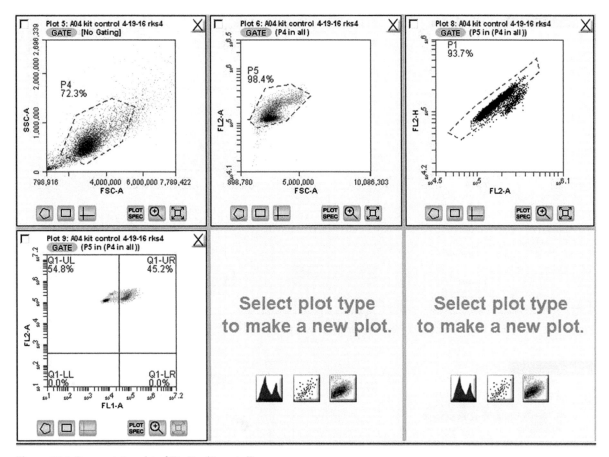

Figure 19.6 Representative plot of "Positive kit control".

2. Data analysis is performed under the "Analyze tab". Each sample must be aligned to "Standard sample" under the "Analyze tab".

19.4.4.2 Alignment Strategy and Data Analysis in the Collect Tab

A. Go to File, open workspace or template. Select the acquisition data saved in the TUNEL template (TUNEL Patient Template).

B. Select an empty well where the standard sample data acquisition file has to be imported.

C. Standard sample should be selected as a sample which should have a known percentage of DNA fragmentation. Go to the "Standard template" and select it.

D. Click on "File import".

E. Select and open workspace.

F. The workspace should be saved as "TUNEL patient acquisition data analyzed, tech initials and date".

G. A single sample is selected as "Standard sample".

H. Select the negative peak of the "Standard sample" and this is used as a reference to be applied to all samples for alignment (Figure 19.8).

I. Click on the histogram for the "Standard sample".

J. Change the X-axis parameter from FSC-A to FL1-A.

K. Right click below the X axis (FL1-A) and select the "Virtual gain" module for alignment.

L. Change the gate to P3 in P1 for plot 5. This gate is the same as plot 4, which is a quadrant gate.

M. Select the vertical line icon at the bottom left of the histogram plot.

N. Align the selected blue line to the center of the histogram to obtain 50 percent cell population on either side (Figure 19.9).

175

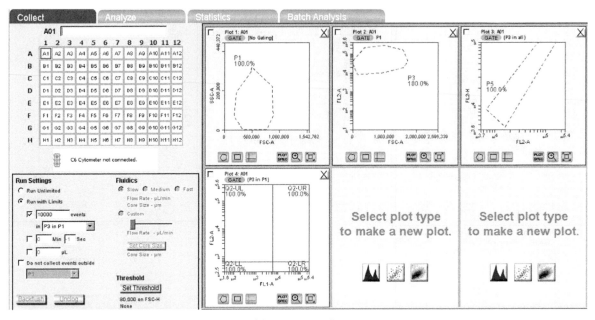

Figure 19.7 Example of template set-up for the analysis of the patient sample.

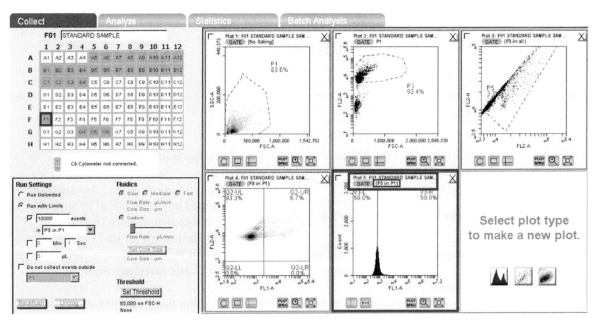

Figure 19.8 Representation of a "Standard sample alignment".

O. Select the sample to be aligned from the grid of wells.

P. Next align the blue line to the center of the peak of the selected sample.

Q. Click the tabs of "Preview" and "Apply".

R. An "Asterix" will appear below the histogram. The star confirms the alignment of the sample (Figures 19.10–19.11).

S. Next hit the close button.

Go to file and hit "Save" after each sample is aligned.

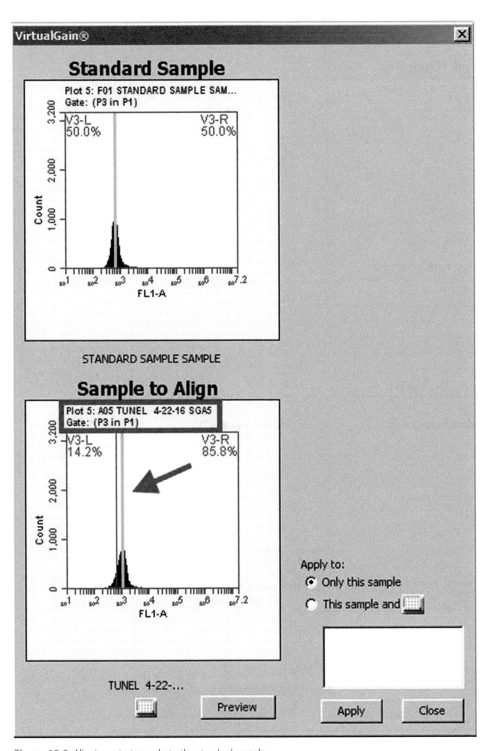

Figure 19.9 Aligning a test sample to the standard sample.

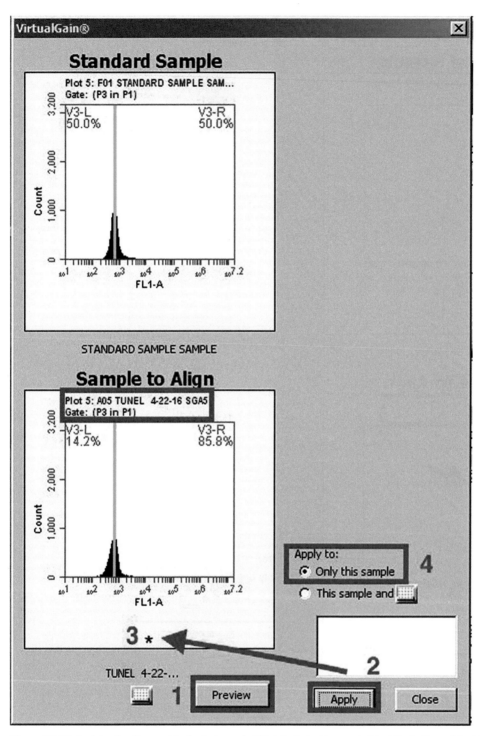

Figure 19.10 Applying the alignment to the test sample. This is indicated by an asterisk at the bottom of the histogram confirming the alignment of the sample to the standard file.

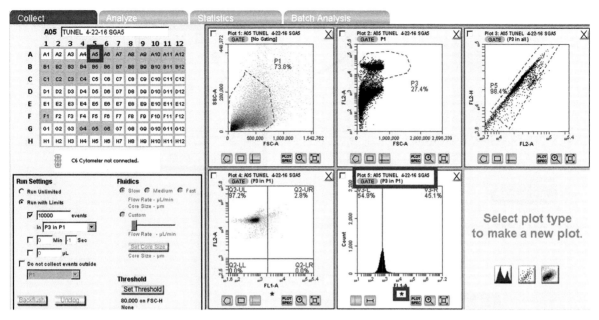

Figure 19.11 Steps showing the alignment of the well with a star saved under the histogram plot.

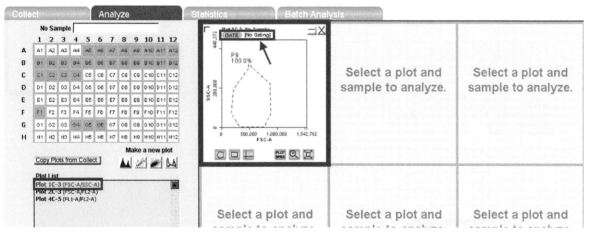

Figure 19.12 Showing the first plot with no gating.

19.4.4.3 Data Analyis in "Analyze" Tab

A. The data acquired in the "Collect" tab is utilized for analysis under the "Analyze" tab within the Accuri C6 software. Open the "Analyze" tab. Create a set of three plots for each sample: FSC-A/SSC-A, FSC-A/FL2-A, and FL1-A/FL2-A.

B. Apply the same gating strategy as used in the "Collect" tab.

C. The first plot "FSC-A/SSC-A" has no gating. The cell population is PX (Figure 19.12).

D. The second plot "FSC-A/FL2-A" will have the gate PX in all events. The cell population is PY (Figure 19.13).

E. The third plot "FL1-A/FL2-A" will have gate of PY in PX in all events (Figure 19.14).

F. Record the percent damage reflected in the upper right quadrant from the "FL1-A/FL2-A" plot (Figure 19.15).

G. Record the preliminary results in the TUNEL Laboratory record form.

179

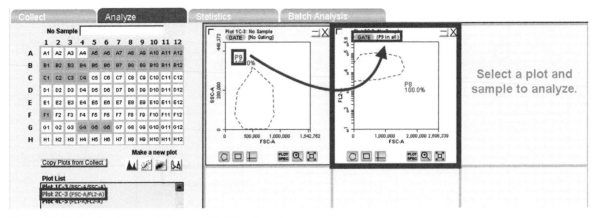

Figure 19.13 Showing the second plot gate with P9 in all events.

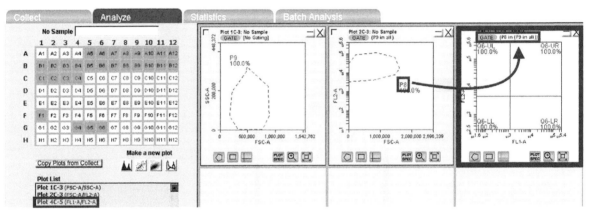

Figure 19.14 Showing the third plot gate showing P8 in P9 in all events.

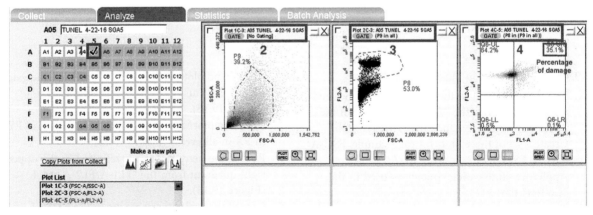

Figure 19.15 Plot in the analyzed mode showing percentage of DNA damage.

19.4.4.4 Final Result Calculation for Sperm DNA Fragmentation Percent Value

A. Calculate the average value of the "Negative samples" where no TdT was added.
B. Subtract the average negative value form the percent damage for each sample recorded from the "FL1-A/FL2-A" in the right upper quadrant of the plot.

19.4.4.5 Reference Values

Test sensitivity, specificity, positive and negative predictive values, and TUNEL cut-off values was calculated using the ROC curve [36]. The SDF is significantly higher (<0.001) in the infertile men than in the controls. Sperm DNA fragmentation at a cut-off value of 16.8 percent is associated with the best specificity of 91.6 percent and a positive predictive value of 91 percent to discriminate infertile men from the controls (Figure 19.16A). At this given cut-off, 91.6 percent of the control population is below this level compared to 67.4 percent of infertile men. The upper limit of SDF in controls is 19.6 percent compared to 68.9 percent in infertile men [36] (Figure 19.16B).

19.4.4.6 Verification of the Validity of the TUNEL Assay Performed

1. The positive kit control sample should have greater than 30 percent of events that are positive for TUNEL.

19.4.4.7 Factors that Can Influence the Protocol and need Special Attention

A. Viscous semen samples: In these samples it is difficult to assess sperm concentration and subsequent sample preparation for TUNEL assay. Viscosity can be reduced by treating with chymotrypsin (5 mg) and incubating the sample for an additional 10 minutes before examining for concentration.
B. Oligozoospermic samples: Samples that have extremely low sperm concentration ($<10 \times 10^{6}$ sperm/mL) will require larger sample volumes. In such cases it is important to remove the seminal plasma to avoid clumping/fixation of the seminal plasma proteins with paraformaldehyde. This will make all the subsequent washing and staining steps difficult. Also, it will likely clog the SIP during the analysis step.
C. Aspiration of the supernatant must be very carefully done as sperm will be lost in each washing and re-suspending step.
D. The reagent volumes that need to be aliquoted for preparing the stain must be carefully calculated and verified as described to avoid over staining or under staining of the samples.
E. It is helpful to give a quick spin to the TdT via to bring the volume to the bottom of the vial.
F. The preparation of the stain and all subsequent steps must be conducted in indirect light or in the dark.

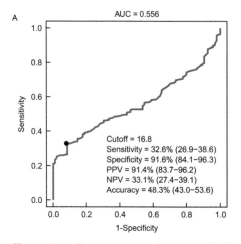
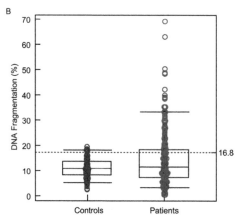

Figure 19.16 Receiver operator characteristic (ROC) curve showing **A:** TUNEL assay cut-off and the area under the curve. Values within the parentheses represent the 95 percent confidence interval and **B:** Distribution of TUNEL test values between controls and infertile men.

G. The incubation step with the stain should not exceed 60 minutes at 37°C.

H. Mix only required "Staining solution" to complete the number of assays prepared per analysis.

I. The "Staining solution" is active for approximately 24 hours at 4°C.

J. The cells must be analyzed within three hours after staining. They will start to deteriorate if left overnight before analysis.

K. Always run the "Kit controls" and "Patient samples" in the "Collect Tab".

L. The gate should be changed to "P3" in "P1" for sample data acquisition.

M. Do not change the settings in the four plots.

N. The test must always be validated to confirm that the test was correctly performed as per the validation criteria provided above.

O. It is important to clean the SIP each time by clicking on the "Back flush" button and following the steps in the manual.

P. The flow cytometer quality control must be performed as recommended for optimal performance of the instrument.

19.4.5 Inter- and Intra-Laboratory and Operator Comparison

Inconsistency and large variability in the results obtained by different techniques is a major challenge in the sperm fragmentation assays. In a study by Ribeiro et al. [36], comparison of the data across two reference laboratories was conducted at Basel, Switzerland and Cleveland Clinic, Ohio, USA. Semen samples from 31 subjects were grouped into three cohorts. Sperm DNA fragmentation data was measured by two experienced operators at two different laboratories using identical semen samples, assay kit, protocol and acquisition settings using identical flow cytometers. No significant differences were observed between the duplicates in any of the experiments performed. By including an additional washing step after fixation in paraformaldehyde, a high correlation was seen between the two laboratories (r=0.94). A strong positive correlation was observed between the average SDF rates (r=0.719). Their study findings confirmed the reproducibility of the TUNEL assay with minimal inter- and intra-laboratory variability and established TUNEL to be a robust test for measuring SDF [36].

19.5 Measurement of DNA Fragmentation by TUNEL Assay Using Microscopy

Although more commonly used in research, the fluorescent microscopy is also used in clinical practice. The TUNEL test is carried out on semen samples using the "In Situ Cell Death Detection Kit" (Roche Diagnostics®, Indianapolis, IN, USA), in which the marker used is FITC. The nuclei of the spermatozoa with double-strand DNA breaks appear green, while those with intact DNA are unstained. For this reason, it's necessary to apply a contrast fluorochrome DAPI (4,6-diamino-2-phenylindol) and the sperm with intact DNA appears blue. Therefore sperm with intact or fragmented DNA can be easily distinguished (Figure 19.17A).

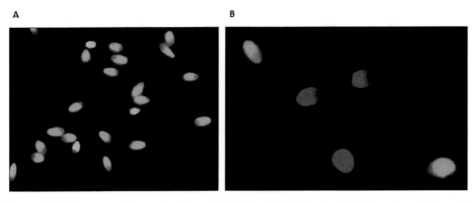

Figure 19.17 Fluroscent microscopic staining with TUNEL and DAPI showing **A:** TUNEL positive cells (apoptotic) cells appearing green compared with blue (non-apoptotic) cells and **B:** TUNEL and propidium iodide staining showing TUNEL positive sperm staining green and TUNEL negative samples staining red.

In this test, 15 μL of sperm sample are smeared onto glass slides, fixed in 4 percent paraformaldehyde for one hour in the dark and at room temperature and then air dried. The fixed slides are rinsed in PBS, pH 7.4, and then permeabilized in sodium citrate solution (Sodium Citrate, distilled H_2O and Triton X-100) on ice for two minutes, rinsed in PBS and air dried. The TdT labeled nucleotide mixture (5 μL of Enzyme solution and 45 μL of Label solution) is added on each slide, and the slides are incubated in a humidified chamber at 37°C for 60 minutes in the dark. Next, the slides are rinsed three times in PBS, with each rinse lasting five minutes, and counterstained with DAPI solution or propidium iodide for five minutes. A total of 500 cells are scored using a fluorescence microscope equipped with Band Pass of 330–380 nm and Long Pass of 420 nm filters. The final percentage of sperm with fragmented DNA (DFI percentage) is referred to as the percentage of TUNEL-positive sperm.

Percentage of DFI:

$$\frac{\text{Green cells (Fragmented DNA)}}{\text{Blue/red cells (Intact DNA)} + \text{Green cells}} \times 100$$

19.5.1 Instrument and Reagents

1. Oscillating arm centrifuge
2. Refrigerated thermostat (4°C)
3. Incubator (37°C)
4. Weighing balance
5. pH meter
6. Epifluorescence microscope with filter for DAPI and FITC
7. Chemical hood

19.5.2 Consumable Materials

1. Slides
2. Cover glasses (24 × 60)
3. Coplin jars
4. Falcon tubes 15 mL

19.5.3 Solutions

1. PBS 1x permeabilizing solution: 0.1 g sodium citrate, 100 μL Triton X-100, 100 mL H_2O
2. DAPI stock solution: 0.1 mg/mL
3. Standard saline concentrate 20×: 3M NaCl, 300 mM Sodium Citrate, pH 7.0

4. DAPI solution: 10 mL SSC 20×, 2 mL DAPI stock, 88 mL of H_2O
5. DABCO (1,4 diazobicycle (2,2,2) octane) solution (1 mL): Tris-HCl 1M (pH 8; 200 μL, glycerol 9 mL, DABCO 0.22 g, H_2O 800 μL).
6. Paraformaldehyde 4 percent

19.5.4 Protocol

1. Centrifuge 1 mL of sample at 300 × g for 15 minutes.
2. Discard the supernatant and resuspend the cell pellet in the same volume of PBS 1×.
3. Centrifuge at 300 g for 15 minutes.
4. Discard the supernatant and resuspend the cell pellet in 50–100 μL of PBS 1×.
5. Streak 10 μL of sample on each slide with an object holder (allow to air dry).
6. Fix the smears in paraformaldehyde for one hour at room temperature and leave to air dry.
7. Immerse slides in 1× PBS for five minutes.
8. Incubate the slides in the permeabilizing solution for two minutes.
9. Rinse the slides in PBS 1× and allow them to air dry.
10. Add the TUNEL reaction mixture (5 μL of Enzyme solution and 45 μL of Label solution) to each slide and place a coverslip.
11. Incubate the slides in a humid chamber for one hour at 37° C in the dark. Avoid exposing the slides to direct light to avoid DNA damage induced by the light itself. Remove the coverslip and wash the slides in PBS 1×.
12. Stain the slides in DAPI solution for five minutes.
13. Rinse the slides in 1× PBS and allow them to air dry.
14. Add 100 μL of DABCO solution; seal with coverslip and apply nail polish on the edges of the coverslip to prevent it from drying.
15. Keep the slides at 4°C in the dark for at least 30 minutes and then observe using fluorescent microscopy.

Another method is to use the APO-DIRECT staining kit (BD Pharmingen).

The staining solution contains reaction mixture, TdT, dUTP labeled with FITC and counterstained with propidium iodide that stains nuclei red (Figure 19.17B).

19.5.5 Reference Values

The sperm DNA damage is quantified as sperm DNA index (DFI percentage). Regardless of the method used to detect the SDF, some threshold values [41] (Table 19.6) are high beyond which the chances of fertilizing an oocyte are close to zero, both through natural conception and ART. However, this technique still lacks a standardized reference value.

19.5.6 Advantages and Disadvantages of Microscopy Method of TUNEL Test

Fluorescent microscopy has been widely used for measuring SDF by TUNEL assay. However, in the last 10 years, the flow cytometry is gaining popularity. Although the flow cytometry seems to be more advanced, many biases due to the inability of this instrument to recognize analyzed cells morphologically, are less explored. On the contrary, the limitations regarding the fluorescence microscopy are well known [69]. The fluorescence microscopy is a highly subjective not-standardized method, related to the operator laboratory experience who has to discriminate the green fluorescent cells from the blue fluorescent ones. This could be a disadvantage of the method but on the contrary it can help avoid the possibility of counting non-sperm cells. In fact, coiled and oval heads of sperm cells are clearly discernable by fluorescence microscopy. The use of fluorescence microscopy is not recommended for quick processing of large numbers of samples as it is a non-automated method. On the other hand, it is recommended for oligozoospermic samples, where flow cytometry may not be able to optimally detect very low sperm concentration.

19.6 Challenges with Current Sperm DNA Fragmentation Protocols

Lack of standardized, reproducible protocols and reference values are among the challenges faced especially when using new or upgraded versions of instruments in reproductive laboratories such as flow cytometry.

Any change in the setting of the reference instrument, including upgrades of hardware or software, may lead to different results and may impact clinicians' decision for treatment. We have reported the standardization of the TUNEL protocol using identical flow cytometers across two laboratories in different continents [36]. This study was conducted under strictly identical controlled conditions where we demonstrated the precision and the accuracy of the TUNEL assay across laboratories.

Recently, a new model of the bench top flow cytometer called C6 Plus was introduced in the market with some improvements over the current C6 flow cytometer model. Some of the features of the BD Accuri C6 Plus (BD Bioscience, San Diego, CA) include redesigned red laser, improved fluidics and enhanced fluorescence sensitivity, reliability with simplified workflow, ready-to-use templates, automated quality control and a small footprint.

We therefore compared TUNEL results of SDF obtained using a standard (C6) flow cytometer with a newer version (C6 Plus) of the same instrument using unadjusted setting and after adjustment with the standard C6. We 1) analyzed the concordance correlation, sensitivity and specificity of the SDF results, 2) established the analytical validity of a new model of flow cytometer utilizing the current flow cytometer as the reference, 3) compared the inter- and intra-observer variability on both flow cytometers and 4) established the agreement between two observers: precision and accuracy of the newer model of the flow cytometer [70].

The cut-off, sensitivity and specificity without any adjustment and after adjustment with the standard flow cytometer was compared. Performance verification was done for normozoospermic samples, samples from infertile men and both positive and negative controls from sperm samples. The two instruments differed significantly in percentage of SDF and correlation between adjusted and unadjusted C6 Plus with the standard C6. After adjustment of the settings, overall concordance became high. We demonstrated a strong agreement between the samples tested on the two flow cytometers after calibration and established the robustness of both instruments (Figures 19.18–19.20). We have established the reproducibility of the two bench top flow cytometers using the standardized staining protocol and demonstrated a clear-cut evidence of robustness of the TUNEL results obtained by the two machines.

19.7 Clinical Interpretation of the TUNEL Result

In a meta-analysis study [33], TUNEL assay was considered the most predictive assay for the miscarriage rate, followed by SCSA. Similar results were obtained

Table 19.6 TUNEL Positivity Using Flow Cytometry or Fluorescence Microscopy Technique

Flow cytometry	TUNEL positive (%) Microscopy	Sample size	Reference
11.07±8.00 (0.79–42.64)	-	140	[42]
7–42 (range)	5–28 (range)	13	[42]
15		43	[43]
–	14.5±1.5 (0.5–75) (swim-up)	150	[44]
–	11.7±7 (low motility sample).	10	[45]
–	35 (15–60); 18 (7–45) (gradient)	25	[46]
–	11 (infertile and ~2.5 (fertile)	52	[47]
20±15 (1.3–64)	–	34	[48]
15% controls	–	97	[49]
–	10.0 (controls)	11	[50]
–	25.4 (infertile) and 10.2 (fertile)	40	[51]
–	7.3±3.5 (pregnancy vs. 13.9±10.8 (no pregnancy (gradient separation)	119	[52]
20.7(1.0–71.7)	–	68	[53]
~15	–	60	[54]
–	10 (patient) and 7 (control) with high motility vs. 33 (patient) and ~25 (control) in low motility samples	34	[15]
–	12–15 (abnormal samples) and 6–7 (normal after gradient separation)	108	[55]
–	~38.4 (miscarriages)	21	[56]
–	10–40 (range) (methanol:ethanol fixed)	6	[57]
10.5 (4–27) (frozen)		18	[58]
40.6 (patients) vs. 13.0 (controls)	12.5±2.2 (0h; washed); 7.6±1.1 (0h; gradient); 1.7±0.8 (0h; swim-up)	7	[59]
40.9±14.3 (patients) and 13.1±7.3 (controls)	8.9±3.7 (patient) and 8.7±3.6 (control)	18	[60]
22.44±29.48 (patients) and 13.1 ±17.56 (controls)	23.6±5.1 (ejaculates) vs. 4.8±3.6 (testicular sperm)	18	[61]
11 (2.5–31) (control)	–	73	[22]
–	–	113	[22]
–	–	15	[22]
–	–	24	[62]
	25.9 (nonsmokers) and 32 (smokers)	108	[63]
	19.5±1.3 (infertile) and 11.1±0.9 (fertile)	67	[64]
39.7±23.1	8.6±3.6 (patient) and 5.4±2.7 (control)	77	[65]
–	40.8±4.9 (low P1/P2) and 21.6±1.7 (normal P1/P2) and 28.3±3.1 (high P1/P2)	79	[66]

Table 19.6 (*cont.*)

Flow cytometry	TUNEL positive (%) Microscopy	Sample size	Reference
	21.0 (8.0–66.0) (pretreatment) 25.0 (10–47)) (post-treatment)	22	[67]
	15.3±10.3	66	[41]
	79.6±13.6 pre-varicocele and 27.5±19.4 (post varicocele)	15	[68]

Data is reported as mean ± SD or range P1 = protamine-1; P2 = protamine-2

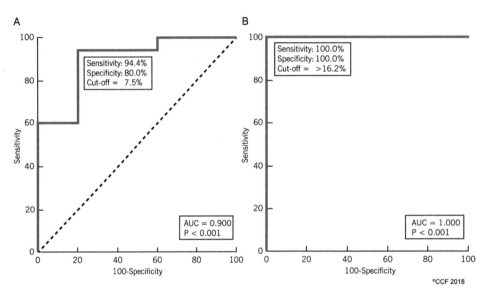

Figure 19.18 Receiver operating characteristic curve showing sensitivity, specificity, and cut-off for C6 Plus in **A:** unadjusted SDF and **B:** after adjustment with the standard C6 flow cytometer.

in another meta-analysis [36] where TUNEL was again shown as the most predictive technique in relation to the birth rate end-point after ARTs. TUNEL assay showed a predictive value in clinical pregnancy after in vitro fertilization (IVF) and ICSI, whereas SCSA and SCD tests showed a "poor" prediction [71]. Therefore, it has the potential of being used as a strong diagnostic tool not only for detecting male infertility but also to understand the predictive ability of many conditions related to achieving pregnancy.

19.8 Advantages and Disadvantages of TUNEL Test by Flow Cytometry

The TUNEL assay using cytometry allows rapid analysis of a large number of sperm in a short period of time and provides a highly sensitive means of defining sperm with fragmented DNA in a more objective, automatic, and precise manner. Therefore, the main advantages are that as objective methods, the detection of sperm fragmented by flow cytometry is highly reproducible and more sensitive for positive cells. However, a few disadvantages could be the presence of M540 bodies that contain fragmented DNA that might affect the SDF determination by flow cytometry, providing a false amount of sperm counted [69].

19.9 Challenges in Measuring DNA Fragmentation by TUNEL Assay

Ribeiro et al. [40] compared the efficacy between the indirect antibody-based labeling system (BrdUTP/

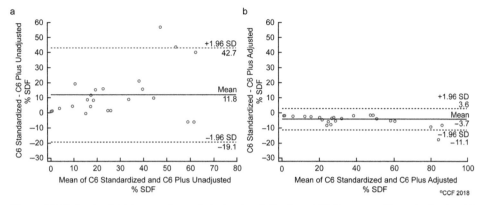

Figure 19.19 Passing Bablok regression analysis showing **A**: Unadjusted C6 Plus versus C6 standardized and **B**: Adjusted C6 Plus versus C6 standardized. The wider deviation of the values from one another can clearly be seen.

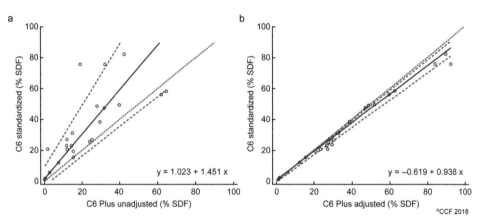

Figure 19.20 Bland-Altman Plots for **A**: Unadjusted C6 Plus versus C6 standardized and **B**: Adjusted C6 Plus versus C6 standardized.

fluorescein-anti-BrdUTP) and the direct labeling system (fluorescein-dUTP). Both labeling systems showed similar staining functions in live spermatozoa. When compared to direct labeling systems, the TUNEL indirect labeling system underestimates the SDF with the differences ranging from 19.2 to 85.3 percent ($p<0.05$). These differences were more pronounced in semen samples where the total motility was less than 40 percent or where weak propidium iodide-stained spermatozoa (PI dimmer spermatozoa) were higher than 14 percent. A correlation was seen between the number of immotile spermatozoa and the intensity of difference between the two labeling systems. The PI dimmer population was labeled to a lesser extent with the indirect TUNEL staining method. Furthermore, compared to direct labeling, indirect labeling only stained a small number from the PI-dimmer population (90.6 percent versus 17.9 percent). Overall, only 30–100 percent of the total number of spermatozoa stained with direct TUNEL labeling system were also stained with the indirect method. The most probable reason for the different staining efficiency of both labeling systems was due to the steric hindrance of the antibody during its binding to the BrdUTP. In addition, condensed chromatin architecture in dead spermatozoa also contributed to the differences in staining.

In earlier studies, measurement of TUNEL assay was highly correlated with sperm vitality [72, 73]. There was a significant difference in the staining efficiency of the dead population of indirect labeling compared to direct labeling (40.1 percent versus 65.7 percent, $p<0.05$). On the other hand, no significant difference was found on staining the number of live spermatozoa using both TUNEL labeling methods (8.9 percent versus 8.3 percent, $p > 0.05$) [36].

19.10 Clinical Scenario

A 29-year-old man presents with secondary infertility of three years' duration. He was evaluated with several conventional semen analyses, the results of which were within reference limits. His wife is 24 years old with a normal fertility evaluation. The couple has a history of three miscarriages, all of which occurred before the twelfth week of gestation. Subsequently, they underwent two IUI cycles (total motile sperm inseminated >5 million) with no clinical pregnancy. The man is otherwise healthy with no significant reproductive or medical/surgical history. This is a case of unexplained infertility, recurrent miscarriage and IUI failure [2]. SDF testing is clearly indicated in this scenario [2], which indeed revealed a SDF percentage of greater than 30 percent [74]. Men

with unexplained infertility present with high SDF [2, 30, 75].

19.11 Conclusion

The TUNEL assay is considered to be the most simple, sensitive and reliable test for assessing SDF with low inter-observer variability. The standardization and optimization of the TUNEL test, with no or little intra-laboratory variation, will increase the positive predictive value and precise use of SDF testing in clinical scenarios to determine molecular factors underlying male infertility. Other laboratories can utilize the methodology and protocol for measuring SDF described here and help further narrow the cut-off values for SDF in infertile men and help increase the utility of this test in the evaluation of the infertile male as well as increase the success rate in infertile couples undergoing ART procedures.

References

1. Agarwal A, Gupta S, Sharma R. (2016) Measurement of DNA fragmentation in spermatozoa by TUNEL assay using bench top flow cytometer. In Agarwal A, Gupta S, Sharma R, eds., *Andrological Evaluation of Male Infertility: A Laboratory Guide.* Geneva: Springer International Publishing, pp. 181–203.

2. Agarwal A, Majzoub A, Esteves SC, Ko E, Ramasamy R, Zini A. Clinical utility of sperm DNA fragmentation testing: practice recommendations based on clinical scenarios. *Trans Androl Urol* 2016; **5**(6): 935.

3. Tremellen K. Oxidative stress and male infertility – a clinical perspective. *Hum Reprod Update* 2008; **14**(3): 243–58.

4. Agarwal A, Mulgund A, Alshahrani S, Assidi M, Abuzenadah AM, Sharma R, Sabanegh E. Reactive oxygen species and sperm DNA damage in infertile men presenting with low level leukocytospermia. *Reprod Biol Endocrinol* 2014; **12**: 126.

5. Sakkas D, Seli E, Bizzaro D Tarozzi N, Manicardi GC. Abnormal spermatozoa in the ejaculate: abortive apoptosis and faulty nuclear remodelling during spermatogenesis. *Reprod Biomed Online* 2003; 7: 428–32.

6. Lewis SE, Aitken RJ. DNA damage to spermatozoa has impacts on fertilization and pregnancy. *Cell Tissue Res* 2005; **322**(1): 33–41.

7. Aitken RJ, Smith TB, Jobling MS, Baker MA, De Iuliis GN. Oxidative stress and male reproductive health. *Asian J Androl* 2014; **16**(1): 31–8.

8. Aitken RJ, De Iuliis GN. On the possible origins of DNA damage in human spermatozoa. *Mol Hum Reprod* 2010; **16**: 3–13.

9. Ollero M, Gil-Guzman E, Lopez MC, Sharma RK, Agarwal A, Larson K, Evenson D, Thomas AJ Jr, Alvarez JG. Characterization of subsets of human spermatozoa at different stages of maturation: implications in the diagnosis and treatment of male infertility. *Hum Reprod* 2001; **16**: 1912–21.

10. Aitken RJ, Sawyer D. The human spermatozoon-not waving but drowning. *Adv Exp Med Biol* 2003; **518**: 85–98.

11. Saleh RA, Agarwal A, Nada EA, El-Tonsy MH, Sharma RK, Meyer A, Nelson DR, Thomas AJ, Jr. Negative effects of increased sperm DNA damage in relation to seminal oxidative stress in men with idiopathic and male factor infertility. *Fertil Steril* 2003; **79**: 1597–1605.

12. De Iuliis GN, Thomson LK, Mitchell LA, Finnie JM, Koppers AJ, Hedges A, Nixon B, Aitken RJ. DNA damage in human spermatozoa is highly correlated with the efficiency of chromatin remodeling and the formation of 8-hydroxy-2′-deoxyguanosine, a marker of oxidative stress. *Biol Reprod* 2009; **81**: 517–24.

13. Sakkas D, Mariethoz E, Manicardi G, et al. Origin of DNA damage in ejaculated human spermatozoa. *Rev Reprod* 1999; **4**: 31–7.

14. Marcon L, Boissonneault G. Transient DNA strand breaks during mouse and human spermiogenesis: new insights in

stage specificity and link to chromatin remodeling. *Biol Reprod* 2004; **70**: 910–18.

15. Weng SL, Taylor SL, Morshedi M, Schuffner A, Duran EH, Beebe S, Oehninger S. Caspase activity and apoptotic markers in ejaculated human sperm. *Mol Hum Reprod* 2002; **8**: 984–91.

16. Matsuda Y, Tobari I, Maemori M, Seki N. Mechanism of chromosome aberration induction in the mouse egg fertilized with sperm recovered from postmeiotic germ cells treated with methyl methanesulfonate. *Mutat Res* 1989; **214**: 165–80.

17. Aitken RJ. Founders' Lecture. Human spermatozoa: fruits of creation, seeds of doubt. *Reprod Fertil Dev* 2004; **16**: 655–64.

18. Steele EK, Lewis SE, McClure N. Science versus clinical adventurism in treatment of azoospermia. *Lancet* 1999; **13** (353): 516–17.

19. O'Connell M, McClure N, Powell LA, Steele EK, Lewis SE. Differences in mitochondrial and nuclear DNA status of high-density and low-density sperm fractions after density centrifugation preparation. *Fertil Steril* 2003; **79**: 754–62.

20. Lewis SE, O'Connell M, Stevenson M, Thompson-Cree L, McClure N. An algorithm to predict pregnancy in assisted reproduction. *Hum Reprod* 2004; **19**: 1385–94.

21. Suganuma R, Yanagimachi R, Meistrich ML. Decline in fertility of mouse sperm with abnormal chromatin during epididymal passage as revealed by ICSI. *Hum Reprod* 2005; **20**: 3101–8.

22. Sergerie M, Laforest G, Bujan L, Bissonnette F, Bleau G. Sperm DNA fragmentation: threshold value in male fertility. *Hum Reprod* 2005; **20**(12): 3446–51.

23. Sharma RK, Sabanegh E, Mahfouz R, Gupta S, Thiyagarajan A, Agarwal A. TUNEL as a test for sperm DNA damage in the evaluation of male infertility. *Urology* 2010; **76**(6): 1380–6.

24. Ribas-Maynou J, Garcia-Peiro A, Fernandez-Encinas A, Abad C, Amengual MJ, Prada E, Navarro J, Benet J. Comprehensive analysis of sperm DNA fragmentation by five different assays: TUNEL assay, SCSA, SCD test and alkaline and neutral Comet assay. *Andrology* 2013; **1**(5): 715–22.

25. Feijo CM, Esteves SC. Diagnostic accuracy of sperm chromatin dispersion test to evaluate sperm deoxyribonucleic acid damage in men with unexplained infertility. *Fertil Steril* 2014; **101**(1): 58–63. e53.

26. Majzoub A, Esteves SC, Gosálvez J, Agarwal A. Specialized sperm function tests in varicocele and the future of andrology laboratory. *Asian J Androl* 2016; **18**(2): 205–12.

27. Ni K, Steger K, Yang H, Wang H, Hu K, Zhang T, Chen B. A comprehensive investigation of sperm DNA damage and oxidative stress injury in infertile patients with subclinical, normozoospermic, and astheno/oligozoospermic clinical varicocoele. *Andrology* 2016; **4**(5): 816–24.

28. Spanò M, Bonde JP, Hjøllund HI, Kolstad HA, Cordelli E, Leter G. The Danish First Pregnancy Planner Study Team. Sperm chromatin damage impairs human fertility. *Fertil Steril* 2000; **73**: 43–50.

29. Zini A, Fischer MA, Sharir S, Shayegan B, Phang D, Jarvi K. Prevalence of abnormal sperm DNA denaturation in fertile and infertile men. *Urology* 2002; **60**(6): 1069–72.

30. Cho CL, Agarwal A. Role of sperm DNA fragmentation in male factor infertility: a systematic review. *Arab J Urol* 2017; **16**(1): 21–34.

31. Rai R, Regan L. Recurrent miscarriage. *Lancet* 2006; **368** (9535): 601–11.

32. Kirkman-Brown JC, De Jonge C. Sperm DNA fragmentation in miscarriage: a promising diagnostic, or a test too far? *Reprod Biomed Online* 2017; **34**(1): 3–4.

33. Practice Committee of the American Society for Reproductive Medicine. The clinical utility of sperm DNA integrity testing: a guideline. *Fertil Steril* 2013; **99**: 673–7.

34. Practice Committee of the American Society for Reproductive Medicine. Evaluation and treatment of recurrent pregnancy loss: a committee opinion. *Fertil Steril* 2012; **98**(5): 1103–11.

35. Zini A. Are sperm chromatin and DNA defects relevant in the clinic? *Syst Biol Reprod Med* 2011; **57**(1–2): 78–85.

36. Sharma R, Ahmad G, Esteves SC, Agarwal A. Terminal deoxynucleotidyl transferase dUTP nick end labeling (TUNEL) assay using bench top flow cytometer for evaluation of sperm DNA fragmentation in fertility laboratories: protocol, reference values, and quality control. *J Assist Reprod Genet* 2016; **33**(2): 291–300.

37. Ribeiro S, Sharma R, Gupta S, Cakar Z, De Geyter C, Agarwal A. Inter- and intra-laboratory standardization of TUNEL assay for assessment of sperm DNA fragmentation. *Andrology* 2017; **5**(3): 477–85.

38. Gupta S, Sharma R, Agarwal A. Inter-and intra-laboratory standardization of TUNEL assay for assessment of sperm DNA fragmentation. *Curr Protoc Toxicol* 2017; **74**: 1–16.

39. Anzar M, He L, Buhr MM, Kroetsch TG, Pauls KP. Sperm apoptosis in fresh and cryopreserved bull semen detected by flow cytometry and its relationship with fertility. *Biol Reprod* 2002; **66**(2): 354–60.

40. Ribeiro SC, Muratori M, De Geyter M, De Geyter C. TUNEL labeling with BrdUTP/anti-BrdUTP greatly underestimates the level of sperm DNA fragmentation in semen evaluation. *PLOS One* 2017; **12**(8): e0181802.

41. Domínguez-Fandos D, Camejo MI, Ballescà JL, Oliva R. Human sperm DNA fragmentation: correlation of TUNEL results as assessed by flow cytometry and optical microscopy. *Cytometry* 2007; **71**: 1011–18.

42. Muratori M, Piomboni P, Baldi E, Filimberti E, Pecchioli P, Moretti E, Gambera L, Baccetti B, Biagiotti R, Forti G, Maggi M. Functional and ultrastructural features of DNA-fragmented human sperm. *J Androl* 2000; **21**: 903–12.

43. Muratori M, Maggi M, Spinelli S, Filimberti E, Forti G, Baldi E. Spontaneous DNA fragmentation in swim-up selected human spermatozoa during long term incubation. *J Androl* 2003; **24**: 253–62.

44. Lopes S, Jurisicova A, Sun J-G, Casper RF. Reactive oxygen species: potential cause for DNA fragmentation in human spermatozoa. *Hum Reprod* 1998; **13**(4): 896–900.

45. Barroso G, Morshedi M, Oehninger S. Analysis of DNA fragmentation, plasma membrane translocation of phosphatidylserine and oxidative stress in human spermatozoa. *Hum Reprod* 2000; **15**: 1338–44.

46. Donnelly ET, O'Connell M, McClure N, Lewis SE. Differences in nuclear DNA fragmentation and mitochondrial integrity of semen and prepared human spermatozoa. *Hum Reprod* 2000; **15**: 1552–61.

47. Gandini L, Lombardo F, Paoli D, Caponecchia L, Familiari G, Verlengia C, Dondero F, Lenzi A. Study of apoptotic DNA fragmentation in human spermatozoa. *Hum Reprod* 2000; **15**: 830–9.

48. Oosterhuis GJ, Mulder AB, Kalsbeek-Batenburg E, Lambalk CB, Schoemaker J, Sergerie M, Ouhilal S, Bissonnette F, Brodeur J, Bleau G. Lack of association between smoking and DNA fragmentation in the spermatozoa of normal men. *Hum Reprod* 2000; **15**: 1314–21.

49. Sergerie M, Ouhilal S, Bissonnette F, Brodeur J, Bleau G. Lack of association between smoking and DNA fragmentation in the spermatozoa of normal men. *Hum Reprod* 2000; **15**: 1314–21.

50. Ramos L, Wetzels AM. Low rates of DNA fragmentation in selected motile human spermatozoa assessed by the TUNEL assay. *Hum Reprod* 2001; **16**: 1703–7.

51. Zini A, Bielecki R, Phang D, Zenzes MT. Correlations between two markers of sperm DNA integrity, DNA denaturation and DNA fragmentation, in fertile and infertile men. *Fertil Steril* 2001; **75**: 674–7.

52. Duran EH, Morshedi M, Taylor S, Oehninger S. Sperm DNA quality predicts intrauterine insemination outcome: a prospective cohort study. *Hum Reprod* 2002; **17**: 3122–8.

53. Sakkas D, Moffatt O, Manicardi GC, Mariethoz E, Tarozzi N, Bizzaro D. Nature of DNA damage in ejaculated human spermatozoa and the possible involvement of apoptosis. *Biol Reprod* 2002; **66**: 1061–7.

54. Shen HM, Dai J, Chia SE, Lim A, Ong CN. Detection of apoptotic alterations in sperm in subfertile patients and their correlations with sperm quality. *Hum Reprod* 2002; **17**: 1266–73.

55. Benchaib M, Braun V, Lornage J, Hadj S, Salle B, Lejeune H, Guérin JF. Sperm DNA fragmentation decreases the pregnancy rate in an assisted reproductive technique. *Hum Reprod* 2003; **18**: 1023–8.

56. Carrell DT, Liu L, Peterson CM, Jones KP, Hatasaka HH, Erickson L, Campbell B. Sperm DNA fragmentation is increased in couples with unexplained recurrent pregnancy loss. *Arch Androl* 2003; **49**: 49–55.

57. Erenpreisa J, Erenpreiss J, Freivalds T, Slaidina M, Krampe R, Butikova J, Ivanov A, Pjanova D. Toluidine blue test for sperm DNA integrity and elaboration of image cytometry algorithm. *Cytometry* 2003; **52**: 19–27.

58. Erenpreiss J, Jepson K, Giwercman A, Tsarev I, Erenpreisa J, Spano M. Toluidine blue cytometry test for sperm DNA conformation: comparison with the flow cytometric sperm chromatin structure and TUNEL assays. *Hum Reprod* 2004; **19**: 2277–82.

59. Lachaud C, Tesarik J, Cañadas ML, Mendoza C. Apoptosis and necrosis in human ejaculated spermatozoa. *Hum Reprod* 2004; **19**: 607–10.

60. Tesarik J, Greco E, Mendoza C. Late, but not early, paternal effect on human embryo development is related to sperm DNA fragmentation. *Hum Reprod* 2004; **19**: 611–15.

61. Greco E, Iacobelli M, Rienzi L, Ubaldi F, Ferrero S, Tesarik J. Reduction of the incidence of sperm DNA fragmentation by oral antioxidant treatment. *J Androl* 2005; **26**: 349–53.

62. Stahl O, Eberhard J, Jepson K, Spano M, Cwikiel M, Cavallin Stahl E, Giwercman A. The impact of testicular carcinoma and its treatment on sperm DNA

integrity. *Cancer* 2004; **100**: 1137–44.

63. Sépaniak S, Forges T, Monnier-Barbarino P. Cigarette smoking and fertility in women and men. *Gynecol Obstet Fertil* 2006; **34**: 945–9.

64. Chohan KR, Griffin JT, Lafromboise M, De Jonge CJ, Carrell DT. Comparison of chromatin assays for DNA fragmentation evaluation in human sperm. *J Androl* 2006; **27**: 53–9.

65. de Paula TS, Bertolla RP, Spaine DM, Cunha MA, Schor N, Cedenho AP. Effect of cryopreservation on sperm apoptotic deoxyribonucleic acid fragmentation in patients with oligozoospermia. *Fertil Steril* 2006; **86**: 597–600.

66. Aoki VW, Emery BR, Liu L, Carrell DT. Protamine levels vary between individual sperm cells of infertile human males and correlate with viability and DNA integrity. *J Androl* 2006; **27**: 890–8.

67. Spermon JR, Ramos L, Wetzels AM, Sweep CG, Braat DD, Kiemeney LA, Witjes JA. Sperm integrity pre- and post-chemotherapy in men with testicular germ cell cancer. *Hum Reprod* 2006; **21**: 1781–6.

68. Sakamoto Y, Ishikawa T, Kondo Y, Yamaguchi K, Fujisawa M. The assessment of oxidative stress in infertile patients with varicocele. *BJU Int* 2008; **101**: 1547–52.

69. Muratori M, Forti G, Baldi E. Comparing flow cytometry and fluorescence microscopy for analyzing human sperm DNA fragmentation by TUNEL labeling. *Cytometry A* 2008; **73**(9): 785–7.

70. Sharma R, Gupta S, Henkel R, Agarwal A. Critical evaluation of two models of flow cytometers for the assessment of sperm DNA fragmentation: an appeal for performance verification. *Asian J Androl* 2019; **21**(5): 438–44.

71. Cissen M, Wely MV, Scholten I, Mansell S, Bruin JP, Mol BW, Braat D, Repping S, Hamer G. Measuring sperm DNA fragmentation and clinical outcomes of medically assisted reproduction: a systematic review and meta-analysis. *PLOS One* 2016; **11**: 165125.

72. Mitchell LA, De Iuliis GN, Aitken RJ. The TUNEL assay consistently underestimates DNA damage in human spermatozoa and is influenced by DNA compaction and cell vitality: development of an improved methodology. *Int J Androl* 2011; **34**(1): 2–13.

73. Muratori M, Tamburrino L, Marchiani S, Cambi M, Olivito B, Azzari C, Forti G, Baldi E. Investigation on the origin of sperm DNA fragmentation: role of apoptosis, immaturity and oxidative stres. *Mol Med* 2015; **21**(1): 109–22.

74. Oleszczuk K, Augustinsson L, Bayat N, et al. Prevalence of high DNA fragmentation index in male partners of unexplained infertile couples. *Androl* 2013; **1**: 357–60.

75. Saleh RA, Agarwal A, Nada EA, et al. Negative effects of increased sperm DNA damage in relation to seminal oxidative stress in men with idiopathic and male factor infertility. *Fertil Steril* 2003; **79**(Suppl. 3): 1597–605.

Chapter 20

DNA Damage: Sperm Chromatin Structure Assay

Sperm Chromatin Structure Assay Test on its Fortieth Anniversary

Don Evenson

20.1 Introduction

The year 2020 is the fortieth anniversary of the introduction of the concept of "sperm DNA fragmentation" as related to human and animal male factor fertility. This concept was introduced by Donald Evenson in a *Science* article (1980) that also introduced the first test for its detection, the Sperm Chromatin Structure Assay (SCSA®). Sperm DNA fragmentation is defined as sperm single and double DNA strand breaks. Experiments on bulls, boars and stallions clearly show that the SCSA test identifies the highest fertile animals. Thousands of measurements on clinical human semen samples also clearly show that when more than 25 percent of sperm (DFI pecentage) in an ejaculate have measurable DNA fragmentation the probability of live birth pregnancy is significantly diminished. SCSA data on percentage DFI and Mean DFI are the same, meaning that the SCSA test measures the total of sperm DNA strand breaks detected with acridine orange staining.

20.2 Sperm Chromatin Structure Assay History 1980–2020

In 2011 John Aitken wrote the Forward to the book *Sperm Chromatin: Biological and Clinical Applications in Male Infertility and Assisted Reproduction*, edited by A. Zini and A. Agarwal. Aitken wrote: "The impetus to study the composition and integrity of sperm chromatin from a clinical perspective can be traced back to the pioneering studies of Don Evenson, who not only initiated research in this area long before it became fashionable but also pioneered one of the major analytical techniques used in assessment of sperm chromatin, the Sperm Chromatin Structure Assay (SCSA). This assay has now become the industry standard against all other techniques."

Going forward to 2017 for an assessment on the value of our anniversary finding there is a quote from C. O'Neill and G. Palermo writing: "Many assays have been introduced into male infertility testing over the past two decades regarding varying aspects of spermatozoal competence. However, none have provided more clinically relevant data and insight into male fertility potential than the study of DNA fragmentation in the male gamete" [1].

Going to PubMed and entering our coined term "Sperm DNA fragmentation" yields 2400 manuscripts. Entering "Sperm Chromatin Structure Assay" yields 804 manuscripts. Our pioneering SCSA clinical paper [2] is among the top three papers ever cited from Human Reproduction. The evidence is clear, the SCSA test has a highly significant impact on the outcome for patients struggling with infertility.

The SCSA test has been extensively evaluated and validated for biochemical and fertility outcome soundness. Sperm from many hundreds of animals exposed to a variety of agents and environmental conditions have been analyzed to understand the SCSA test. On this fortieth anniversary of the SCSA test it can be solidly stated that the SCSA test is the most statistically robust assay for understanding the concepts of sperm DNA fragmentation.

20.3 The Sperm Chromatin Structure Assay Test

The original SCSA test [3] used heating of sperm (100^0C/five minutes) to open the sperm nuclear DNA strands at sites of single (ss) and double (ds) DNA breaks. These DNA strand breaks are captured by staining with fluorescent acridine orange (AO). AO intercalated into ds DNA fluoresces green while AO stained ss DNA collapses into a crystal that upon

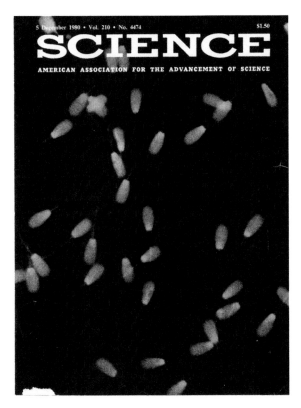

Figure 20.1 Cover of *Science* (1980) showing AO stained heated bull sperm.

20.4 The Sperm Chromatin Structure Assay Test Protocol

Switching from heating of sperm to the new acid denaturation protocol is done as per the following and has been described [5–7]. Individual frozen semen samples are thawed in a 37^0C water bath just until all ice has melted and then immediately diluted with TNE buffer (0.01M TRIS, 0.15 M NaCl, 1 mM EDTA, 4°C) to a final concentration of $1–2 \times 10^6$ sperm/mL. A 200 μL sperm suspension is admixed with 400 μL acid solution (0.1 percent Triton X-100, 0.15 M NaCl, and 0.08 N HCl, pH 1.20, 4°C) for 30 seconds followed by addition of 1.20 mL of acridine orange (AO) staining solution (containing 6 μg chromatographically purified AO (Polysciences Inc., Warrington, Pennsylvania) per mL of AO buffer (370 mL of stock 0.1 M citric acid, 630 mL of stock 0.2 M Na2HPO4 disodium hydrogen phosphate , 1 mM disodium EDTA. 0.15 M NaCl, pH 6.0, 4°C) as previously described in detail [6, 7]. Individual samples are placed into a flow cytometer (for our lab an Ortho Diagnostics L30 flow cytometer (FCM)) and after ~2 minutes of hydrodynamic equilibration of sample and sheath flow, 5000 sperm are measured at rates of ≤250 cells/second. All samples are measured independently twice. The mean values of the two independent measurements are then calculated. These mean data are processed through SCSAsoft® software (or equivalent) to produce a clinical report. These reports are sent back to the clinics via a secured WEB address.

Figure 20.2 shows SCSA raw data obtained by the acid denaturation protocol and processed though our SCSAsoft software.

Very importantly, all semen samples are measured by **exactly** the same strict protocol. Prior to measurements, laser focus is accomplished by maximizing red and green fluorescence values of fluorescent polystyrene beads [7]. Also, a positive (high percentage DFI) and a negative (low percentage DFI) semen sample are measured to verify the results as previously established. Then a reference semen sample from a set made up with hundreds of samples of small aliquots stored in LN_2 are used to set the red and green photomultipliers tubes to the same (±5/1024 channels) X, Y coordinates; approximately 540/1024 green versus 130/1024 red. This setting allows the capture of high DNA stainable (HDS) sperm. When one set of reference samples is nearly depleted, another set is

exposure to 488 nm light has a metachromatic shift from green to red fluorescence as seen in the *Science* cover (Figure 20.1).

While many have tried to quantitate sperm DNA fragmentation with light microscopy of AO stained sperm [4], it is now clear that due to many technical problems this can not reliably by done by light microscopy [5] but is, however, very accurately accomplished by flow cytometry [2, 6].

This *Science* article [3] showed the increased shift from green to red fluorescence in sperm from sub-infertile bulls and humans. Sub-fertile bulls and infertility clinic patients had 2.6x and 1.6x increased mean alpha t (Mean DFI) respectively, relative to highly fertile bulls and men. These data were very encouraging for the prospect of using the SCSA test in the human infertility clinic; however, before using this new test in the highly sensitive area of human infertility, this test was evaluated in numerous ways including toxicology, reproductive biology and animal fertility experiments.

193

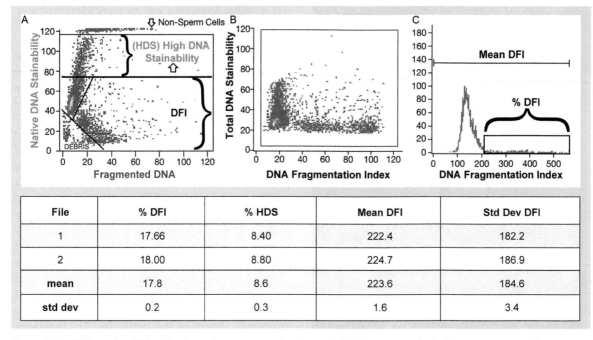

Figure 20.2 SCSA test data. **A)** Raw data from a flow cytometer showing each of 5000 sperm as a single dot on a scattergram. Y axis = green fluorescence with 1024 gradations (channels) of DNA stainability. X axis = red fluorescence with 1024 gradations of red fluorescence (ss DNA). Axes shown are 1024/10. Dotted line at Y = 75 marks the upper boundary of DNA staining of normal sperm chromatin; above that line are sperm (dots) with partially uncondensed chromatin allowing more DNA stainability (HDS sperm). Bottom left corner shows gating out of seminal debris. **B)** Raw data from left panel are converted by SCSAsoft® software (or equivalent) to red/red + green fluorescence. This transforms the angled sperm display in left panel to a vertical pattern that is often critical for accurately delineating the percentage of sperm with fragmented DNA. Y axis = total DNA stainability versus X axis = red/red + green fluorescence (DFI). **C)** Frequency histogram of data from middle panel showing computer gating into percentage DFI and Mean DFI. Bottom box. SCSAsoft calculations of mean of two independent measures of: percentage DFI, percentage HDS, mean DFI and SD DFI. **Note:** Mean DFI are presented here with range from 0 to 1024 flow cytometer channels. Some studies have shown this in a range from 0 to 1; e.g. 0.22.

File	% DFI	% HDS	Mean DFI	Std Dev DFI
1	17.66	8.40	222.4	182.2
2	18.00	8.80	224.7	186.9
mean	17.8	8.6	223.6	184.6
std dev	0.2	0.3	1.6	3.4

made, even if from a different individual with different mean red (X) and green (Y) values. This is accomplished by first measuring the previous reference sample, then the new reference semen sample is measured at the same red/green photomultiplier gains and noting the new mean red and green fluorescence values. In this fashion, samples measured years ago can be measured again with the new reference sample and obtain the near exact same results [7].

20.5 Examples of Sperm Chromatin Structure Assay Validation Experiments

20.5.1 Toxicology

Triethylenemelamine, a trifunctional alkylating agent, has a highly negative effect on mammalian spermatogenesis as seen in Figure 20.3. For the purpose of this chapter, two important factors were learned about the SCSA test from our study on TEM treated mice [8].

1. Fresh sperm and frozen/thawed sperm produce the same near exact results.
2. Measurements made of freshly isolated sperm at repeated times following toxicant exposure provided the same results as when aliquots of the frozen and stored samples were measured months later; thus showing that the flow cytometer variables can be repeated with exacting results.

20.5.2 Human Air Pollution

Since the 1950s the residents of Teplice, Czech Republic, had been exposed to high levels of air pollution generated from the combustion of high-sulfur coal used for local industry and home heating. The air pollution was severe during the winter when climate inversion smog conditions existed. Infertility and miscarriage were a significant problem. The Czech Republic government and the US EPA came in to evaluate the problem. The study protocol had semen

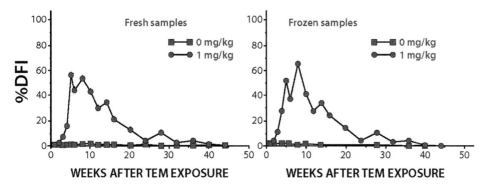

Figure 20.3 Epididymal sperm from mice treated with triethylenemelamine (TEM) and over 45 weeks harvested with one fresh sample measured at the time of isolation and frozen/thawed aliquots measured months later.

SCSA and Air Pollution

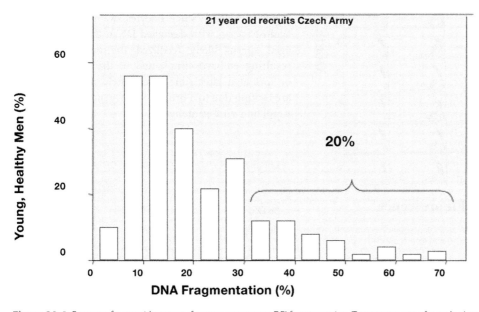

Figure 20.4 Percent of men with extent of sperm percentage DFI fragmentation. Twenty percent of men had pathological (>30 percent DFI) levels of DNA fragmentation.

sample testing of young men over two years that included both winter-time smog and summer-time clean air exposure. Figure 20.4 shows that the Teplice donors had very poor SCSA percentage DFI data during wintertime smog exposure [9]. While the great majority of semen samples should normally have been in the 5–10 percent DFI range, the majority of these samples were above that level, with 20 percent being in the pathological range above 30 percent DFI.

Interestingly, semen samples from Teplice men exposed to the winter-time air pollution had an increase of sperm motility.

20.5.3 Reproductive Biology

Analysis of monthly semen samples obtained over eight consecutive months from donor men [10] showed that although SCSA data are heterogeneous

195

among men, individual men provide highly repeatable SCSA data from month to month as seen in Figure 20.5.

Experimental studies on animal reproduction have some great advantages over human studies that require more ethical standards. One of the best means to evaluate the fertility potential of sperm from different animals is done with heterospermic insemination. For example, equal numbers of motile sperm can be mixed from e.g. a black and white bull, and that mixture used to inseminate 100 cows. If 80 black and 20 white calves are born that would clearly show the superiority of the sperm from the black bull. Figure 20.6 shows that SCSA data of percentage DFI and SD DFI are highly correlated with the known competitive index of bulls [11].

Another study [12] with boars provided data showing that SCSA data are significantly correlated with the number of successful pregnancy outcomes. Also, boars with poorer percentage DFI had fewer pigs/litter likely due to death of embryos as seen in Table 20.1. Semen from 18 sexually mature boars with known fertility information was bred to 1867 females. Boar fertility was defined by farrow rate (FR) and average total number of pigs born (ANB) per litter of gilts and sows mated to individual boars. Fertility data were compiled for 1867 matings across the 18 boars (Table 20.1).

It is of great interest to note the significant correlations between DFI values and average number of piglets per liter. Since oocytes do not discriminate against sperm with damaged DNA, these DNA damaged sperm likely fertilized the oocytes and the resulting embryos implanted in the female only to be lost at a later time when likely needed proteins are lacking due to a broken DNA/gene(s) required for supplying vital proteins.

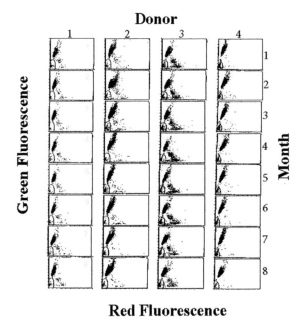

Donor

Green Fluorescence

Month

Red Fluorescence

Figure 20.5 Sperm Chromatin Structure Assay cytograms of semen samples from four donors over eight consecutive months of collections.

Table 20.1 Boar Fertility and Average Pigs Born versus Sperm Chromatin Structure Assay Percentage DFI and Mean DFI

	FR	APB
% DFI	−0.55[a]	−0.54[a]
SD DFI	−0.67[b]	−0.54[c]

[a] $P < 0.01$ [b] $P < 0.002$ [c] $P < 0.02$

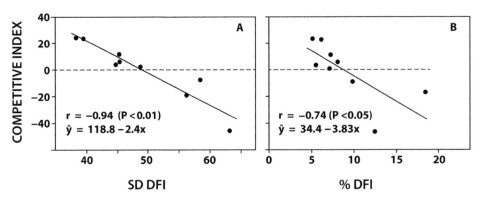

A — $r = -0.94$ $(P < 0.01)$; $\hat{y} = 118.8 - 2.4x$

B — $r = -0.74$ $(P < 0.05)$; $\hat{y} = 34.4 - 3.83x$

COMPETITIVE INDEX

SD DFI

% DFI

Figure 20.6 Bull heterospermic competitive index versus SCSA SD DFI and SCSA percentage DFI of bulls with different phenotypes.

20.6 Sperm Chromatin Structure Assay for Humans

20.6.1 Sperm Chromatin Structure Assay and Pregnancy by Intercourse

The first definitive study for SCSA-defined clinical utility was done in the "Georgetown study" [2]. This study uniquely evaluated 165 couples, without known female infertility factors, who had time sensitive intercourse over 12 menstrual cycles. During the first three months biochemical testing for pregnancy was performed. SCSA data from male partners of 73 couples (group 1) who achieved pregnancy during months 1–3 were compatible with "high fertility". The SCSA values from 118 semen samples from 40 couples achieving pregnancy in months 4–12 were significantly (p<0.01) higher than those from couples achieving pregnancy within three menstrual cycles. Also, the 89 semen samples obtained from 32 couples not achieving pregnancy by month 12 had highly significant (p<0.001) increase in SCSA values. Finally, the 115 semen samples from men attending an infertility clinic had highly significant (p<0.001) increases in SCSA values; the percentage DFI was 115 percent greater from these men in comparison to couples achieving pregnancy within three months (Table 20.2).

20.6.2 High DNA Stainable Sperm

Since AO stained histone complexed DNA stains 2.3× more than protamine complexed DNA [13], this HDS sperm fraction with increased histones is easy to detect with the SCSA test (Figure 20.7). Flow cytometer sorted HDS population of human sperm showed that these sperm nuclei are more rounded, consistent with lack of full sperm chromatin maturity [5, 14]. These sorted HDS sperm were negative for pH 10 Comets and thus they contained no DNA strand breaks (percentage DFI) [5]. These

sorting experiments also showed that SCSA defined moderate level DFI sperm had DNA strand breaks but also a totally normal morphology [5,14], meaning that picking up a sperm for ICSI with a normal morphology is not a guarantee of normal DNA integrity.

Abnormal sperm nuclear condensation involves a complex sequence of events including topological rearrangements, transition of DNA binding proteins, transcriptional alterations, nucleosomal structure loss and abnormal condensation of chromatin resulting in disturbances in the organization of genomic material in the sperm nuclei and decreasing sperm functional ability. Ultimately this reduces normal fertilization, affects early embryonic development and interferes with the primary mission of the sperm DNA which is reliable transmission of paternal genetic information.

Interestingly, while it is known that abnormally high levels of HDS lead to early embryo death and miscarriage [2, 15, 16], the rationale for this is controversial with suggestions that it is related to increased aneuploidy [15, 16]. Alternatively, it is more likely related to abnormality of tertiary chromatin structure, thereby causing an abnormal read out of early embryo proteins needed for embryo growth and differentiation [17, 18]. Interestingly, while percentage DFI increases with age of men the percentage HDS goes down with age [16, 19].

20.6.3 Sperm Chromatin Structure Assay and Clinical Assisted Reproductive Technology Lab Pregnancies

1. **IUI.** The subsequent studies of Bungum et al. [20] showed that DFI >25 percent reduced IUI pregnancy success to almost nil.
2. **IVF/ICSI.** The study of Oleszczuk et al. [21] summarized SCSA outcomes on 1633 IVF and ICSI cycles. The percentage DFI values were

Table 20.2 Sperm Chromatin Structure Assay Outcomes from the Georgetown Study and Infertility Clinic

Pregnancy Outcomes	n	X DFI	SD DFI	% DFI	%HDS
PG in 3 months	73	234.6	137.9	11.2	8.95
PG 4–12 months	40	255.1[**]	157.9[**]	15.5[**]	8.78
No Pregnancy	31	270.3[***]	173.7[***]	17.2[***]	15.03[***]
Infertility Clinic	115	308.6[***]	194.2[***]	24.0[***]	

placed into four intervals: DFI<10 percent (reference group), 10 percent≤DFI≤20 percent, 20percent<DFI≤30 percent, DFI>30 percent. For the three latter intervals, the following outcomes of IVF/ICSI procedures were analyzed in relation to the reference group: fertilization, good quality embryo, pregnancy, miscarriage, and live births. In the standard IVF group, a significant negative association between DFI and fertilization rate was found. When calculated per ovum pick up (OPU), odds ratios (ORs) for at least one good quality embryo (GQE) were lower in the standard IVF group if DFI>20 percent. OR for live birth calculated per OPU was significantly lower in the standard IVF group if DFI>20 percent (OR, 0.61; 95 percent CI: 0.38–0.97; p=0.04). No such associations were seen in the ICSI group. OR for live birth by ICSI compared to IVF were statistically significantly higher for DFI>20 percent (OR, 1.7; 95 percent CI: 1.0–2.9; p=0.05). OR for miscarriage was significantly increased for DFI>40 percent (OR, 3.8; 95 percent CI: 1.2–12; p=0.02). These results suggest that ICSI may be a preferred method of in vitro treatment in cases with high DFI. Extensive SCSA data on infertility

patients have shown that when a patient has <20 percent DFI, such semen sample with regards to sperm DNA integrity is consistent with normal pregnancy by intercourse or IUI unless other classical semen analysis shows one or two abnormal scores which decrease the odds for pregnancy [22]. Decreasing odds are present with >20 percent DFI and at 25 percent DFI the odds become poor for pregnancy by intercourse or IUI. At 30 percent DFI, reasonable success requires

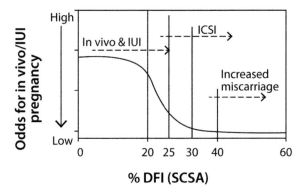

Figure 20.7 Odds for live birth versus percentage DFI.

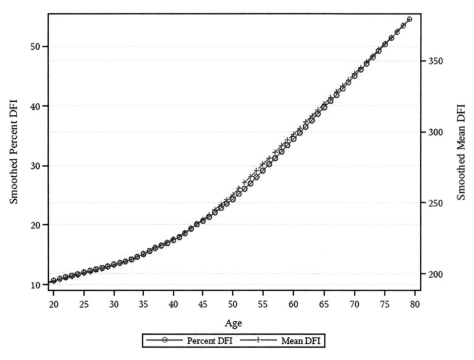

Figure 20.8 Percentage DFI versus Mean DFI (n=3K human semen samples).

ICSI. At 40 percent DFI the odds become very poor for pregnancy and increased odds for miscarriage. Values above 50 percent may rarely achieve pregnancy, but the odds are indeed poor. Figure 20.7 graphically summarizes the live birth thresholds for SCSA: the 20–25 percent DFI has been considered the "grey zone" [21–22], suggesting that fertility problems may start to occur when SCSA percentage DFI reaches this level. It is noted, however, that our SCSA diagnostic center has seen natural full-term pregnancy with up to 68 percent DFI. This observation illustrates that these percentage DFI clinical thresholds are statistical values and not absolute values.

Figure 20.7 summarizes the decreasing statistical chances of a full-term successful pregnancy with increasing SCSA percentage DFI of the male partner. Success begins to drop off at 15–20 percent DFI. Twenty-five percent DFI is considered the statistical threshold for in vivo and IUI fertilization and when IVF/ICSI should be used in the ART lab. Greater than 40 percent DFI significantly increases the risk for miscarriages.

20.7 Comparison of Percentage DFI versus Mean DFI

Percentage DFI is determined by visual computer gating of the sperm (dots) that correspond to increased red fluorescence due to single (ss) and double (ds) DNA strand breaks. Mean DFI is the measure in FCM channels (0–1024) of increased red fluorescence of the entire sperm population. As seen in Figure 20.8 the SCSA data show both the percentage DFI and Mean DFI.

For the first years of SCSA reporting the Mean DFI was used [e.g. 20, 22] to express the level of sperm DNA damage in the measured samples. Since it was easier for reproductive medicine personnel to understand percentage DFI, i.e. percent good versus percent bad sperm, we changed our quantitation of DNA damage to use of percentage DFI in both our research manuscripts and clinical reports. The question has been asked whether the percentage DFI accounts for the entirety of total DNA strand breaks. Figure 20.8 shows that the curves of percentage DFI and Mean DFI are the same thereby proving that the percentage DFI method accounts for the total of the sperm DNA breaks.

It is highly recommended that all users of the SCSA test use percentage DFI since the use of Mean DFI requires highly strict attention to being certain that the green and red fluorescence values of reference semen samples are the same for measurements of all clinical samples. It is known from published cytograms that some laboratories are not consistent in placing the reference sample with exactly the same (±5 channels) photomultiplier (PMT) gains for red and green fluorescence. Thus, it is strongly suggested that only percentage DFI be used to characterize SCSA-derived sperm DNA integrity.

20.8 Sperm Chromatin Structure Assay Testing with Different Flow Cytometers in Different Locations

Since there are a variety of flow cytometers worldwide it was important to determine whether different types of instruments could produce the same results. Figure 20.9

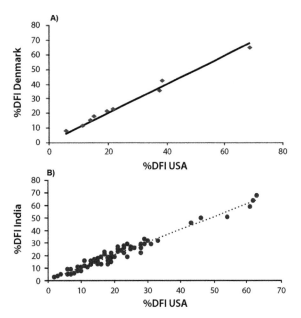

Figure 20.9 Correlations between SCSA data obtained on three continents. **A)** Correlation between SCSA percentage DFI on ten frozen/thawed human samples on two different brands of flow cytometers (Cytofluorograf 30; Ortho Diagnostics) at SCSA Diagnostics, Inc. in South Dakota, USA and (FACScan, Beckton Dickenson) at the University of Copenhagen, Denmark. (Correlation: $R^2=0.961$). **B)** Correlation between SCSA percentage DFI on 57 frozen/thawed human samples on two different brands of flow cytometers (Cytofluorograf 30; Ortho Diagnostics) at SCSA Diagnostics, Inc. in South Dakota and a Beckman Coulter flow cytometer in the Andrology Lab, Coimbatore, India. (Correlation: $R^2=0.9812$)

199

shows that data on frozen/thawed semen samples from humans measured on different types of flow cytometers in three countries are nearly exactly the same.

20.9 Conclusions

The SCSA test has proven to be a very rapid, highly reliable and statistically robust test to measure sperm DNA integrity as related to pregnancy outcomes. The SCSA test is considered to measure the total of sperm DNA fragmentation. It is the most direct DNA fragmentation assay in that starting with a fresh or frozen/thawed raw semen sample, SCSA data on 5000 sperm can be obtained in less than 10 minutes. Using raw semen samples assures that all cell types present are measured, and none lost or biochemically changed by experimental manipulations. Somatic cells are also measured as non-sperm cells as seen in Figure 20.2. Being assured that frozen/thawed samples produce the exact data as fresh samples means that semen samples obtained anywhere in the world can be frozen and shipped by air carriers such as Federal Express to a lab with expertise in SCSA testing. Likewise, samples frozen for various reasons, such as cryopreservation in sperm banks, can be retrieved and measured.

Importantly for the human infertility clinic, SCSA thresholds of sperm DNA fragmentation have been determined as seen in Figure 20.7 allowing couples striving for a pregnancy to help understand whether the male partner's sperm DNA quality is adequate to have a good probability of pregnancy success.

References

1. O'Neill CL, Palermo GD. A worldwide profile of the utilization of sperm DNA fragmentation testing in relation to reproductive outcome. *Transl Androl Urol* 2017; **6**: S320–S321.

2. Evenson DP, Jost LK, Zinaman MJ, Clegg E, Purvis K, de Angelis P, Clausen OP. Utility of the sperm chromatin structure assay (SCSA) as a diagnostic and prognostic tool in the human fertility clinic. *Hum Reprod* 1999; **14**: 1039–49.

3. Evenson DP, Darzynkiewicz Z, Melamed MR. Relation of mammalian sperm chromatin heterogeneity to fertility. *Science* 1980; **210**: 1131–3.

4. Tejada RI, Mitchell JC, Norman A, Marik JJ, Friedman S. A test for the practical evaluation of male fertility by acridine orange (AO) fluorescence. *Fertil Steril* 1984; **42**: 87–91.

5. Evenson DP. The Sperm Chromatin Structure Assay (SCSA®) and other sperm DNA fragmentation tests for evaluation of sperm nuclear DNA integrity as related to fertility. *Anim Reprod Sci* 2016; **169**: 56–75.

6. Evenson DP, Larson K, Jost LK. The sperm chromatin structure assay (SCSATM): clinical use for detecting sperm DNA fragmentation related to male infertility and comparisons with other techniques. *J Andrology* 2002; **23**: 25–43.

7. Evenson D. (2011) Sperm Chromatin Structure Assay (SCSA®): detailed protocol. In Zini A and Agarwal A, eds., *Sperm Chromatin: Biological and Clinical Applications in Male Infertility and Assisted Reproduction*. New York: Springer-Verlag, pp. 487–97.

8. Evenson DP, Baer RK, Jost LK. Long term effects of triethylenemelamine exposure on mouse testis cells and sperm chromatin structure assayed by flow cytometry. *Environ Mol Mutagen* 1989; **14**: 79–89.

9. Rubes J, Selevan S G, Evenson DP, Zudova D, Vozdova M, Zudova Z, Robbins WA, Perreault S D. Episodic air pollution is associated with increased DNA fragmentation in human sperm without other changes in semen quality. *Hum Reprod* 2005; **20**(10): 2776–83.

10. Evenson DP, Jost L, Baer R, Turner T, Schrader, S. Individuality of DNA denaturation patterns in human sperm as measured by the sperm chromatin structure assay. *Reprod Toxicol* 1991; **5**: 115–25.

11. Ballachey BE, Hohenboken WD, Evenson DP. Heterogeneity of sperm nuclear chromatin structure and its relationship to fertility of bulls. *Biol of Reprod* 1987; **36**: 915–25.

12. Didion BA, Kasperson KM, Wixon R, Evenson DP. Boar fertility and sperm chromatin structure status. *Retrosp Rep J Androl* 2009; **30**: 1–6.

13. Evenson DP, Darzynkiewicz Z, Jost L, Janca F, Ballachey B. Changes in accessibility of DNA to various fluorochromes during spermatogenesis. *Cytometry* 1986; **7**: 45–53.

14. Evenson DP, Tritle D. Characterization of SCSA resolved sperm populations by Comet assay and image analysis. IFFS 8th World Congress on Fertility and Sterility Abstract 2004.

15. Jerre E, Bungum M, Evenson D, Giwercman A. Sperm chromatin structure assay high DNA stainability sperm as a marker of early miscarriage after

intracytoplasmic sperm injection. *Fert Steril* 2019; **12**: 46–53.

16. Wyrobek AJ, Eskenazi B, Young S, Arnheim N, Tiemann-Boege I, Jabs EW, Glaser RL, Pearson FS, Evenson D. Advancing age has differential effects on DNA damage chromatin integrity, gene mutations, and aneuploidies in sperm. *Proc Natl Acad Sci* 2006; **103**: 9601–6.

17. Menezo Y, Clement P, Amar E. Evaluation of sperm DNA structure, fragmentation and decondensation: an essential tool in the assessment of male infertility. *Transl Androl Urol* 2017; **6**(Suppl. 4): S553–S556.

18. Cornet D, Cohen M, Clement A, Amar E, Fournols L, Clement P, Neveux P, Ménézo Y. Association between the MTHFR-C677T isoform and structure of sperm DNA. *J Assist Reprod Genet* 2017; **34**: 1283–8.

19. Evenson DP, Djira G, Kasperson K, Christianson J. Relationships between age of 25K men attending infertility clinics and SCSA defined sperm DNA and chromatin integrity. *Fertil Steril* 2020; **114**: 311–20.

20. Bungum M, Humaidan P, Axmon A, et al. Sperm DNA integrity assessment in prediction of assisted reproduction technology outcome. *Hum Reprod* 2007; **22**: 174–9.

21. Oleszczuk A, Giwercman A, Bungum M. Sperm chromatin structure assay in prediction of in vitro fertilization outcome. *Andrology* 2016; **4**: 290–6.

22. Erenpreiss J, Elzanaty S, Giwercman A. Sperm DNA damage in men from infertile couples. *Asian J Androl* 2008; **10** (5): 786–90.

23. Evenson DP. Evaluation of sperm chromatin structure and DNA strand breaks is an important part of clinical male fertility assessment. *Transl Androl Urol* 2016; **5**: 935–50.

Chapter 21

DNA Damage: COMET Assay

Luke Simon, Benjamin R. Emery, Douglas T. Carrell

21.1 Introduction

Sperm are highly specialized cells, evolved to function as vehicles for the transport of the paternal genome to the oocyte. The sperm cell is characterized by a distinct head, mid-piece and tail, structured for a streamlined function. The sperm head consists of the haploid paternal genome (23 chromosomes), packed in a specific tight manner with the help of specialized proteins called protamines. The mid-piece consists of the centrosome and mitochondria, organelles that provide energy for sperm propulsion from the tail. The unique sperm structure, complimented with its motility, helps the sperm to swim through the male and female reproductive tract and penetrate the egg. Therefore, the primary function of the sperm is to successfully deliver the paternal genome to the oocyte.

Abnormalities in the form of DNA strand breaks, Y chromosome microdeletions, alterations in chromosome number, and distorted epigenetic regulation have been reported in mature sperm and such sperm carrying the abnormal sperm chromatin are known to be delivered to the oocyte [1]. Hence, in recent years the characterization of such sperm chromatin abnormalities has gained importance in an effort to establish a molecular association to male reproductive health. A number of research groups worldwide have studied sperm DNA fragmentation, and DNA strand breaks are considered as the common property of sperm and are widely associated with male reproductive health and assisted reproductive treatment success [2]. There are a variety of tests available to measure the level of DNA strand breaks in sperm and the most commonly used tests are the Comet assay, Terminal deoxyuridine Nick End Labelling (TUNEL) assay, Sperm Chromatin Structure Assay (SCSA), and the Sperm Chromatin Dispersion (SCD) Assay or Halo test. These tests could be broadly classified into direct methods (Comet and TUNEL assays), and indirect methods (SCSA and SCD assays) of sperm DNA strand breaks measurement [3]. Each of these assays determines different aspects of sperm DNA strand breaks. In this chapter, we discuss in detail the Comet assay and its clinical importance.

21.2 The Principle of the Comet Assay

The principle of the assay is based on the separation of broken DNA strands under the influence of an electric field facilitated by the charge and size of the broken strands [4]. Following separation, the large strands of intact DNA remain in the comet's head, whereas single- and double-stranded broken DNA fragments migrate into the comet's tail. Therefore, the sperm with high levels of DNA strand breaks show an intense comet tail and increased comet tail length [5]. Additional parameters have been used to increase the efficiency of the test such as the diameter of the nucleus, olive tail moment, and comet tail length [5].

Unlike in somatic cells, the sperm chromatin is organized in a specific manner with the help of protamines and such compact structure prevents the complete access to the DNA strand breaks.

In order to expose the broken DNA strands from the sperm nucleus, the Comet assay involves the following steps: sperm cells are mixed with agarose and layered on a microscopic slide. Detergents and a high salt concentration are used to lyse their cell membranes, and remove nuclear proteins (protamines and histones), which relax the DNA into a supercoiled nucleoid structure. The slides are then incubated in a neutral or an alkaline buffer: in the neutral buffer only DNA with double-strand damage is measured due to the lack of the separation of double-strand DNA, while in the alkaline buffer, single- and double-strand breaks are detectable due to the unwinding of the strands [5]. The nucleoids are then subjected to an electrophoretic field resulting in the migration of the broken strands of DNA through the agarose, resulting in a comet like structure when visualized using a fluorescent DNA binding dye. The non-fragmented DNA remains in the comet's head, whereas the fragmented DNA migrates, forming the comet's tail [5].

21.3 Advantages and Disadvantages of the Comet Assay

The Comet assay is inexpensive and on average it costs about one USD in chemicals and supplies to analyze a sample. It is considered as one of the most sensitive techniques available to measure sperm DNA damage. The alkaline Comet assay can be used in various cell types including sperm. Unlike other assays, the Comet assay requires only a few cells, approximately $<6 \times 10^4$ cells per slide. The results of each comet analyzed correspond to the level of DNA damage from individual cells [5].

In human sperm, the DNA is packed with specialized proteins called protamines. Complete decondensation or the removal of protamines is required to expose the fragmented DNA strands and such a step could be obtained only using Comet assay. The significance of the Comet assay in assessing male infertility and the clinical association with assisted reproductive treatment outcomes are discussed in Section 21.7 of this chapter.

There are a few disadvantages of the Comet assay. The assay lacks standardized protocols, which makes it difficult to fully understand and relate the results of different laboratories. The assay condition is known to damage the alkaline-labile sites, making it difficult to discriminate between endogenous and induced DNA breaks. Unlike sperm, somatic cells contain excess levels of RNA, in such case DNA damage can be overestimated by the Comet assay due to the presence of residual RNA which can increase the background intensity during analysis [6]. The assay is also criticized for underestimation of DNA damage due to entangling of DNA strands. In scenarios where the chromatin decondensation of sperm is incomplete, then the level of DNA damage will be underestimated. Overlapping comet tails decrease the accuracy of the assay, small tail fragments may be lost, and excessively small fragments are difficult to visualize [7]. The assay is laborious, can have a high level of inter-laboratory variation, and hence it is not commonly used under clinical settings [8].

21.4 Methodology of the Comet Assay

This is a modified and improved protocol commonly used [9]. All steps are performed at room temperature unless otherwise specified.

1. Prepare normal melting point (NMP) agarose gel (0.5 percent gel) in phosphate-buffered saline (PBS) and low melting point (LMP) agarose gel (0.25 percent gel) in PBS. Heat flasks in the microwave or burner to completely melt the agarose. Place the NMP gel in the 45°C water bath and the LMP gel in the 37°C water bath, until use.

2. Carefully pipette 200 μL of NMP agarose gel onto the fully frosted surface of the glass slide and immediately cover with a 24 × 50 mm coverslip. Leave the slides on the bench for 15 minutes to allow the agarose to solidify. The function of the NMP agarose layer is to hold the LMP agarose (containing sperm) firmly to the slide surface.

3. Adjust the concentration of sperm to 6×10^6/mL using PBS. Place, 10 μL of the sperm sample into a 0.5 mL Eppendorf tube. After the NMP agarose is solidified, add 75 μL of LMP agarose to the sperm in tube, mix gently using a pipette, add dropwise on top of the layer of NMP agarose gel and immediately cover with a coverslip. Allow the gel to solidify on the bench for 15 minutes. The LMP agarose acts as a platform to hold the sperm cells during the experimental process for electrophoresis.

4. Incubate the agarose slides without coverslip in lysis buffer (2.5 M NaCl, 100 mM Na$_2$EDTA, and 10 mM Tris–HCl, pH 10) with 1 percent Triton X-100 for one hour at 4°C. The function of the lysis buffer is to remove the cell wall of the sperm.

5. After lysis, remove the slides out of the jar, add dithiothreitol (DTT) to obtain a final concentration of 0.5 mM/mL, mix well and incubate for 30 minutes at 4°C. Following incubation with DTT, remove the slides out of the jar, add lithium diiodosalicyclate (LIS) to obtain a final concentration of 0.2 mM/mL, mix well and incubate for 90 minutes. Decondensation of sperm chromatin takes place with the help of DTT and LIS. During this process, the sperm nuclear proteins are denatured facilitating the decondensation process.

6. Remove the slides from the jar and place them in a horizontal gel electrophoresis tank with the gel surface facing upwards. For the alkaline Comet

assay, add freshly prepared alkaline electrophoresis buffer (300mM NaOH and 1mM EDTA, pH 13.0) and incubate the slides for 20 minutes. The high pH conditions help to unwind the double-strand DNA facilitating the exposure of single- and double-strand DNA breaks.

The neutral Comet assay is performed with neutral buffer (300 mM NaOAc and 100 mM Tris-HCl, pH 8.3), during which only double-strand DNA strand breaks are accessed due to the lack of the separation of DNA strands.

7. Electrophoresis is performed with alkaline buffer or neutral buffer corresponding to the type of assays. The electrophoresis is performed for 10 minutes by applying a current at 25 V (0.714 V/cm) adjusted to 300 mA by adding or removing (±1–20 mL) buffer in the tank. During this step, the broken DNA strands migrate towards the anode based on their size. Smaller fragments move faster than the larger fragments through the LMP agarose.

8. Following electrophoresis, drain the slides of any electrophoresis buffer, place them on a tray and flood them with three changes of neutralization buffer (0.4M Tris; pH 7.5) for five minutes each. This step reduces the pH of the gel towards neutral conditions in order to facilitate the binding of ethidium bromide (EtBr) stain to DNA fragments.

9. Drain the slides thoroughly to remove the neutralization buffer. Add 50 µL of fresh EtBr solution (20 µg/mL) to each slide and cover with a coverslip. View the slides using a fluorescence microscope with appropriate Comet software. Analyze 50–100 comets per slide.

The intact DNA stays in the Comet's head and the broken DNA fragments migrate into the Comet's tail, which can be visualized based on the intensity of fluorescence emitted by the Comets.

The comet software is designed to convert the intensity of fluorescence into parameters such as percent head DNA, percent tail DNA, tail extent moment, olive tail moment, and tail length. Most studies in the existing literature have used the percent tail DNA as the classic parameter to describe the level of fragmentation in the sperm cell [2, 10, 11, 12, 13]. The level of DNA fragmentation can be expressed in a numerical continuous value by obtaining a mean across all the comet's tail DNA of a given sample.

Alternately, each comet can be converted into a binary value based on the level of DNA fragmentation. For example, each Comet can be classified into damaged sperm (if the percent tail DNA exceeds 25 percent), resulting in the expression of the percentage of damaged or normal sperm present in a given sample [2, 13, 14].

21.5 Threshold Values

The level of DNA fragmentation measured by the alkaline Comet assay is always greater than the neutral Comet assay for a given sample as the alkaline version measures both single- and double-strand DNA breaks, whereas the neutral Comet assay measures only the double-strand DNA breaks. As a result, most studies in the existing literature have used alkaline Comet assay as a test to measure sperm DNA damage compared to the neutral version. Therefore, in this chapter we will discuss the clinical importance of DNA fragmentation as measured by the alkaline Comet assay.

Studies using the alkaline Comet assay have established two critical threshold values, first a diagnostic value to determine male infertility, determined by comparing the level of DNA fragmentation in the sperm of fertile and infertile men. A threshold value of 25 percent mean DNA fragmentation has been established to diagnose male infertility [2].This study reported that 95 percent of the fertile population had sperm DNA fragmentation below 25 percent, whereas only 10 percent of the infertile group had sperm DNA fragmentation below 25 percent, while the mean DNA fragmentation of sperm from infertile men was 57.92 ±2.67 percent and that of donors was 12.47±1.67 percent (p<0.001) [2]. Using this threshold value of 25 percent DNA fragmentation for the diagnosis of male infertility, the OR (95 percent CI) was 117.3 (12.73–2731.83). Men with DNA fragmentation more than this threshold value had a relative risk for infertility of 8.75 (95 percent CI: 4.48–17.08), with an area under the ROC of 0.970 cm^2, 63.6 percent sensitivity and 98.5 percent specificity [2].

A second threshold value was established in [14] to determine the success of assisted reproductive treatment (ART) by comparing the level of sperm DNA fragmentation in couples who were successful following ART with those who were unsuccessful. This study shows that the mean percentage of sperm DNA fragmentation was significantly higher in sperm from non-pregnant couples compared with that from pregnant couples undergoing in vitro fertilization (IVF) in both the native semen (51.7±23.6 percent versus 39.5±17.9 percent; p=0.004) and the density gradient centrifugation (DGC) prepared sperm for clinical use (36.8±21.6 percent versus 26.9±14.6 percent; p=0.01). Using the threshold values of 56 percent for the native semen and 44 percent for the DGC sperm, the odds ratios (95 percent CI) calculated for clinical pregnancies were 4.52 (1.79–11.92) and 6.20 (1.74–26.30), respectively.

In a later study, Simon et al. [15] established another threshold value using the parameter percentage of sperm with DNA fragmentation. In this clinical study, 82 percent sperm with DNA fragmentation (or 18 percent sperm with normal DNA) was established as a threshold to have high prognostic value to determine the chances of a clinical pregnancy, in vitro. Using this threshold value of 82 percent sperm DNA fragmentation, the OR (95 percent CI) to determine a clinical pregnancy was 7.00 (3.62–13.94). Men with DNA fragmentation higher than this threshold value had a relative risk for an unsuccessful clinical pregnancy of 1.89 (95 percent CI: 1.51–2.38), with 85.3 percent sensitivity and 45.0 percent specificity. The threshold value of 82 percent of sperm with DNA fragmentation is comparable to the threshold value of 56 percent mean Comet DNA fragmentation published previously by [14].

21.6 Laboratory and Clinical Interpretation of Threshold Values

The threshold value of 82 percent sperm with DNA fragmentation and the 56 percent threshold of mean sperm DNA fragmentation in the native semen established for the alkaline Comet assay is significantly higher than the threshold values used for SCSA and TUNEL assays [14]. This can be attributed to the sensitivity of the alkaline Comet assay, where in each sperm, the assay can measure variable levels of DNA fragmentation ranging from 0 to 100 percent. In sperm absent of DNA fragmentation – 100 percent of the DNA remains in the comet's head, whereas in sperm with extensive DNA fragmentation the entire nuclear DNA migrates to the comet's tail, leading to absence of comet's head [5].

The biology and structural organization of the sperm nucleus restricts the complete evaluation of sperm DNA fragmentation. The sperm nuclear DNA is crystalline in nature due to the supercoils of negatively charged DNA strands around positively charged protamines resulting in a highly compact DNA-protein complex. The SCSA and TUNEL assays permeabilize the cell wall to reach the nuclear DNA, which may not be sufficient for the evaluation of complete DNA fragmentation [13]. However, the sensitivity of the alkaline Comet assay to measure sperm DNA fragmentation can be attributed to its elaborate methodology [16]. During the Comet protocol, the sperm cells are lysed for an hour (step 4) resulting in the complete removal of cell wall. The decondensation of DNA (step 5) for two hours facilitates the removal of nuclear proteins. During this step the chemicals DTT and LIS reduce the disulphide bonds of protamines and nucleo-histones, thereby inducing relaxation of supercoiled DNA. The unwinding of the double-stranded DNA into single-strand at high pH conditions (step 6) facilitates the exposure of single-strand DNA breaks. These steps result in the complete exposure of double- and single-strand breaks throughout the entirety of relaxed chromatin, in contrast to other assays where perhaps more peripheral DNA strand breaks are determined [5].

The alkaline Comet assay has the ability to show a distinct distribution of damaged sperm populations ranging from 0 to 100 percent, which could be depicted graphically. The study by Simon et al. [5] demonstrated the distribution of sperm with DNA fragmentation by categorizing the scattering into three distinct patterns (A, B and C), based on the level of DNA fragmentation exhibited by the sperm population when depicted on a graphical plot. In type A distribution plot, the peak of sperm population lies between 0 and 25 percent, in type B distribution plot (25–75 percent) and in type C distribution plot (>75 percent). This study [5] reported that all the fertile donors exhibited type A distribution, while the infertile patient populations exhibited type A (45 percent), type B (41 percent) and type C (14 percent) distribution. Type B distribution could be further categorized into two types: B1 when the peak is between 26 and 50 percent damage and B2 when the peak is between 51 and 75 percent. The same study also showed that 66 percent of couples with type A distribution plot were successful after ART, whereas couples with type B1, B2 and C distribution plots achieved 56 percent, 44 percent and 33 percent clinical pregnancy, respectively [5]. Such distinct distribution patterns of sperm DNA fragmentation can be established only using the alkaline Comet assay as a result of its elaborated methodology to expose the DNA fragmentation present within the nucleus.

21.7 Clinical Significance of the Alkaline Comet Assay

DNA fragmentation is known to be more prevalent in the sperm of infertile men and may contribute to their declined fertility status. An increase in the level of DNA fragmentation in infertile men can be attributed to abnormal histone to protamine exchange, abnormal protamine content and ratio, and reduced antioxidant activity in the seminal plasma [17]. Dorostghoal et al. [18] reported that infertile men showed significantly higher percentage of sperm with fragmented DNA in comparison with fertile subjects using the neutral Comet assay. With the help of the alkaline Comet assay, Simon et al. [2] reported a significant difference in DNA fragmentation of sperm from infertile men compared to fertile donors. A recent meta-analysis including 28 studies drawn across all four sperm DNA fragmentation assays showed a significant increase in DNA fragmentation of sperm from infertile men [19]. This meta-analysis concluded that measurement of sperm DNA fragmentation is relevant for male infertility and higher accuracy in detecting sperm function compared to the conventional semen parameters [19].

A literature search resulted in the identification of nine studies associating sperm DNA fragmentation measured by the alkaline Comet assay with fertilization rate (Tables 21.1 and 21.2). The systematic review suggested that all studies including IVF cycles reported a significant inverse relationship between sperm DNA fragmentation and fertilization rate, but no such association was observed with studies using only ICSI cycles. The differential adverse effect of sperm DNA fragmentation on IVF and ICSI fertilization may be due to the fact that conventional IVF occurs "naturally" as a result of sperm-oocyte interaction, whereas during ICSI treatment this natural selection process is bypassed due to the manual selection and injection of morphologically normal and motile sperm by the embryologists, which may increase the probability of selecting sperm with low DNA fragmentation [20, 21]. Based on the available literature, we can conclude that sperm DNA fragmentation may be associated with IVF fertilization rate but not with ICSI fertilization rates.

The systematic review identified nine studies that associated sperm DNA fragmentation measured by the alkaline Comet assay with embryo quality and development following ART (Tables 21.1 and 21.2). Of these, seven studies reported an adverse effect, while two studies showed no effect. Interestingly, all studies involving IVF treatment showed an adverse effect of sperm DNA fragmentation on embryo quality, whereas two of the three studies involving ICSI treatment showed no effect. The available literature shows that sperm DNA fragmentation detected by the alkaline Comet assay was significantly associated with poor embryo quality in 78 percent of the studies in comparison to other assays, TUNEL, SCSA and SCD assays [24]. This association may be due to the increased sensitivity of the comet assays, where both single- and

Table 21.1 Summary of Studies Associating Sperm DNA Fragmentation Measured by the Alkaline Comet Assay with Fertilization Rate and Embryo Quality

	IVF		ICSI		IVF + ICSI	
	Studies (n)	Cycle (n)	Studies (n)	Cycle (n)	Studies (n)	Cycle (n)
Studies reporting no effect on fertilization rate	0	0	4	243	1	60
Studies reporting adverse effect on fertilization rate	3	362	0	0	1	238
Studies reporting no effect on embryo quality	0	0	2	138	0	0
Studies reporting adverse effect on embryo quality	4	402	1	28	2	298

IVF: in vitro fertilization; ICSI: intracytoplasmic sperm injection

Table 21.2 Description of Studies Associating Sperm DNA Fragmentation with Fertilization Rate and Embryo Quality

Study	ART	(n)	DF vs. FR	Day of ET	EQ marker	DF vs. EQ
[21]	ICSI	77	Non-significant	2		NA
[10]	IVF+ICSI	60	Non-significant	2	Development	Significant
[22]	ICSI	28	Non-significant	2	Development	Significant
[14]	IVF	219	Significant	2 or 3	Grade	Significant
	ICSI	116	Non-significant	2 or 3	Grade	Non-significant
[2]	IVF	70	Significant	2 or 3	Grade	Significant
[17]	IVF	73	Significant	2 or 3	Grade	Significant
	ICSI	22	Non-Significant	2 or 3	Grade	Non-Significant
[15]	IVF+ICSI	238	Significant	5	Grade and development	Significant
[23]	IVF	40	NA	3	Grade	Significant

IVF: in vitro fertilization; ICSI: intra-cytoplasmic sperm injection; ET: embryo transfer; EQ: embryo quality; DF: DNA fragmentation; FR: fertilization rate; NA: not available; n: number of cycles.

Table 21.3 Meta-Analysis Summary: Odds Ratios of Studies on Sperm DNA Fragmentation and Clinical Pregnancies Following Assisted Reproductive Technologies

ART	Number of studies (cycles)	Fixed effects model		Random effects model		Percentage of variation across studies I^2 (%)	Test of Heterogeneity p value
		OR (95%CI)	p value	OR (95%CI)	p value		
Combined all ART	7 (798)	3.34 (2.32–4.82)	<0.001	3.56 (1.78–7.09)	<0.001	65.5	0.008
IVF	3 (367)	5.86 (2.97–11.53)	<0.001	8.39 (2.16–32.55)	0.002	67.8	0.044
ICSI	2 (149)	1.84 (0.92–3.68)	0.085	1.84 (0.92–3.68)	0.085	0.0	0.669
IVF+ICSI	2 (282)	3.36 (1.92–5.86)	<0.001	2.27 (0.46–11.26)	0.315	81.0	0.018

ART: assisted reproduction technology; OR: odds ratio; CI: confidence interval

double-strand breaks are measured and the intensity of broken DNA in the comet tail is directly proportional to the level of actual damage. An increase in sperm DNA fragmentation could affect normal embryonic development by interfering with a variety of cellular processes, including DNA repair mechanisms, transcription, and cell cycle control [25].

A recent meta-analysis studied the effect of sperm DNA fragmentation assays on clinical pregnancies after ART [24]. A total of 56 studies were included in the meta-analysis, of which seven studies used the alkaline Comet assay to measure sperm DNA fragmentation, consisting of 798 ART treatment cycles.

The combined OR estimates for all the studies using the alkaline Comet assay were statistically significant (p<0.001) using both the fixed effects model and the random effects model (Tables 21.3 and 21.4). The relationship between sperm DNA fragmentation and clinical pregnancy by type of assisted reproduction stated a statistically significant correlation with IVF treatment type only and mixed studies including IVF + ICSI treatment. Based on the results, the meta-analysis concluded that there is sufficient evidence in the existing literature suggesting that sperm DNA fragmentation has a negative effect on clinical pregnancy following IVF and/or ICSI treatment [24].

Table 21.4 Diagnostic Properties of Studies on Sperm DNA Fragmentation Measured Using Alkaline Comet Assay and Clinical Pregnancy after Assisted Reproductive Technologies

Study	ART	(n)	RR	95% CI	Z Statistics	p value	OR	95% CI	Z Statistics	p value	Sensitivity	Specificity	NPV	PPV
[14]	IVF	219	1.24	1.11–1.39	3.68	<0.001	4.33	1.82–10.31	3.31	0.001	48.65	82.05	25.20	92.78
	ICSI	116	1.22	0.92–1.62	1.36	0.174	1.73	0.82–3.66	1.43	0.153	67.47	45.45	42.55	70.00
[2]	IVF	70	2.82	1.7–4.68	4.04	<0.001	76	0.06–637.59	3.99	0.001	80.00	95.00	65.92	97.56
[17]	IVF	73	1.30	1.04–1.76	2.24	0.025	4.5	1.28–15.89	2.34	0.019	62.07	73.33	33.33	90.00
	ICSI	22	1.39	0.71–2.67	0.97	0.331	2.67	0.42–16.83	1.04	0.297	66.67	57.14	44.44	76.92
[15]	IVF+ICSI	238	2.11	1.61–2.76	5.46	<0.001	4.74	2.53–8.86	4.87	<0.001	45.00	85.27	66.67	70.67
[10]	IVF+ICSI	60	0.98	0.69–1.37	0.14	0.889	0.92	0.27–3.10	0.14	0.888	57.89	40.00	27.27	70.97
Combining all studies		**798**	**2.55**	**2.01–3.24**	**4.27**	**<0.001**	**3.92**	**2.83–5.43**	**8.23**	**<0.001**	**75.09**	**56.52**	**81.69**	**46.76**

IVF: in vitro fertilization; ICSI: intra-cytoplasmic sperm injection; ART: assisted reproductive technology; OR: odds ratio; CI: confidence interval; RR: relative risk; NPV: negative predictive value; PPV: positive predictive value; n: number of cycles.

The meta-analysis [24] reported a statistically significant odds ratio to determine a successful clinical pregnancy using the alkaline Comet assay and a high negative predictive value (82 percent) for a clinical pregnancy, but the positive predictive value to determine a clinical pregnancy was moderate (47 percent). One explanation for such a moderate relationship between the two parameters may be due to patient inclusion factors, where most of the studies have included couples with female factors, and therefore the effect of sperm DNA damage on pregnancy outcome is compromised by female infertility factors. In studies where patients with female infertile factor were eliminated, the odds to predicting a successful pregnancy have significantly increased irrespective to the type of DNA fragmentation testing method [2, 26].

21.8 Clinical Scenario where the Alkaline Comet Assay Could Be Useful

21.8.1 As a Biomarker Independent to Semen Analysis

DNA fragmentation is a common property of the sperm. Once the DNA fragmentation occurs, sperm lack the ability to repair the strand breaks, and therefore the damage occurring to sperm chromatin is an irreversible change. Sperm DNA fragmentations measured by the alkaline Comet assay are shown to be higher in patients with infertility issues [2] and are associated with abnormal semen parameters [2, 14, 27]. Studies using the SCSA reported that measurement of sperm DNA fragmentation is a good biomarker for time and an excellent predictor of natural conception [28]. Sperm DNA fragmentation is also a useful biomarker for various end points during ARTs, such as fertilization rate, embryo quality, development and clinical pregnancy, and live birth rate [29, 30]. Despite moderate correlations between semen parameters and sperm DNA fragmentation, measurement of single- and double-strand DNA breaks using the alkaline Comet assay could be an additional parameter included with the semen analysis.

21.8.2 Diagnosis of Male Infertility and Counseling for Infertile Couples

In 20–30 percent of couples attending the clinic for infertility diagnostics or treatment, male factor is the primary cause for their infertility and contributes to another 30–40 percent of infertile couples as the secondary cause, with addition to the female factors. Therefore, male factor infertility is present in half of all couples with infertility issues, however, to date, the traditional semen analysis is the only test to determine their infertility status. A large portion of infertile men are presented with a normal semen profile, suggesting that a definitive diagnosis of male infertility cannot be performed only on the basis of semen analysis. However, most studies comparing sperm DNA fragmentation between fertile and infertile men have suggested that DNA fragmentation measured using the alkaline Comet assay and other assays could be a useful biomarker for male infertility diagnosis [2, 28]. Therefore, sperm DNA fragmentation can be considered as an additional parameter to determine male infertility along with the traditional semen analysis. In couples where the male partner has extensive DNA fragmentation, counseling to improve their reproductive health and strategies to reduce the level of sperm DNA fragmentation should be provided.

21.8.3 Counseling Infertile Couples Planning to Choose Assisted Treatment

The question still remains whether ICSI would be a beneficial treatment of choice if the male partner presents with an increased level of sperm DNA fragmentation. When sperm DNA fragmentation is above the threshold value of the alkaline Comet assay, ICSI treatment results in increased pregnancy rates compared to IVF treatment [14]. In a study by Simon et al. [30], the authors identified 15 studies in the literature that simultaneously measured sperm DNA fragmentation (using the four major assays) in IVF and ICSI groups separately, and correlated the clinical outcomes with sperm DNA fragmentation. This analysis included a total of 5564 treatment cycles, separated into 3853 cycles obtained after IVF treatment and 1711 cycles after ICSI treatment. In addition, the cycles were segregated into above and below the threshold value with respect to the DNA fragmentation measurement assays. The results show that pregnancy rates were comparable between IVF and ICSI treatment when DNA fragmentation was below the threshold value, 34.19 percent for IVF and 37.15 percent for ICSI treatment (Chi Sq.=2.847; df=1; p=0.0915). However, when the clinical pregnancies were analyzed when sperm DNA fragmentation was above the threshold value, then ICSI had a higher clinical pregnancy rate (32.14 percent) compared to IVF (16.41 percent) treatment (Chi Sq.=20.815; df=1; p<0.0001). This study shows that pregnancy rates were significantly higher after ICSI treatments, when sperm DNA fragmentation is above the threshold value [30].

A comprehensive large study by Simon et al. [13] comparing the quality of 2210 embryos (observed on day 2, 3 and 5) obtained from IVF or ICSI insemination at different levels of sperm DNA fragmentation, reported that the quality of ICSI embryos are significantly higher than IVF embryos when patients are presented with high sperm DNA fragmentation. This study reported that in patients with an intermediate level of sperm DNA fragmentation (31–70 percent) as measured by the alkaline Comet assay, ICSI cycles consistently resulted in an increased percentage of good quality embryos on day 2, 3 and 5 compared to the IVF cycles. However, no such variations in embryo quality were observed between IVF and ICSI cycles, when sperm DNA fragmentation was low (<30 percent) or high (>70 percent). This report suggests there may be a modest improvement in the embryo quality following ICSI treatment when men are presented with increased sperm DNA fragmentation, and such improvement in embryo quality could translate into increased clinical pregnancy rates. However, an increase in pregnancy rate following ICSI treatment may be attributed to a lower proportion of couples presented with female factor infertility. It can also be postulated that selection of physiologically motile and morphologically normal sperm for ICSI insemination by the embryologists increases the probability of choosing sperm with low DNA fragmentation, as motility and morphology are associated with sperm DNA fragmentation [27]. Therefore, it is possible that couples with increased sperm DNA fragmentation have a better chance of having good embryos and successful pregnancy following ICSI treatment compared to IVF treatment.

21.8.4 Cases Presented with Unexplained Infertility

It is well known that 25–30 percent of couples undergoing ARTs are suffering from unexplained or idiopathic infertility. These cases can be defined as men having no obvious history of fertility problems and physical conditions or endocrine issues, and having a

normal semen analysis, yet experiencing infertility issues. In a study reported by Simon et al. [29], 147 unexplained infertile men were screened for sperm DNA fragmentation using the alkaline Comet assay; 84 percent of these patients had DNA fragmentation above the 25 percent threshold value used to determine men's fertility status. A study using the SCSA reported that 26 percent of men diagnosed with unexplained infertility had DNA fragmentation index above the SCSA threshold value [31]. Similarly, other studies using SCD and TUNEL assays have reported an increased level of sperm DNA fragmentation in men presented with unexplained infertility [32]. Collectively, the results obtained from the alkaline Comet assay and other assays suggest that to some extent sperm DNA fragmentation may interfere with men's reproductive health and measurement of sperm DNA fragmentation may help to identify men with fertility problems even when they are presented with normal semen analysis, as reported as unexplained infertility.

21.9 Conclusion

The primary function of the sperm is to transport the haploid paternal genetic material through the male and female reproductive tract and deliver it to the oocyte. Therefore, abnormalities in the sperm function may hinder the delivery of sperm to the oocyte. However, in the case of assisted reproduction procedure, the sperm is delivered near the oocyte (IVF) or delivered into the oocyte (ICSI). In such a case, it may not be reasonable to expect any of the semen parameters to predict ART success, but the integrity of the sperm chromatin delivered to the oocyte gains significant importance to account for its success. Among the tests used to measure the integrity of sperm chromatin, the alkaline Comet assay is extremely reliable, cost-efficient, able to predict outcomes, and has the potential to assist clinicians in decision-making. Unlike other assays, the methodological aspects of the Comet assay, involving lysis and decondensation, for the identification of DNA strand breaks embedded in the sperm nucleus, reveal the complete level of DNA fragmentation in the sperm. Therefore, the level of DNA strand breaks measured by the alkaline Comet assay are higher when compared to other assays, and have a strong correlation with IVF fertilization rate, embryo quality and development, and have the capability to predict the success of ARTs.

In addition, sperm DNA fragmentation can assist clinicians to evaluate male infertility and help them in choosing an appropriate type of assisted reproductive treatment. Based on the reviews discussed in this chapter, we support the notion that sperm DNA fragmentation measured by the alkaline Comet assay should be added to the conventional semen analysis for a complete diagnosis of male reproductive health.

References

1. Aitken RJ, de Iuliis GN. On the possible origins of DNA damage in human spermatozoa. *Mol Hum Reprod* 2010; **16**: 3–13.

2. Simon L, Lutton D, McManus J, Lewis SEM. Sperm DNA damage measured by the alkaline Comet assay as an independent predictor of male infertility and IVF success. *Fertil Steril* 2011a; **95**: 652–7.

3. Panner Selvam MK, Agarwal A. A systematic review on sperm DNA fragmentation in male factor infertility: laboratory assessment. *Arab J Urol* 2018; **16**(1): 65–76.

4. Singh NR, Stephens RE. X-ray-induced DNA double-strand breaks in human sperm. *Mutagenesis* 1998; **13**(1): 75–9.

5. Simon L, Aston KI, Emery BR, Hotaling J, Carrell DT. Sperm DNA damage output parameters measured by the alkaline Comet assay and their importance. *Andrologia* 2017a; **49**: e12608.

6. Shamsi MB, Kumar R, Dada R. Evaluation of nuclear DNA damage in human spermatozoa in men opting for assisted reproduction. *Indian J Med Res* 2008; **127**: 115–23.

7. Shamsi MB, Imam SN, Dada R. Sperm DNA integrity assays: diagnostic and prognostic challenges and implications in management of infertility. *J Assist Reprod Genet* 2011; **28**: 1073–85.

8. Olive PL, Wlodek D, Durand RE, Banáth JP. Factors influencing DNA migration from individual cells subjected to gel electrophoresis. *Exp Cell Res* 1992; **198**: 259–67.

9. Hughes CM, Lewis SEM, McKelvey-Martin V, Thompson W. Reproducibility of human sperm DNA measurements using the alkaline single cell gel electrophoresis assay. *Mutat Res* 1997; **374**: 261–8.

10. Morris ID, Ilott S, Dixon L, Brison DR. The spectrum of DNA damage in human sperm assessed by single cell gel electrophoresis (Comet assay) and its relationship to fertilization and embryo development. *Hum Reprod* 2002; **17**(4): 990–8.

11. Piperakis SM. Comet assay: a brief history. *Cell Biol Toxicol* 2009; **25**: 1–3.

12. Ribas-Maynou J, Fernandez-Encinas A, García-Peiro A, Prada E, Abad C, Amengual MJ, Navarro J, Benet J. Human semen cryopreservation: a sperm DNA fragmentation study with alkaline and neutral Comet assay. *Andrology* 2014; **2**: 83–7.

13. Simon L, Murphy K, Shamsi MB, Liu L, Emery B, Aston KI, Hotaling J, Carrell DT. Paternal influence of sperm DNA integrity on early embryonic development. *Hum Reprod* 2014b; **29**(11): 2402–12.

14. Simon L, Brunborg G, Stevenson M, Lutton D, McManus J, Lewis SEM. Clinical significance of sperm DNA damage in assisted reproductive outcome. *Hum Reprod* 2010; **25**(7): 1594–608.

15. Simon L, Liu L, Murphy K, Ge S, Hotaling J, Aston KI, Emery B, Carrell DT. Comparative analysis of three sperm DNA damage assays and sperm nuclear protein content in couples undergoing assisted reproduction treatment. *Hum Reprod* 2014a; **29**: 904–17.

16. Simon L, Carrell DT. (2011d) Sperm DNA damage measured by Comet assay. In Carrell DT and Aston KI, eds., *Spermatogenesis and Spermiogenesis: Methods and Protocols*. New Jersey: Humana Press, pp. 137–46.

17. Simon L, Castillo J, Oliva R, Lewis S. The relationship between human sperm protamines, DNA damage and assisted reproductive outcomes. *Reprod Biomed Online* 2011b; **23**: 724–34.

18. Dorostghoal M, Kazeminejad SR, Shahbazian N, Pourmehdi M, Jabbari A. Oxidative stress status and sperm DNA fragmentation in fertile and infertile men. *Andrologia* 2017; **49**(10): e12762.

19. Santi D, Spaggiari G, Simoni M. Sperm DNA fragmentation index as a promising predictive tool for male infertility diagnosis and treatment management – meta-analyses. *Reprod BioMed Online* 2018; **37**(3): 315–25.

20. Sakkas D. Novel technologies for selecting the best sperm for in vitro fertilization and intracytoplasmic sperm injection. *Fertil Steril* 2013; **99**: 1023–9.

21. Lewis SEM, O'Connell M, Stevenson M, Thompson-Cree L, McClure N. An algorithm to predict pregnancy in assisted reproduction. *Hum Reprod* 2004; **19**: 1385–94.

22. Nasr-Esfahani MH, Salehi M, Razavi S, Anjlmshoa M, Rozahani S, Moulavi F, Mardani M. Effect of sperm DNA damage and sperm protamine deficiency on fertilization and embryo development post-ICSI. *RBM Online* 2005; **11**: 198–205.

23. Tomsu M, Sharma V, Miller D. Embryo quality and IVF treatment outcome may correlate with different sperm comet parameters. *Hum Reprod* 2002; **17**: 1856–62.

24. Simon L, Zini A, Ciampi A, Dyachenko A, Carrell DT. A systematic review and meta-analysis to determine the effect of sperm DNA damage measured by different assays on IVF and ICSI outcomes. *Asian J Androl* 2017b; **19**: 80–90.

25. Bazrgar M, Gourabi H, Yazdi PE, Vazirinasab H, Fakhri M, Hassani F, Valojerdi MR. DNA repair signalling pathway genes are overexpressed in poor-quality pre-implantation human embryos with complex aneuploidy. *Eur J Obstet Gynecol Reprod Biol* 2014; **175**: 152–6.

26. Giwercman A, Lindstedt L, Larsson M, Bungum M, Spano M, Levine RJ, Rylander L. Sperm chromatin structure assay as an independent predictor of fertility in vivo: a case-control study. *Int J Androl* 2010; **32**: 221–7.

27. Simon L, Lewis SEM. Effects of progressive motility and sperm DNA damage on fertilization rates in vitro: is one better than the other? *Syst Biol Reprod Med* 2011c; **57**(3): 133–8.

28. Evenson DP, Jost LK, Marshall D, Zinaman MJ, Clegg E, Purvis K, de Angelis P, Claussen OP. Utility of the sperm chromatin structure assay as a diagnostic and prognostic tool in the human fertility clinic. *Hum Reprod* 1999; **14**: 1039–49.

29. Simon L, Proutski I, Stevenson M, Jennings D, McManus J, Lutton D, Lewis SEM. Sperm DNA damage has negative association with live birth rates after IVF. *Reprod Biomed Online* 2013; **26**: 68–78.

30. Simon L, Carrell DT, Zini A. (2018) Sperm DNA tests are clinically useful. In Zini A. and Agarwal A., eds., *A Clinician's Guide to Sperm DNA and Chromatin Damage*. New York: Springer International Publishing, pp. 431–67.

31. Oleszczuk K, Augustinsson L, Bayat N, Giwercman A, Bungum M. Prevalence of high DNA fragmentation index in male partners of unexplained infertile couples. *Andrology* 2013; **1**: 357–60.

32. Feijo CM, Esteves SC. Diagnostic accuracy of sperm chromatin dispersion test to evaluate sperm deoxyribonucleic acid damage in men with unexplained infertility. *Fertil Steril* 2014; **101**: 58–63.

Chapter 22

DNA Damage: Halo Sperm Test

Jaime Gosálvez, José Luís Fernández

22.1 Introduction

Fertility, pregnancy and childbirth are connected and inseparable realities that ultimately need to combine to result in a "baby at home"; each one of these phenomena possesses their own suite of challenges and limitations. From a biological viewpoint, the factors contributing to a successful "baby at home" are male factors (mainly sperm quality) and female factors (mainly oocyte quality and endometrial receptivity). Any failure or disability in one of these competences shall likely contribute to the reduced probability of having a "baby at home". However, in modern times a new factor is playing a crucial role in this scenario, the so called "Artificial Reproduction Techniques" (ART). Thus, it is becoming increasingly possible for reproductive biologists and clinicians to apply a range of technologies to transform a biologically infertile couple to an assisted fertile one. To this purpose, a series of novel technologies, some of them with ethical implications at the time of their use on a routine basis, have and will continue to have a remarkable potential impact on fertility treatments [1].

Infertility associated with a male factor has been estimated to affect approximately 50 percent of infertile couples [2, 3], but when semen parameters are in the normal range, as defined by the World Health Organization (WHO), a reliable diagnosis of infertility associated to male factor remains elusive. Given this issue, any new technique that is able to shed some light to elucidate what might be described as a "third factor of infertility", would be of substantive value to helping couples achieve a successful pregnancy. This is one of the reasons why Sperm DNA Fragmentation (SDF) is considered a promising diagnostic tool for the management and diagnosis of male infertility with both research and clinical applications [4].

High levels of SDF in the ejaculate are associated with an increased time to conception, impaired fertilization, decreased early embryo development, higher miscarriage rates and recurrent pregnancy loss after ART [4, 5, 6, 7, 8]. Thus, the detection of anomalous levels of SDF can serve as an additional marker of fertility potential and a predictor of the success of pregnancy. A significant proportion of men with normal semen profiles are still considered infertile [3], suggesting that other semen parameters also contribute to understanding unexplained infertility; clearly sperm DNA damage and associated DNA modifications are important potential sperm parameters that have a role here [9].

Since the proposal by Evenson that flow cytometry be used as a valuable methodology to assess SDF [5], a series of alternative techniques have subsequently emerged. These include the TUNEL assay, the Comet assay (with different variants) and the Sperm Chromatin Dispersion (SCD) test. All of these techniques are considered reliable methodologies providing consistent results on the sperm DNA quality of donors and patients. All of them offer the possibility to assess DNA quality in fresh, processed or cryopreserved samples. In this paper, we review some aspects of the SCD test and derived results of its application in clinical practice, including the rationale of the technique and implications in different fields of ART.

22.2 Methodological Basis of the Sperm Chromatin Dispersion Test

The SCD test was serendipitously discovered when using the DNA Breakage Detection-Fluorescence In Situ Hybridization (DBD-FISH), a technique that is a very sensitive assay in determining DNA breaks. From a conceptual viewpoint, DBD-FISH is a straightforward methodology. Unfixed cells, which are enclosed in an inert thin microgel on a slide, are incubated with an alkaline DNA denaturing solution and with lysing solutions to remove proteins. The alkaline solution is a main step in the DNA unwinding assays and classically employed to evaluate ionizing radiation induced DNA breaks. High pH conditions denatures the DNA starting from the end of the DNA breaks (5′–3′ free ends), producing stretches of single-stranded DNA that may be quantified by different approaches.

Nuclear proteins pack the DNA molecules in the nuclear volume, while the lysing solutions remove proteins and membranes from the cell and the nucleus. Subsequently, after extensive nuclear protein removal, DNA is unpackaged producing a peripheral halo of chromatin loops that spread from the central remnant core. These are remnant cores known as nucleoids and they remain retained within the microgel after the whole process. Single-stranded DNA motifs produced by the alkaline unwinding treatment from the DNA breaks may then be detected under fluorescence microscopy by hybridization of fluorescent labeled DNA probes. The higher the number of DNA breaks, the higher the amount of single-stranded DNA motifs produced by the denaturing solution, the higher the amount of hybridized probe and the visualized fluorescence (Figure 22.1A,B). The hybridized DNA probe can be quantified by digital image analysis software (Figure 22.1C–F). The system is sensitive enough to assess DNA breaks in the whole genome or within specific DNA sequence domains such as repetitive DNA sequences or single gene copies [10]; (Figure 22.1G,H). DBD-FISH evaluates

possible differences in sensitivity to DNA damaging agents in different regions of the genome.

When the DBD-FISH protocol was applied to native human sperm cells, without exposure to any damaging agent, it was observed that a certain and variable proportion of spermatozoa, depending on the ejaculate used, appeared strongly labeled when using a whole genome DNA probe, showing an intense fluorescence. These sperm were interpreted and presenting with a very high amount of DNA breakage, i.e. DNA fragmentation; the rest of the sperm showed a slight labeling, mainly within specific regions of the nucleoid. Counterstaining of the DNA revealed that the nucleoids from sperm with non-fragmented DNA presented the typical central core and peripheral halo of spread DNA loops (Figure 22.2A). Surprisingly, those sperm strongly labeled after the DBD-FISH protocol, i.e. containing fragmented DNA, did not show peripheral halos or these were small by comparison but they presented a high level of hybridized DNA probe (Figure 22.2B).

As a direct correlation between the presence of halo and DNA-labeling intensity can be established, the long hybridization step could then be omitted resulting in a more efficient procedure. The rationale of the DBD-FISH was simplified and sperm enclosed in the microgel are then simply incubated with an unwinding solution to denature DNA presenting free ends and

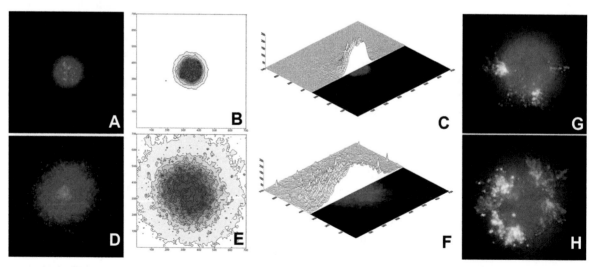

Figure 22.1 DNA Breakage Detection-Fluorescence In Situ Hybridization (DBD-FISH) in somatic cells. **A)** DBD-FISH using a whole DNA genomic probe on a somatic cell in absence of DNA damage. **B,C)** Flat (B) and 3D planimetry (C) of Figure 21.1A. **D)** DBD-FISH using a whole DNA genomic probe on a somatic cell in absence of DNA. **E,F)** Flat (E) and 3D planimetry (F) of Figure 22.1D. DBD-FISH using restrictive human centromeric DNA probes satellite 1 (red) and satellite 2 (green) of chromosome 1 in untreated **(G)** and irradiated **(H)** cells. Note the difference in amount of hybridized DNA probe according with the expected level of DNA damage.

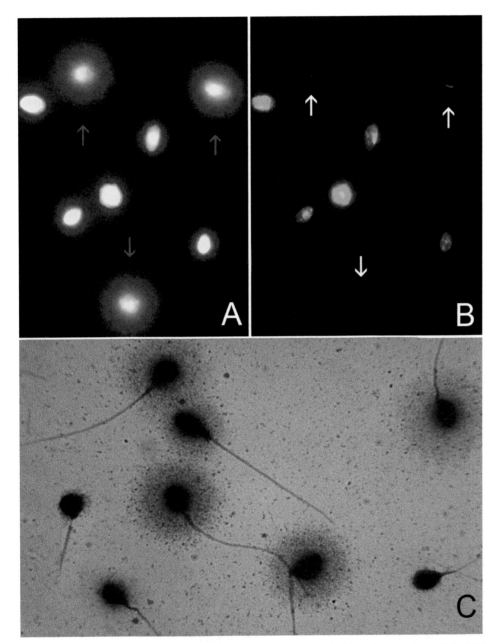

Figure 22.2 Visualization of different sized haloes depending on the level of DNA damage observed after DNA denaturation and protein depletion. **A)** Spermatozoa stained for fluorescence microscopy. Red arrows indicate those spermatozoa without DNA damage. **B)** Same image as Figure 22.2A but after DBD-FISH. Note that spermatozoa with large haloes are free of hybridization (white arrows) while those with small haloes in Figure 22.2A show large signals of hybridization. **C)** SCD test but visualized under bright filed microscopy.

later with lysing solutions to remove proteins. Finally, the resulting nucleoids can be stained and visualized even using bright field microscopy (Figure 22.2C). Spermatozoa exhibiting small halo or no halo correspond to sperm with fragmented DNA while those presenting a large halo of dispersed chromatin were considered as those presenting non-fragmented DNA molecules. This simplified assay was coined the "Sperm Chromatin Dispersion test" [11].

The reality is that sperm DNA damage affects every cell continuously and it is expected that different levels of damage are therefore likely to present

215

differentially. Within the context of interpreting results of the SCD test, these differences are characterized with the visualization of a series of different sized haloes after staining (Figure 22.3A,B) and with the help of digital image analysis, different cell subpopulations can be discriminated [12]; (Figure 22.3C).

Following this initial development, the procedure was refined, designing an exclusive lysing solution, specific to human sperm, that removes protamines while keeping the sperm tails visible. This was possible by exchanging the alkaline solution with an acidic solution. The main advantage of using acid denaturation is that it is less strong than the alkaline one to denature from DNA ends on the DNA damaged molecule. Spermatozoa with fragmented DNA produce single-stranded DNA stretches that after

protein removal give rise to small or no haloes. Spermatozoa without DNA fragmentation practically do not denature the DNA and after protein depletion, the peripheral haloes are larger than those observed after using the stronger alkaline solution. The use of a controlled acid denaturation improves the contrast between sperm with and without fragmented DNA; furthermore, the technique allows for better nucleoid staining not only by fluorochromes but also by standard dyes like Wright or Diff-Quik staining procedures, allowing the use of the basic bright-field microscope for visualization of the haloes [13]. The actual SCD protocol, including the scoring of 300–500 sperm, may be accomplished in less than an hour. The assay has now been standardized as a commercialized kit (Halosperm®; Halotech DNA SL, Madrid, Spain), being user-friendly, not technically

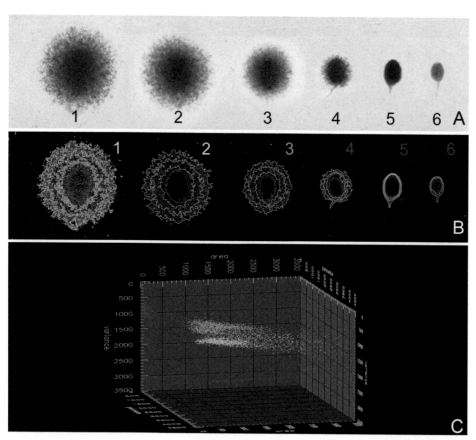

Figure 22.3 Different sized haloes in spermatozoa processed with the SCD test. **A)** 1–2: large haloes = no fragmented sperm; 3: medium-sized halo = no fragmented sperm; 4: small halo = fragmented sperm; 5 and 6: no halo and degraded sperm respectively = fragmented sperm. **B)** Color planimetry to show density differences in the different nucleoids. **C)** Multidimensional plot obtained using morphometric variables (area, perimeter and associated variances) to show the differential clustering obtained. Color code in Figure 22.3C corresponds to color number in Figure 22.3B.

demanding and easy to be implemented at any laboratory to obtain reliable and consistent results.

Different approaches validate the ability of the SCD test to determine SDF. First at all, the sequential DBD-FISH technique performed in each specific sperm (Figure 22.2), confirms that those spermatozoa without haloes or with small haloes contain massive DNA breakage. Moreover, the SCD-processed sperm may also be sequentially incubated for enzymatic labeling of DNA breaks, either with the terminal deoxynucleotidyl transferase (TdT; TUNEL assay) or the Klenow fragment of the DNA polymerase (Klenow-end labeling) or just using the DNA polymerase (ISNT: In Situ Nick Translation). As is the case with the DBD-FISH procedure, DNA breakage labeling by the different DNA polymerases is only observed in the sperm nucleoids without haloes or with a small halo. Other important proof of evidence is the incubation of sperm with DNA damaging agents. Treatment with DNase I or with free radicals such as hydrogen peroxide or sodium nitroprusside (SNP), results in the sperm displaying small or no haloes [14]. Finally, the SCD test strongly correlates with the results of other procedures to determine SDF, like the Sperm Chromatin Structure Assay (SCSA), TUNEL assay and the single-cell gel electrophoresis (SCGE)/Comet assay [15, 16, 17].

22.3 Advanced Applications of the Sperm Chromatin Dispersion Test

From a technical viewpoint, the SCD test may also be coupled with other techniques of interest for basic and clinical research. Staining with a mix of fluorochromes with different affinities and emission wavelengths may reveal different DNA characteristics of SCD-processed sperm. For example, DNA may be stained with a DNA interacting fluorochrome such as propidium iodide or Gel-Red, whereas proteins/protein remnants may be stained by 2,7-dibrom-4-hydroxy-mercury-fluorescein. Using this fluorochrome combination and a dual-band excitation-emission block filter, the nucleoids (mainly DNA) fluoresce red, while sperm tails (mainly proteins) fluoresce green (Figure 22.4A). This staining facilitates that somatic cells, like leukocytes, which may be present in the semen sample, can be easily discriminated from surrounding spermatozoa. Somatic cells show large round nucleoids without a prominent halo of dispersed chromatin. These cells exhibit a mixture of red and green fluorescence

emissions due to the presence of DNA and histones retained in the nucleus. Under these staining conditions, somatic cells can be easily differentiated from the sperm heads (Figure 22.4B).

This approach provides some advantages in certain clinical situations such as patients with leukocytospermia [18] or identification of testicular sperm where the number of somatic cells is high because of the invasive characteristics of sperm retrieval. Testicular samples often contain debris and other cell types like spermatogonia, spermatids or Sertoli cells making the discrimination from spermatozoa problematic. This situation can be extreme in some patients such as those presenting with Kartagener's syndrome or varicocele [19, 20], but even in these patients, somatic cells can be easily distinguished using a combination of fluorochromes targeting DNA and proteins with different emission spectra.

Sperm DNA Fragmentation assessment in severe oligozoospermic samples is not possible with procedures based on flow cytometry, which require a relatively high amount of cells to be processed. The SCD procedure is also very effective when studying testicular sperm from biopsies or puncture-aspiration, spermatozoa isolated with restrictive selection systems such as MACS, PICSI or microfluidic based devices. The SCD can also be used to assess SDF in just one selected sperm, as in the case of IMSI [12]; (Figure 22.4C–F) or very few selected spermatozoa such us those captured after PICSI or MACS [21, 22].

Evaluation of modified DNA bases on SCD processed slides may be accomplished through incubation with specific antibodies. When SCD-processed sperm are incubated with antibodies binding to 8-oxoguanosine (8-oxoG), the presence of DNA fragmentation and the presence of oxidative damage can be simultaneously determined [23]. Additionally, the DNA methylation level, using an antibody that binds to 5-methylcytosine, can also be assessed in different spermatozoa after being processed with the SCD test (figure 10 in [24]).

Specific DNA sequences may be identified in SCD-processed nucleoids by standard FISH [25, 26]. To this purpose, dehydrated nucleoids are carefully denatured, trying to avoid loss of DNA from the haloes, and hybridized with specific DNA probes. Counterstained nucleoids reveal presence or absence of DNA fragmentation through evaluation of halo size, whereas the enumeration of signals from

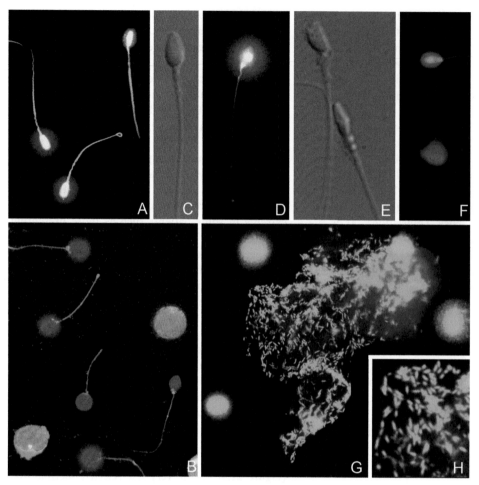

Figure 22.4 The SCD test used for different purposes. **A)** Simultaneous visualization of the sperm head and flagellum in a normal ejaculate. **B)** Testicular sperm. Discrimination between somatic (yellow cells without flagellum) and spermatozoa (red cells with flagellum). **C–F)** Use of SCD to assess sperm DNA damage in individualized spermatozoa. **C)** Intra-cytoplasmic morphologically selected sperm injection (IMSI) selected sperm showing normal head morphology and absence of DNA damage **(D)**. **E)** Two selected spermatozoa showing head abnormalities. **F)** Same spermatozoa as in 22.4B but showing DNA damage. **G)** SCD visualizing different spermatozoa and presence of bacteria associated to a leukocyte. **H)** Detailed enlargement of Figure 22.4G.

chromosome specific hybridization of DNA sequences indicates the presence or absence of aneuploidies. This strategy allows identification of DNA damage and presence of aneuploidies in the same sperm.

It is interesting to highlight that bacteria, when they are present at the ejaculate, are only partially affected by the lysing solutions used in the SCD protocol. Because of this chromatin relaxation, they remain more perceptible and produce a much more efficient fluorochrome-DNA interaction. The final result is that bacteria can be identified when they are present at the ejaculate whether they are free or endosymbiotic (Figure 22.4G,H); [27].

One peculiarity of the SCD test is the ability to distinguish a special kind of sperm with fragmented DNA, the "degraded" subtype. This is a sperm without halo but presenting an irregular or faint stained nucleoid and corresponds to a strongly damaged sperm containing both massive single- and double-strand DNA breaks [28]. In semen samples from men with varicocele, this "degraded" type has been found to be increased in proportion with respect to the whole population of sperm with fragmented DNA (sperm degradation index: SDI; [20]). A degradation index (considering this as the proportion of degraded sperm within the fragmented population) of >0.33 may predict the presence of varicocele, even when these are subclinical, with an accuracy of 94 percent [20].

22.4 Sperm DNA Fragmentation and Reproductive Outcome

A value of 30 percent SDF is regarded as one of the most accepted cut-off values of SDF that discriminates low from high levels of damaged DNA. Evenson and colleagues have suggested this value in different papers using the SCSA technique [6, 29]. The SCD technique was adapted to produce near equivalent results to those obtained with the SCSA technique [13]. However, discrepancies exist among the cut-off values when compared with other techniques such as TUNEL (lower values than 30 percent) or the alkaline comet assay (higher values than 30 percent). Probably, this is mostly related to the resolution capacity of each technique to capture the entire DNA damage present in the sperm, rather than with the results of reproductive outcome obtained. What is important is that all the techniques show good correlation at the time of determining variable levels of SDF existing among different patients [16, 30].

Numerous studies have reported a close correlation between SDF and clinical outcomes using different strategies for fertilization such as intrauterine insemination, in vitro fertilization and intracytoplasmic sperm injection [7, 31, 32, 33, 34, 35, 36]. While in general, a negative correlation has been found when SDF values are plotted against rates of fertilization, embryo quality and development, implantation rates, and pregnancy, this association is not perfect and some investigations point out to a quasi-neutral role of SDF in reproductive outcome [37, 38, 39]. One of the most inclusive studies to correlate SDF and pregnancy outcome was a multicenter survey including 622 couples [40]; these type of studies, at least, eliminate confounding factors such as variability of the technique to assess SDF, or inclusion criteria. Vélez de la Calle et al. [40] reported that the correlation between pregnancy and SDF was not as high as that reported in other studies, although they found a significant positive correlation for SDF and reduced rate of oocyte fertilization, embryo quality, and rate of blastocyst implantation.

One of the possible explanations for these discrepancies is that the assessment of SDF is usually performed in neat sperm and this is not the actual sample that will be used for fertilization purposes. In fact, the samples that will be used for fertilization are those obtained after performing different sperm selection techniques on the ejaculated sample. Each technique to select sperm presents different levels of skill and efficiency to remove damaged sperm [41]. Additionally, the ineludible negative impact of iatrogenic damage is rarely considered as an important modulator of SDF with respect to time. Another confounding factor is the quality of the embryo selected to be transferred. When different oocytes are fertilized but only one is transferred, this is a form of selection and this can mask the net effect of SDF on reproductive outcome. Then, the question would be: if a selected embryo fails to implant or develop, is this reflective of the other fertilized but not-transferred oocytes?

Understanding the actual role of SDF on reproductive outcome requires a consistent experimental model that is able to minimize confounding factors. The use of donated oocytes to be fertilized with the semen sample of the partner minimizes the role of female factor. This can be a good experimental strategy to understand the true role of male factor in reproductive outcome; nevertheless, even under these conditions, confounding factors cannot be discarded. For example, the receptive female is contributing to these factors with respect to her endometrial receptivity or other physiological characteristics that may be compromised, especially taking into consideration that the majority of these females are attending an ovodonation program for different abnormal physiological reasons. Using this experimental model, we performed a prospective study where each male partner was controled at different levels; SDF was assessed both at 30 minutes after ejaculation and at the time of fertilization. All the samples were processed with swim-up for sperm selection and used for ICSI. Fixing these conditions, receiver operator characteristics (ROC) showed that SDF cut-off values for pregnancy were 24.8 percent for neat sperm, while for swim-up processed samples these values decrease to 17.5 percent. Interestingly, prediction of pregnancy from ejaculated samples or swim-up processed samples were quite similar showing a sensitivity and specificity of 77 percent and 73 percent, respectively. These results show that while increased levels of SDF have a negative impact in reproductive outcome, the predictive values of SDF can be different if we only use as reference fresh ejaculated samples or samples that have been processed [12].

22.5 Assessing Sperm DNA Longevity with the Sperm Chromatin Dispersion Test

In those cases where ICSI, IVF or IUI are used for the purpose of fertilization, the sperm must be kept alive in in vitro conditions until the oocyte is reached. This unpretentious statement has crucial implications if we want to achieve a successful fertilization. The ejaculate is maintained in vitro for liquefaction, sperm capacitation, sperm selection and sperm-oocyte interaction. Altogether, these steps may impair the environment where the sperm is maintained free of non-desirable modifications at different levels. For many years now, it has been well known that sperm quality declines over time following ejaculation and semen characteristic such as membrane quality and sperm motility decrease after ejaculation, even when using the best sperm preservation environments; this produces a serious decline in the abilities of sperm to achieve reproductive outcome. We know now that DNA quality does not escape this general rule and DNA quality declines after ejaculation. This decline is different when comparing the sperm of individuals within one species or when different species are compared [42, 43, 44], or when cryopreserved samples are compared with fresh ones [45].

One important aspect of the dynamic assessment of DNA fragmentation for ART is taking into account the negative impact of iatrogenic damage caused by exposure of sperm to a panoply of changing ex vivo conditions. If the time elapsed between SDF assessment and fertilization is not considered, then it is not surprising that there is often not a strong correlation of these variables and we see mixed conclusions about the predictability of SDF and infertility. In a recent paper, and using a highly sensitivity technique to assess DNA damage as the two-tail Comet assay, our group has called attention to this particular issue. Cryopreserved human samples increase in single-strand DNA breaks after only 30 minutes post-thawing [47], and in most cases, we would generally not consider this potential DNA damage as a possible effector of pregnancy loss; perhaps we have underestimated this problem, especially if the post-thaw sperm are left longer before use in ART procedures.

Sperm DNA longevity can be conceptualized and partially modeled in the laboratory imitating what goes on in the female reproductive tract. The physiological temperature in the female reproductive tract is around 36°C, so if we examine changing values of SDF along a determined period of incubation at this temperature, we may detect genomes predisposed to assume higher levels of DNA damage than others do over time. With the level of resolution of the SCD technique it can be determined that SDF shows changing values after only two hours of incubation [46]. The rate of sperm DNA fragmentation (increase of SDF per time unit) is variable among individuals but is also highly dependent on the storage conditions or environmental influence. When thawed-cryopreserved samples are tested, an increase of SDF of about 8 percent in some individuals is appreciated after 24 hours of incubation. However, in other cases, this increase reaches 80 percent of the spermatozoa [46]. If the semen sample is to be used for IVF or IUI, the baseline level of SDF as diagnosed in the patient probably will change during co-incubation of intrauterine inoculation. In routine IVF, oocytes are co-incubated with sperm overnight. Some aspects about the negative impact of iatrogenic DNA damage were reported some years ago [48] using sperm samples that were delivered between different ART clinics. The main conclusion of that paper was that miscarriage improved after co-incubation of sperm-oocyte for short periods of time in those cases where sperm was delivered between different centers. It has been reported that this period of co-incubation may cause problems in normal embryo development. To avoid this trouble, short periods of co-incubation may be recommended to achieve better rates of fertilization in IVF conditions [48, 49].

While in humans, problems for embryo development related with an increased incidence of SDF occurring during co-incubation need to be demonstrated, we do have evidence of this situation in animal models. In the case of rabbits using the same females to be inseminated with males presenting high or low rates of SDF, it was found that the rate of stillborn pups was significantly higher in females inseminated by males with a high rate of SDF when compared to those with low rate of SDF. Moreover, the risk of stillborn animals was low when males with low rates of SDF were used. This risk increased dramatically after inseminating the same females with animals presenting with a high rate of SDF [50]. It is interesting to highlight, that using zebra-fish as an experimental model, when sperm DNA damage is controled under in vitro conditions and used for fertilization purposes, fertilization rates are less affected than the embryo viability rates [28]; this finding agrees with the high correlation of embryo loss associated with high levels of SDF reported in humans.

The concept of sperm DNA longevity can also be applied to donor sperm banks in order to select those individuals exhibiting the highest level of DNA stability. In a prospective study, it was found that donors exhibited a sperm DNA longevity 2.5 times higher than that observed in a cohort of patients. Static values of SDF after thawing indicated that a level of SDF of about 11 percent identify donors within a general population with 71 percent sensitivity and 84 percent specificity. On the other hand, a dynamic SDF increase of 2.3 units per hour might identify the donors with 70 percent sensitivity and 66 percent specificity [51].

22.6 Improving Sperm DNA Quality for Assisted Reproductive Technologies

The mere detection of increased levels of SDF is not paramount in solving the infertility problem, but once abnormal levels are detected, we may use different approaches to reduce these altered levels of SDF. These procedures open a new space in ART that are linked to the concept of personalized medicine since they not only try to identify the problem, but also to test and fix the most efficient methodology to obtain the most competitive sperm for fertilization associated to each patient. In a previous review, we have summarized some of the available strategies to reduce high levels of sperm DNA damage when observed in the neat ejaculate [52]. Some of these strategies are extremely useful because they are not invasive or based on supplements administration, but try to interpret and mimic what nature is doing at the time of ejaculation.

22.6.1 Recurrent Ejaculations

Ejaculatory abstinence duration is one of the non-invasive strategies that may allow us to decrease high levels of SDF. At the epididymis, there is a potential ROS capacity that may produce DNA damage; equally, active mechanisms of DNA repair are not available to the spermatozoon. Ejaculation abstinence for long periods before collecting sperm may seem like a way of increasing the proportion of good quality sperm, but this is likely to be a misleading strategy. In fact, we have shown that recurrent ejaculations every 24 hours for 72 hours resulted in a significant decrease in SDF [24]; other studies have observed an equivalent response of the ejaculate [53]. In these cases, DNA quality improved even further when these same samples were processed using density gradient centrifugation. This is most likely linked to the fact, that recurrent ejaculation produces an increase in immature sperm that are most efficiently selected using DGC because the cell surface area (including the cytoplasmic droplet) presented to gradient media is higher than that offered by compact mature sperm cells. As a general pattern, patients with a high level of SDF should undergo recurrent ejaculation every 24 hours for 3–4 days with a final period of abstinence of 12 hours. This can be combined with sperm selection using DGC and fertilization with ICSI. This combination results in a significant increase in pregnancy rate [54, 55].

22.6.2 Ejaculate Fractionation

Fractionation of the ejaculate is also a relatively simple strategy that may decrease the level of SDF observed at the whole ejaculate. In most clinics, the ejaculate to be processed for fertilization is not fractionated. However, a whole ejaculation consists of different semen fractions that are successively released during natural intercourse and they present different characteristics in composition with respect to their biological role [56, 57]. In those mammalian species so far studied, it is evident that the level of SDF is consistently lower in the first fraction when compared with that of the second fraction or in the whole collected ejaculate [58, 59]. Consequently, in cases where a high level of SDF is observed in a routine spermiogram, the use of the first ejaculated fraction, followed by the standard sperm selection techniques, is likely to produce a reduction in the levels of SDF.

22.6.3 Sperm Selection Techniques

At ejaculatation, not all spermatozoa have reached equivalent functional characteristics and the percentage of spermatozoa having full fertilization capacity is highly variable among individuals [60, 61, 62]. This situation may change after sperm selection, since one of the aims of sperm selection is to concentrate a subgroup of spermatozoa presenting good motility, morphology, and in the era of ICSI, mainly good DNA quality, since the rest of the sperm characteristics are less significant for fertilization. While the most common sperm selection techniques are swim-up and density gradient centrifugation, in more recent years, a series of new and highly selective strategies such as MACS, IMSI, PICSI or techniques based on microfluidics have been employed [63, 64]. In general, the main aim of using these techniques is focused on improving the final concentration of spermatozoa presenting with good DNA quality, but in some circumstances, this is not the case and certain parameters such as motility can be negatively affected after sperm selection [63]. The level of SDF selection observed in some patients after processing the neat samples with swim-up or density gradient centrifugation can also be higher in the selected samples than the one observed in the original ejaculate [22].

Some of these undesired results may be related to the technical complexity and/or manual ability of the operator [65], but also with the time of sperm processing after collection, which may cause iatrogenic sperm damage [24, 46]. The patient profile coupled to the appropriate sperm selection technique may also be contributing to this variability. For example, using a two-tail Comet assay, both single- and double-strand DNA breaks can be detected. If this experimental approach is used, we have observed that while swim-up and density gradient centrifugation do not show statistical differences to eliminate double-strand DNA damage, density gradient centrifugation appears to be more competent than-swim up at the time of selecting spermatozoa with lower levels of single-strand DNA breakage [41].

In summary, all available sperm selection techniques may reduce the proportion of sperm with DNA damage, but determination of the best option associated to each patient is still elusive and we may need to concentrate part of our efforts to be more precise and individually patient orientated with our application of these skills. SDF can be used to confidently demonstrate if the processing technique associated to a patient has been effective or not in improving the general characteristic of the ejaculate.

22.6.4 Plasma Removal and Sperm Concentration

At ejaculation, spermatozoa are imperatively collected with seminal plasma. In reality, during ejaculate collection for ART purposes, we are creating a mixture of fluids emerging from different glands that are not mixed during natural intercourse. However, during sperm collection for ART, the ejaculate is collected as the accumulation of a series of different ejaculated fractions. This is one of the reasons why the influence of maintaining seminal plasma mixed with sperm is controversial. Thus, some studies associate a protective role of the seminal plasma with some form of antioxidant capacity that can be beneficial to the spermatozoa present in the neat ejaculate [66]. Nevertheless, in terms of DNA quality, it can also be demonstrated that rapid elimination of seminal plasma after ejaculation and restitution with an appropriate media produces beneficial effects on sperm DNA longevity [67].

Moreover, to improve the whole final characteristics of the selected sample that will be used for fertilization and to avoid the impact of iatrogenic damage, elimination of the seminal plasma can be coupled with a final adjustment of sperm concentration tending to produce samples with less than 10 million of spermatozoa per mL [67]. It is known that variable sperm concentration is obtained in the whole ejaculate when different individuals are compared. In the field of cryopreservation, commercial doses of sperm have a smaller number of spermatozoa than those of the original ejaculate, and sperm concentration recommended for insemination may also vary when different mammalian species are compared [68, 69]. Thus, the question with respect to ART should focus on what is the optimal sperm concentration to maintain sperm alive for longer and still produce effective fertilization? In the era of ICSI, sperm concentration is no longer considered a bottleneck for fertilization, but in more traditional approaches (such as IVF and IUI) this may be an important issue [67]. Evidence currently exists that both motility and membrane integrity improve with increased dilution of the sample. In bulls, for example, the lower the sperm concentration, the higher the proportion of viable cells with active acrosomes [70]. The influence of sperm concentration on sperm DNA longevity was first tested in an experimental model such as ram, where sperm concentrations are extremely high. It was demonstrated that within the same ejaculate, sperm DNA longevity is greater at low sperm concentrations [71]. An equivalent experimental model in humans showed that in vitro DNA longevity decreases when sperm concentration is above 10 million [67]. Subsequently, for ICSI where sperm concentration is not a limiting factor, the use of sperm concentrations lower that 10×10^6 mL^{-1} improved DNA stability. In general, the sperm concentration obtained at the first fraction is high compared with the second one and this may negatively interfere with seminal characteristics by reducing its effectivity at the time of reproductive outcome. Thus, for ART purposes the synergistic coupling of using the first ejaculated fraction with an appropriate sperm concentration may be a worthy strategy to prevent sperm damage while the samples are manipulated in vitro.

22.6.5 Use of Testicular Sperm for Intra-Cytoplasmic Sperm Injection

Under clinical situations such as azoospermia or severe oligozoospermia, the possibility exists to obtain immature sperm directly from the testis; these samples, after in vitro maturation, have the physiological capacity to produce syngamy. Interestingly, sperm obtained directly from the testicle present lower levels of DNA damage compared to their ejaculated counterparts [72, 73]. The magnitude of SDF reduction in the testis compared to the ejaculated sample can be as high as 80 percent [74]. In addition, results indicate that ICSI outcomes were significantly better in the group of patients using testicular sperm when compared to the group of similar characteristics where only ejaculated sperm and ICSI was used [74]. Testicular recovered sperm also reduces early miscarriage when compared with equivalent cohorts of patients when ejaculated sperm is used [74].

22.6.6 Other Strategies

Sperm DNA Fragmentation tends to be lower in donors and normozoospermic males than in infertile patients although there is still significant variation in the levels of SDF when different ejaculates of the same individual are assessed [75]. Taking this into account, the establishment of a mini-cryopreserved sperm bank using samples from different ejaculates of the same patient where SDF levels are systematically assessed would allow selecting the specimens with lower SDF to be used at the time of fertilization. The different levels of SDF can be compared with the fresh sampleobtained on the day of fertilization and in the case that this value is very high, a sample presenting a lower SDF value in personalized cryo-banking could be used. This approach may have interest because different tactics for sperm selection can be used in different ejaculates trying to decrease the levels of SDF. Benefits of these personalized mini sperm banks are attractive since they can be variably combined with recurrent ejaculations, use of the first ejaculated fraction, as well as multiple techniques for sperm selection.

Finally, we would like to draw attention to the possibility of using flow cytometry to decrease SDF. Flow cytometry has been used to separate X- and Y-bearing sperm and this technique has produced viable offspring in some mammalian species [76]. In humans, the method has been applied in some countries, where legally allowed, for sex selection [77]. While the possibility of using this technique to decrease SDF has not been tested in humans after semen processing, in animal models such as bulls, where the technique is used on a routine basis, it has been demonstrated that sperm sorting reduces the proportion of sperm containing a fragmented DNA molecule compared with the original ejaculate [44]. In this case, the simple targeting of dead/alive cells to discriminate unviable spermatozoa and separate them from the viable ones give rise to a significant reduction in the levels of SDF. Not all spermatozoa presenting with DNA damage are removed but a reduction of approximately 60 percent can be achieved. The main problem of using this technical strategy is that the methodology is aggressive and gives rise to a decrease of sperm DNA longevity [45]. This strategy, if possible, needs further investigation to be used on a routine basis.

22.7 Conclusion

The sperm chromatin dispersion test can be considered a quick and standardized alternative to other available techniques to assess sperm DNA fragmentation. The rationale of the technique can be used not only for human sperm samples but is also functional, with methodological adaptations to produce congruent results in a wide range of animal species. The technique shows good correlation with SDF values obtained with other techniques such as TUNEL, Comet assay or SCSA. The procedure offers predictive results of fertilization, embryo quality, pregnancy and live birth in an equivalent range to other alternative techniques. In addition, the SCD test provides some capabilities that are not inherent to the other alternative technologies. We highlight the capacity of the SCD to be used in patients with extremely low sperm counts, such as severe oligozoospermia, testicular sperm, MACs, IMSI, PICSI selected sperm or sperm processed with microfluidics. The simultaneous assessment of SDF and DNA base modifications such as the level of methylation, presence of 8-oxoguanine or detection of aneuploidies, can also be performed on SCD processed slides. The assessment of sperm DNA longevity is closely connected with the presence of iatrogenic damage and can also mimic the behavior of sperm DNA in the female reproductive tract. One of the main advantages of the SCD technique is that it provides an open interface to assess SDF, in a simultaneous and synergistic combination with other diagnostic tools to accomplish the best DNA quality in the male gamete that will be used for the purposes of fertilization.

References

1. Gleicher N. Expected advances in human fertility treatments and their likely translational consequences. *J Transl Med* 2018; **16**: 149.

2. Boivin J, Bunting L, Collins JA, Nygren KG. International estimates of infertility prevalence and treatment-seeking: potential need and demand for infertility medical care. *Hum Reprod* 2007; **22**: 1506–12.

3. Kothandaraman N, Agarwal A, Al-Qahtani MHE. Pathogenic landscape of idiopathic male infertility: new insight towards its regulatory networks. *Genomic Med* 2016; **1**: 16023.

4. Santia D, Spaggiaria G, Simonia M. Sperm DNA fragmentation index as a promising predictive tool for male infertility diagnosis and treatment management-meta-analyses. *Reprod BioMed Online* 2018; **37**: 315–26.

5. Evenson DP, Darzynkiewicz Z, Melamed MR. Relation of mammalian sperm chromatin heterogeneity to fertility. *Science* 1980; **210**: 1131–3.

6. Evenson DP, Wixon R. Data analysis of two in vivo fertility studies using sperm chromatin structure assay-derived DNA fragmentation index vs. pregnancy outcome. *Fertil Steril* 2008; **90**: 1229–31.

7. Zini A, Meriano J, Kader K, Jarvi K, Laskin CA, Cadesky K. Potential adverse effect of sperm DNA damage on embryo quality after ICSI. *Hum Reprod* 2005; **20**: 3476–80.

8. Castilla JA, Zamora S, Gonzalvo MC, Luna del Castillo JD, Roldan-Nofuentes JA, Clavero A, Björndahl L, Martínez L. Sperm chromatin structure assay and classical semen parameters: systematic review. *Reprod BioMed Online* 2010; **20**: 114–24.

9. Tang Q, Pan F, Yang J, Fu Z, Lu Y, Wu X, Han X, Chen M, Lu C, Xia Y, Wang X, Wu W. Idiopathic male infertility is strongly associated with aberrant DNA methylation of imprinted loci in sperm: a case-control study. *Clin Epigenet* 2018; **10**: 134.

10. Fernández JL, Goyanes VJ, Ramiro-Díaz J, Gosálvez J. Application of FISH for in situ detection and quantification of DNA breakage. *Cytogenet Cell Genet* 1998; **82**: 251–6.

11. Fernández JL, Muriel L, Rivero MT, Goyanes V, Vazquez R, Alvarez JG. The sperm chromatin dispersion test: a simple method for the determination of sperm DNA fragmentation. *J Androl* 2003; **24**: 59–66.

12. Gosálvez J, Caballero P, López-Fernández C, Ortega L, Guijarro JA, Fernández JL, Johnston SD, Nuñez-Calonge R. Can DNA fragmentation of neat or swim-up spermatozoa be used to predict pregnancy following ICSI of fertile oocyte donors? *Asian J Androl* 2013; **15**: 812–18.

13. Fernández JL, Muriel L, Goyanes V, Segrelles E, Gosálvez J, Enciso M, LaFromboise M, De Jonge C. Simple determination of human sperm DNA fragmentation with an improved sperm chromatin dispersion (SCD) test. *Fertil Steril* 2005; **84**: 833–42.

14. Santiso R, Tamayo M, Gosálvez J, Johnston SJ, Mariño A, Fernández C, Losada C, Fernández JL. DNA fragmentation dynamics allows the assessment of cryptic sperm damage in humans: evaluation of exposure to ionizing radiation, hyperthermia, acidic pH and nitric oxide. *Mutation Res* 2012; **734**: 41–9.

15. Chohan KR, Griffin JT, Lafromboise M, De Jonge CJ, Carrell DT. Comparison of chromatin assays for DNA fragmentation evaluation in human sperm. *J Androl* 2006; **27**: 53–9.

16. Ribas-Maynou J, Garcia-Peiro A, Fernández-Encinas A, Abad C, Amengual MJ, Prada E, Navarro J, Benet J. Comprehensive analysis of sperm DNA fragmentation by five different assays: TUNEL assay, SCSA, SCD test and alkaline and neutral Comet assay. *Andrology* 2013; **1**:715–22.

17. Aamir J, Talkad MS, Ramaiah K. Evaluation of sperm DNA fragmentation using multiple methods: a comparison of their predictive power for male infertility. *Clin Exp Reprod Med* 2019; **46**: 14–21.

18. Rodriguez B, et al. Varicocele, leukocytospermia and its impact on the spermatic DNA fragmentation. *Revista*

Internacional de Andrología 2012; **10**(1): 3–10.

19. Nuñez R, López-Fernández C, Arroyo F, Caballero P, Gosálvez J. Characterization of sperm DNA damage in Kartagener´s syndrome with recurrent fertilization failure: case revisited. *Sex Reprod Health* 2010; **1**: 73–5.

20. Esteves SC, Gosálvez J, López-Fernández C, Núñez-Calonge R, Caballero P, Agarwal A, Fernández JL. Diagnostic accuracy of sperm DNA degradation index (DDSi) as a potential noninvasive biomarker to identify men with varicocele-associated infertility. *Int Urol Nephrol* 2015; **47**: 1471–7.

21. Parmegiani L, Cognigni GE, Bernardi S, Troilo E, Ciampaglia W, Filicori M. "Physiologic ICSI", Hyaluronic acid (HA) favors selection of spermatozoa without DNA fragmentation and with normal nucleus, resulting in improvement of embryo quality. *Fertil Steril* 2010; **93**: 598–604.

22. González-Martínez M, Sánchez-Martín P, Dorado-Silva M, Fernández JL, Girones E, Johnston SD, Gosálvez J. Magnetic-activated cell sorting is not completely effective at reducing sperm DNA fragmentation. *J Assist Reprod Genet* 2018; **35**: 2215–21.

23. Santiso R, Tamayo M, Gosálvez J, Meseguer M, Garrido N, Fernández JL. Simultaneous determination in situ of DNA fragmentation and 8-oxoguanine in human sperm. *Fertil Steril* 2010; **93**: 314–18.

24. Gosálvez J, González-Martínez M, López-Fernández C, Fernández JL, Sánchez-Martín P. Shorter abstinence decreases sperm deoxyribonucleic acid fragmentation in ejaculate. *Fertil Steril* 2011; **96**: 1083–6.

25. Muriel L, Goyanes V, Segrelle E, Gosálvez J, Alvarez J, Fernández JL. Increased aneuploidy rate in sperm with fragmented DNA as determined by the Sperm Chromatin Dispersion (SCD) test and FISH analysis. *J Androl* 2007; **28**: 38–49.

26. Kim SW, Jee BC, Kim SK, Kim SH. Sperm DNA fragmentation and sex chromosome aneuploidy after swim-up versus density gradient centrifugation. *Clin Exp Reprod Med* 2017; **44**: 201–6.

27. González-Marín C, Roy R, López-Fernández C, Diez B, Carabaño MJ, Fernández JL, Kjelland ME, Moreno JF, Gosálvez J. Bacteria in bovine semen can increase sperm DNA fragmentation rates: a kinetic experimental approach. *Animal Reprod Sci* 2011; **123**: 139–48.

28. Gosálvez J, López-Fernández C, Hermoso A, Fernández JL, Kjelland ME. Sperm DNA fragmentation in zebrafish (Danio rerio) and its impact on fertility and embryo viability. Implications for fisheries and aquaculture. *Aquaculture* 2014; **433**: 173–82.

29. Evenson DP, Wixon R. Clinical aspects of sperm DNA fragmentation detection and male infertility. *Theriogenology* 2006; **65**: 979–91.

30. Simon L, Liu L, Murphy K, Ge S, Hotaling J, Aston KI, Emery B, Carrell DT. Comparative analysis of three sperm DNA damage assays and sperm nuclear protein content in couples undergoing assisted reproduction treatment. *Hum Reprod* 2014; **29**: 904–17.

31. Bungum M, Humaidan P, Axmon A, Spano M, Bungum L, Erenpreiss J, Giwercman A. Sperm DNA integrity assessment in prediction of assisted reproduction technology outcome. *Hum Reprod* 2007; **22**: 174–9.

32. Frydman N, Prisant N, Hesters L, Frydman R, Tachdjian G, Cohen-Bacrie P, Fanchin R. Adequate ovarian follicular status does not prevent the decrease in pregnancy rates associated with high sperm DNA fragmentation. *Fertil Steril* 2008; **89**: 92–7.

33. Avendano C, Franchi A, Duran H, Oehninger S. DNA fragmentation of normal spermatozoa negatively impacts embryo quality and intracytoplasmic sperm injection outcome. *Fertil Steril* 2010; **94**: 549–57.

34. Simon L, Brunborg G, Stevenson M, Lutton D, McManus J, Lewis SE. Clinical significance of sperm DNA damage in assisted reproduction outcome. *Hum Reprod* 2010; **25**: 1594–608.

35. Speyer BE, Pizzey AR, Ranieri M, Joshi R, Delhanty JD, Serhal P. Fall in implantation rates following ICSI with sperm with high DNA fragmentation. *Hum Reprod* 2010; **25**: 1609–18.

36. Nuñez-Calonge R, Caballero P, López-Fernández C, Guijarro JA, Fernández JL, Johnston SD, Gosálvez J. An improved experimental model for understanding the impact of sperm DNA fragmentation on human pregnancy following ICSI. *Reprod Sci* 2012; **19**: 1163–8.

37. Gandini L, Lombardo F, Paoli D, Caruso F, Eleuteri P, Leter G, Ciriminna R, Culasso F, Dondero F, Lenzi A, Spanò M . Full-term pregnancies achieved with ICSI despite high levels of sperm chromatin damage. *Hum Reprod* 2004; **19**: 1409–17.

38. Muriel L, Garrido N, Fernández JL, Remohi J, Pellicer A, de los Santos MJ, Meseguer M. Value of the sperm deoxyribonucleic acid fragmentation level, as measured by the sperm chromatin dispersion test, in the outcome of in vitro fertilization and intracytoplasmic sperm injection. *Fertil Steril* 2006; **85**: 371–83.

39. Esbert M, Pacheco A, Vidal F, Florensa M, Riqueros M, Ballesteros A, Garrido N, Calderón G. Impact of sperm DNA fragmentation on the outcome of IVF with own or

donated oocytes. *Reprod BioMed Online* 2011; **23**: 704–10.

40. Vélez de la Calle JF, Muller A, Walschaerts M, Clavere JL, Jimenez C, Wittemer C, Thonneau P. Sperm deoxyribonucleic acid fragmentation as assessed by the sperm chromatin dispersion test in assisted reproductive technology programs: results of a large prospective multicenter study. *Fertil Steril* 2008; **90**: 1792–9.

41. Enciso M, Iglesias M, Galán I, Sarasa J, Gosálbez A, Gosálvez J. The ability of sperm selection techniques to remove single- or double-strand DNA damage. *Asian J Androl* 2011; **13**: 764–8.

42. López-Fernández C, Crespo F, Arroyo F, Fernández JL, Arana P, Johnston SD, Gosálvez J. Dynamics of sperm DNA fragmentation in domestic animals II: the stallion. *Theriogenology* 2007; **68**: 1240–50.

43. López-Fernández C, Fernández JL, Gosálbez A, Arroyo F, Vázquez JM, Holt WV, Gosálvez J. Dynamics of sperm DNA fragmentation in domestic animals III. Ram. *Theriogenology* 2008; **70**: 898–908.

44. Gosálvez J, López-Fernández C, Fernández JL, Gouraud A, Holt WV. Relationships between the dynamics of iatrogenic DNA damage and genomic design in mammalian sperm from eleven species. *Mol Reprod Dev* 2011a; **78**: 951–61.

45. Gosálvez J, Núñez R, Fernández JL. López-Fernández C, Caballero P. Dynamics of sperm DNA damage in fresh versus frozen-thawed and gradient processed ejaculates in human donors. *Andrologia* 2011b; **43**: 373–7.

46. Gosálvez J, Cortés-Gutierrez EI, López-Fernández C, Fernández JL, Caballero P, Nuñez R. Sperm deoxyribonucleic acid fragmentation dynamics in fertile donors. *Fertil Steril* 2009; **92**: 170–3.

47. Gosálvez J, Sánchez R, Alvarez JG. Single- and double-strand DNA breaks after incubation of thawed cryopreserved human spermatozoa. *Fertil Steril* 2019 (in press).

48. Dalzell LH, McVicar CM, McClure N, Lutton D, Lewis SE. Effects of short and long incubations on DNA fragmentation of testicular sperm. *Fertil Steril* 2004; **82**: 1443–5.

49. Bungum M, Bungum L, Humaidan P. A prospective study, using sibling oocytes, examining the effect of 30 seconds versus 90 minutes gamete co-incubation in IVF. *Hum Reprod* 2006; **21**: 518–23.

50. Johnston SD, López-Fernández C, Arroyo F, Gosálbez A, Cortés Gutiérrez EI, Fernández JL, Gosálvez J. Reduced sperm DNA longevity is associated with an increased incidence of still born; evidence from a multi-ovulating sequential artificial insemination animal model. *J Assist Reprod Genet* 2016; **33**: 1231–8.

51. Tvrdá E, López-Fernández C, Sánchez-Martín P, Gosálvez J. Sperm DNA fragmentation in donors and normozoospermic patients attending for a first spermiogram: static and dynamic assessment. *Andrologia* 2018a; **50**: e12986.

52. Gosálvez J, Agarwal A, Esteves SC. Strategies to diminish DNA damage in sperm samples used for ART. In A. Zini and A. Agarwal, eds., *A Clinician's Guide to Sperm DNA and Chromatin Damage.* Cham, Switzerland: Springer, pp. 571–87.

53. Pons I, Cercas R, Villas C, Braña C, Fernández-Shaw S. One abstinence day decreases sperm DNA fragmentation in 90% of selected patients. *J Assist Reprod Genet* 2013; **30**: 1211–18.

54. Marshburn PB, Alanis MC, Matthew MLS. A short period of abstinence before intrauterine insemination is associated with higher pregnancy rates. *Fertil Steril* 2009; **93**: 286–8.

55. Sánchez-Martín P, Sánchez-Martín F, González-Martínez M, Gosálvez, J. Increased pregnancy after reduced male abstinence. *System Biol Reprod Sci* 2013; **59**: 256–60.

56. Cohen J, Euser R, Schenck PE, Brugman FW, Zeilmaker GH. Motility and morphology of human spermatozoa in split ejaculates. *Andrologia* 1981; **13**: 491–8.

57. Mortimer D. Biochemistry of spermatozoa and seminal plasma. In *Practical Laboratory Andrology.* New York: Oxford University Press, pp. 89–109.

58. Hebles M, Dorado M, González-Martínez M, Sánchez-Martín P. Seminal quality in the first fraction of ejaculate. *Syst Biol Reprod Med* 2014; **30**: 1–4.

59. de la Torre J, Sánchez-Martín P, Gosálvez J, Crespo F. Equivalent seminal characteristics in human and stallion at first and second ejaculated fractions. *Andrologia* 2016; **49**: 1–5.

60. Mann T, Lutwak-Mann C. Biochemistry of spermatozoa: chemical and functional correlations in ejaculated semen. Andrological aspect. In T. Mann, C. Lutwak-Mann, eds., *Male Reproductive Function and Semen.* London: Springer, pp. 195–268.

61. Holt WV, Van Look KJ. Concepts in sperm heterogeneity, sperm selection and sperm competition as biological foundations for laboratory tests of semen quality. *Reproduction* 2004; **127**: 527–35.

62. Santolaria P, Soler C, Recreo P, Carretero T, Bono A, Berné JM, Yániz JL. Morphometric and kinematic sperm subpopulations in split ejaculates of

normozoospermic men. *Asian J Androl* 2016; **18**: 831–4.

63. Said TM, Land JA. Effects of advanced selection methods on sperm quality and ART outcome: a systematic review. *Hum Reprod Update* 2011; **17**: 719–33.

64. Sikka SC, Hellstrom WJG. Current updates on laboratory techniques for the diagnosis of male reproductive failure. *Asian J Androl* 2016; **18**: 392–401.

65. López-Fernández C, Johnston SD, Gosálbez A, Fernández JL, Álvarez JG, Gosálvez J. Inter-center variation in the efficiency of sperm DNA damage reduction following density gradient centrifugation. *Nat Sci* 2013; **5**: 15–20.

66. Bansal AK, Bilaspuri GS. Impacts of oxidative stress and antioxidants on semen functions. *Vet Med Int* Article ID 686137; http://dx.doi.org/10.4061/2011/686137

67. Tvrdá E, Arroyo F, Gosálvez J. Dynamic assessment of human sperm DNA damage I: the effect of seminal plasma-sperm co-incubation after ejaculation. *Int Urol Nephrol* 2018b; **50**: 1381–8.

68. Auger J, Eustache F, Ducot B, Blandin T, Daudin M, Diaz I, Matribi SE, Gony B, Keskes L, Kolbezen M, Lamarte A, Lornage J, Nomal N, Pitaval G, Simon O, Virant-Klun I, Spira A, Jouannet P. Intra- and inter-individual variability in human sperm concentration, motility and vitality assessment during a workshop involving ten laboratories. *Hum Reprod* 2000; **15**: 2360–8.

69. Lüpold S, Fitzpatrick JL. Sperm number trumps sperm size in mammalian ejaculate evolution. *Proc Biol Sci* 2015; **282**(1819): 20152122.

70. Januskauskas A, Söderquist L, Håård MG, Håård MC, Lundeheim N, Rodriguez-Martinez H. Influence of sperm number per straw on the post-thaw sperm viability and fertility of Swedish red and white A.I. bulls. *Acta Vet Scand* 1996; **37**: 461–70.

71. López-Fernández C, Johnston SD, Fernández JL, Wilson RJ, Gosálvez J. Fragmentation dynamics of frozen-thawed ram sperm DNA is modulated by sperm concentration. *Theriogenology* 2010; **74**: 1362–70.

72. Greco E, Scarselli F, Iacobelli M, Rienzi L, Ubaldi F, Ferrero S, Franco G, Anniballo N, Mendoza C, Tesarik J. Efficient treatment of infertility due to sperm DNA damage by ICSI with testicular spermatozoa. *Hum Reprod* 2005; **20**: 226–30.

73. Moskovtsev SI, Jarvi K, Mullen JB, Cadesky KI, Hannam T, Lo KC. Testicular spermatozoa have statistically significantly lower DNA damage compared with ejaculated spermatozoa in patients with unsuccessful oral antioxidant treatment. *Fertil Steril* 2010; **93**: 1142–6.

74. Esteves SC, Sanchez-Martín F, Sanchez-Martín P, Schneider DT, Gosálvez J. Comparison of reproductive outcome in oligozoospermic men with high sperm DNA fragmentation undergoing intracytoplasmic sperm injection with ejaculated and testicular sperm. *Fertil Steril* 2015; **104**: 1398–1405.

75. Rylander L, Wetterstrand B, Haugen TB, Malm G, Malm J, Bjørsvik C, Henrichsen T, Sæther T, Giwercman A. Single semen analysis as a predictor of semen quality: clinical and epidemiological implications. *Asian J Androl* 2009; **11**: 723–30.

76. Johnson LA, Flook JP, Hawk HW. Sex preselection in rabbits: live births from X and Y sperm separated by DNA and cell sorting. *Biol Reprod* 1989; **41**: 199–203.

77. Karabinus DS, Marazzo DP, Stern HJ, Potter DA, Opang CI, Cole ML, Johnson LA, Schulman JD. The effectiveness of flow cytometric sorting of human sperm (MicroSort®) for influencing a child's sex. *Reprod Biol Endocrinol* 2014; **12**: 106.

Chapter 23

DNA Damage: Fluorescent In-Situ Hybridization

Sezgin Gunes

23.1 Fluorescent In-Situ Hybridization

Several sperm DNA integrity and chromatin quality assays have been developed and used for the detection of sperm DNA fragmentation and chromosomal aberrations [1, 2]. The Comet assay is one of the most commonly used single cell gel electrophoresis methods first developed by Östling and Johanson [3]. Damaged or fragmented sperm DNA is separated from undamaged DNA by electrophoresis. Fluorescent in situ hybridization (FISH) is a hybridization method that provides specific identification of selected DNA sequences and is frequently used for cytogenetic analysis of spermatozoa. These two methods were combined as the Comet-FISH technique first by Santos and colleagues in 1997 [4]. The Comet-FISH technique is a combination of two well-known methods, the Comet assay and FISH, and is a useful detection tool for screening of whole and region-specific DNA damage [5, 6]. In addition, the analysis of labeled DNA sequences and whole chromosomes of interest and identification of region-specific DNA and overall damage and repair in single cells is possible [7, 8]. Therefore, the modification of these assays interpolates hybridization with specific fluorescent-labeled probes to selected DNA sequences of interest after unwinding and electrophoresis [6] and developed a standardized Comet assay for human sperm with additional information for telomeres or special DNA sequences of interest. Thus, specific gene sequences can be detected using the Comet-FISH technique [9].

23.1.1 Sperm Aneuploidy Screening with Fluorescent In-Situ Hybridization

Aneuploidies are numerical chromosomal aberrations of a cell/organism and these aneuploidies are the major causes of early pregnancy loss, mental retardation, developmental disorders, and infertility [10].

Aneuploidies arise from non-disjunction of sister chromatids and anaphase lagging (Figure 23.1). FISH is a molecular cytogenetic assay, which is used for detecting and measuring of sperm aneuploidy and based on binding of fluorescently labeled primers specifically to each chromosome in the sperm sample and visualization of the samples under a fluorescent microscope. A decrease or increase in the fluorescent signals indicates aneuploidy [11].

Infertile men with aneuploidy in their somatic cells usually have impaired spermatogenesis. Therefore, these chromosomal aberrations could also be observed as sperm chromosome abnormalities [12]. Although a full detection of sperm aneuploidy should comprise all autosome and sex chromosomes, non-lethal chromosomes as well as chromosomes compatible with survival may be sufficient for sperm aneuploidy detection. These chromosomes are 13, 18, 21, X and Y [13].

Previously, sperm aneuploidy was detected using karyotype analysis. However, nowadays, it is detected using the FISH technique in sperm nuclei or using sequencing technology such as next-generation sequencing assays [14]. Sarrate and Anton [15] have described the sperm FISH assay in five steps. These steps are sample (epididymal, ejaculated or testicular sperm) processing with fixation of the cells, decondensation, annealing, post-annealing washes and visualization. Briefly, sperm chromosomes are fixed and decondensate on the slide. Fluorescently labeled DNA probes specific for the chromosomes that shall be analyzed are hybridized. After the hybridization, slides are washed and finally analyzed by means of fluorescent microscopy.

Standardized evaluation criteria must be used for correct assessment of sperm aneuploidy. Every normal spermatozoon must give one blue, green and red signal corresponding to chromosome 18, X and Y, respectively. In addition, green and red signals must be differentiated for chromosomes 13 and 21,

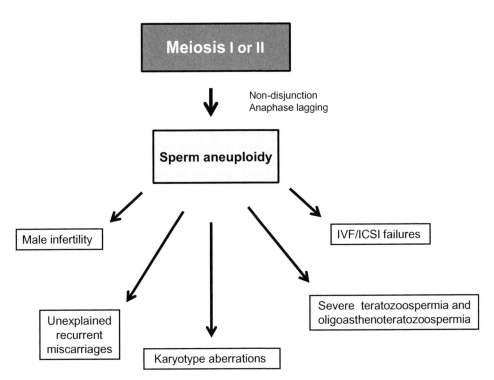

Figure 23.1 Sperm aneuploidy mechanisms and consequences.

respectively, in each normal spermatozoa as well [15]. To avoid variation of the results, sperm heads without a well-defined boundary or overlapped spermatozoa must not be counted. In the evaluation of disomic and diploidic spermatozoa, the intensity of the signal should be separated and be equal [16].

Sperm FISH analysis gives a predication of the frequency of sperm chromosomal aberrations including disomy, nullisomy, and diploidy. However, there is no concurrence on statistical analysis of sperm FISH results. Recently, a study suggested a non-parametric Wilcoxon Rank Sum test for the statistical analysis of sperm FISH results including disomy, nullisomy, diploidy and a number of 13 chromosomes (1, 2, 9, 13, 15, 16, 17, 18, 19, 21, 22, X, and Y) in human sperm nuclei from 14 fertile males using automatized FISH. In this manner, fertile males have been classified as normal or altered regarding the sperm aneuploidy with application of this approach [17]. The main limitation of this analysis is the difficulty of evaluation of all chromosomes of spermatozoa. Evaluation of clinically relevant chromosomes (13, 18, 21, X and Y) is sufficient to reveal the presence of meiotic defects [18].

Nonetheless, sperm DNA FISH analysis is recommended for men whose partners have a history of recurrent pregnancy loss (RPL) or IVF failures [11]. Hence, sperm with sex chromosome, chromosome 13 or 21 and chromosome 18 aneuploidies were found to be 2.7-, 3.3- and 6-times more frequent in men whose partners have a history of RPL compared with fertile men. In total, 40 percent of normozoospermic controls showed sperm aneuploidy in all evaluated chromosomes. Sex chromosome and sperm aneuploidy were found to be higher in men with abnormal strict morphology compare with those of men with normal morphology (>4 percent) (57 percent versus 28 percent). Additionally, no association between sperm DNA fragmentation and sperm aneuploidy studied group has been reported [19].

23.1.1.1 Indications for the Fluorescent In-Situ Hybridization Analysis in Spermatozoa

Before performing sperm FISH analysis, it is useful to select, which patients should undergo the analysis. Sperm FISH analysis is indicated in men with normal semen parameters whose partners suffer from RPL [19].

229

Several studies revealed a significant relation between sperm aneuploidy and decreased sperm count, motility and morphology. Thus, FISH evaluation of spermatozoa for infertile men with low sperm count [18, 20] and abnormal sperm morphology [19] have been suggested as useful methods. Rubio et al. [20] investigated the association between semen parameter and numerical chromosomal abnormalities in 63 men [20]. The rate of disomy and diploidy of chromosomes 18 and 21 and sex chromosomes (average 0.28 percent) have been found to be significantly higher in patients with oligoasthenoteratozoospermia (OAT) ($<20 \times 10^6$ spermatozoa/mL [WHO 1999]) compared to normozoospermic men (0.1 percent of diploidy). Results were found to be more prominent in patients with severe oligozoospermia ($<5 \times 10^6$ spermatozoa/mL) (0.45 percent). Similarly, a small study including nine severe OAT patients and four proven fertile donors showed higher autosomal disomy (0–5.4 percent versus 0.05–0.2 percent), disomy of the sex chromosome (1.6–4.9 percent versus 0.15 percent) and also diploidy (0.4–9.6 percent versus 0.04 percent) than the controls [22].

The most frequent chromosome aberration of spermatozoa of infertile males is diploidy of sex chromosomes, 24,XY and 24,YY. Therefore, a second group of candidates for FISH analysis of spermatozoa are men with 47,XXY and 47,XYY karyotypes. Men with 47,XXY and 47,XYY karyotypes produce more diploidy of sex chromosomes compared to men with normal karyotype [23].

Since spermatozoa have to be obtained from the epididymis or testicle, men with non-obstructive azoospermia (NOA) are also candidates for sperm FISH analysis. Several studies have found higher frequency of aneuploidy in testicular spermatozoa compared with those of ejaculated spermatozoa from normal controls [24, 25, 26, 27]. However, the results were found to be contradictory regarding aneuploidy frequency in spermatozoa retrieved from testicle or epididymis. The aneuploidy rate of chromosomes 18, 21,X and Y was found to be significantly ($p<0.0001$) higher in testicular spermatozoa of men with NOA (11.4 percent) than that observed in epididymal sperm of men with obstructive azoospermia (1.8 percent) and in ejaculated spermatozoa of healthy men (1.5 percent), respectively [27]. Similarly, Rodrigo et al. [28] observed no difference in the aneuploidy rate between the epididymal and ejaculated spermatozoa.

Recent studies have reported that chromosomal aberrations of human spermatozoa in older men are more often structural rearrangements than aneuploidies [29]. Indeed, the analysis of sperm from men older than 50 years demonstrated significantly higher percentages of sperm with damaged DNA, elevated global aneuploidy rates, and a significantly ($p\leq0.05$) increased number of embryos with trisomy in IVF/ICSI cycles [30, 31]. Moreover, paternal aging not only leads to several alterations in the male endocrine system including lower androgen and higher follicle stimulating hormone (FSH) levels, but also to variations in testicular structure and volume leading to changes in sperm production and quality, elevated sperm DNA fragmentation [29, 31]]. Consequently, several studies showed that men with NOA, severe OAT, severe teratozoospermia [32, 33] are good candidates for FISH analysis. Similarly, sperm samples retrieved from the testes are reported to be prone to aneuploidy compared to those retrieved from the epididymis [27, 28]. Nevertheless, men from female partners with unexplained RPL or recurrent implantation failure (RIF) may benefit from sperm aneuploidy screening [17]. However, data on the reproductive outcome after performing this examination are still missing [23].

23.1.2 Genetic Counseling in Men with Sperm Aneuploidies

The progress of assisted reproductive technologies including IVF and ICSI helps infertile men with abnormal semen parameters to father a child. Gametes from these men demonstrate increased rates of chromosomal aberrations compared with fertile men. Furthermore, higher rates of aneuploidy have been reported after preimplantation genetic diagnosis (PGD) in embryos obtained after IVF/ICSI with sperm from men with OAT and higher chromosomal alterations [18].

Genetic counseling is necessary to help these couples to understand the nature and consequences of sperm chromosomal aberrations. Likewise, genetic counseling for these patients may provide appropriate treatment and management options to increase their chances to fertilize oocytes and decrease the risk of recurrent miscarriages.

A family history of infertility, RPL, birth defects, intellectual disability, possible consanguinity and ethnic information is obtained by drawing a three-generation pedigree. Genetic counselors advise couples that the general frequency of birth defects and intellectual disabilities is about 3 percent in all pregnancies regardless of maternal age, ethnicity, or family history. Subsequently, couples are counseled for the risk of trisomy 21 (Down syndrome) and other aneuploidies related to maternal age, reproductive risks related to family history and ethnic background [11].

An inverse correlation was found between sperm aneuploidy frequency and sperm quality [34]. Sperm morphology aberrations such as multinucleate, macrocephalic, and multi-flagellate sperm were found to be related with increased sperm disomy, diploidy and polyploidy [34, 35, 36].

Sperm FISH evaluation reveals aneuploidy of a single chromosome or a global increase of aneuploidy in all evaluated chromosomes. Balanced chromosomal translocations lead to an increase in aneuploidy of a single chromosome and are known causes of infertility, repeated miscarriages and IVF failure [11]. Patients carrying balanced chromosomal translocations, including both reciprocal and Robertsonian translocations, may show variable sperm production phenotypes ranging from normozoospermia to azoospermia. Reciprocal translocations are rearrangements between two non-homologous chromosomes. Likewise, Robertsonian translocations are centric fusions of two acrocentric chromosomes. Diagnostically, PGD is recommended for men with both reciprocal and Robertsonian chromosomal translocations. Several studies demonstrated that the live birth rate might increase from 4.9 percent to more than 80 percent if PGD is used [37, 38].

Males with numerical karyotype abnormalities including non-mosaic Klinefelter's patients [39] and Y-chromosome microdeletions are prone to develop spermatozoa with sex chromosome aneuploidy [40]. Likewise, fertile men who have fathered a child with paternally derived aneuploidy, men whose partner suffers from RPL, infertile oligozoospermic men, and even men with normal karyotypes are also at elevated risk of producing chromosomally abnormal spermatozoa [41]. Nicopoullos et al. [42] investigated the aneuploidy rates of chromosomes 13, 18, 21, X/Y in infertile men who achieved unsuccessful and successful ICSI outcome using FISH. In this study, the total aneuploidy rate (2.37 percent versus. 1.18 percent, p=0.01; unsuccessful and successful ICSI) and aneuploidy rate of chromosomes 18, X/Y and 18 + X/Y (1.48 percent versus 0.67 percent, p=0.005; unsuccessful and successful ICSI) have been found to be significantly higher in infertile men who achieve unsuccessful ICSI compared with successful ones.

23.2 Conclusion

It needs to be understood that all males at reproductive age produce aneuploid spermatozoa to some amount. However, the incidence of sperm aneuploidy and diploidy is higher in males with altered seminal parameters. Y-chromosome microdeletions, chemotherapy, varicocele, lifestyle and occupation may lead to aneuplody during meiosis I or II in spermatogenesis. Studies have demonstrated that sperm aneuploidy and diploidy is related to male infertility, repeated implantation failure (RIF), pregnancy loss after IVF/ICSI cycles, recurrent abortion and miscarriages, and elevated aneuploidies rates in live births. To better understand the clinical significance of higher sperm aneuploidy, further studies are necessary with larger and well designed patient and control groups.

References

1. Shamsi MB, Imam SN, Dada R. Sperm DNA integrity assays: diagnostic and prognostic challenges and implications in management of infertility. *J Assist Reprod Genet* 2011; **28**(11): 1073–85. doi:10.1007/s10815-011-9631-8

2. Simon L, Liu L, Murphy K, Ge S, Hotaling J, Aston KI, . . . Carrell DT. Comparative analysis of three sperm DNA damage assays and sperm nuclear protein content in couples undergoing assisted reproduction treatment. *Hum Reprod* 2014; **29**(5): 904–17. doi:10.1093/humrep/deu040

3. Ostling O, Johanson KJ. Bleomycin, in contrast to gamma irradiation, induces extreme variation of DNA strand breakage from cell to cell. *Int J Radiat Biol Relat Stud Phys Chem Med* 1987; **52**(5): 683–91. doi:10.1080/09553008714552201

4. Santos SJ, Singh NP, Natarajan AT. Fluorescence in situ hybridization with comets. *Exp Cell Res* 1997; **232**(2): 407–11. doi:10.1006/excr.1997.3555

5. Glei M, Hovhannisyan G, Pool-Zobel BL. Use of Comet-FISH in the study of DNA damage and repair: review. *Mutat Res* 2009; **681**(1): 33–43. doi:10.1016/j.mrrev.2008.01.006

6. Mondal M, Guo J. Comet-FISH for ultrasensitive strand-specific

detection of DNA damage in single cells. *Methods Enzymol* 2017; **591**: 83–95. doi:10.1016/bs.mie.2017.03.023

7. Glei M, Schlormann W. Analysis of DNA damage and repair by comet fluorescence in situ hybridization (Comet-FISH). *Methods Mol Biol* 2014; **1094**: 39–48. doi:10.1007/978-1-62703-706-8_4

8. Horvathova E, Dusinska M, Shaposhnikov S, Collins AR. DNA damage and repair measured in different genomic regions using the comet assay with fluorescent in situ hybridization. *Mutagenesis* 2004; **19**(4): 269–76. doi:10.1093/mutage/geh030

9. Shaposhnikov S, El Yamani N, Collins AR. Fluorescent in situ hybridization on comets: FISH comet. *Methods Mol Biol* 2015; **1288**: 363–73. doi:10.1007/978-1-4939-2474-5_21

10. Hassold T, Hunt P. To err (meiotically) is human: the genesis of human aneuploidy. *Nat Rev Genet* 2001; **2**(4): 280–91. doi:10.1038/35066065

11. Kohn TP, Kohn JR, Darilek S, Ramasamy R, Lipshultz L. Genetic counseling for men with recurrent pregnancy loss or recurrent implantation failure due to abnormal sperm chromosomal aneuploidy. *J Assist Reprod Genet* 2016; **33**(5): 571–6. doi:10.1007/s10815-016-0702-8

12. Bernardini L, Martini E, Geraedts JP, Hopman AH, Lanteri S, Conte N, Capitanio GL. Comparison of gonosomal aneuploidy in spermatozoa of normal fertile men and those with severe male factor detected by in-situ hybridization. *Mol Hum Reprod* 1997; **3**(5): 431–8. doi:10.1093/molehr/3.5.431

13. Templado C, Uroz L, Estop A. New insights on the origin and relevance of aneuploidy in human spermatozoa. *Mol Hum Reprod* 2013; **19**(10): 634–43. doi:10.1093/molehr/gat039

14. Colaco S, Sakkas D. Paternal factors contributing to embryo quality. *J Assist Reprod Genet* 2018; **35**(11): 1953–68. doi:10.1007/s10815-018-1304-4

15. Sarrate Z, Anton E. Fluorescence in situ hybridization (FISH) protocol in human sperm. *J Vis Exp* 2009; **31**: 1405. doi:10.3791/1405

16. Blanco J, Gabau E, Gomez D, Baena N, Guitart M, Egozcue J, Vidal F. Chromosome 21 disomy in the spermatozoa of the fathers of children with trisomy 21, in a population with a high prevalence of Down syndrome: increased incidence in cases of paternal origin. *Am J Hum Genet* 1998; **63**(4): 1067–72. doi:10.1086/302058

17. Garcia-Mengual E, Trivino JC, Saez-Cuevas A, Bataller J, Ruiz-Jorro M, Vendrell X. Male infertility: establishing sperm aneuploidy thresholds in the laboratory. *J Assist Reprod Genet* 2019; **36**(3): 371–81. doi:10.1007/s10815-018-1385-0

18. Sanchez-Castro M, Jimenez-Macedo AR, Sandalinas M, Blanco J. Prognostic value of sperm fluorescence in situ hybridization analysis over PGD. *Hum Reprod* 2009; **24**(6): 1516–21. doi:10.1093/humrep/dep037

19. Ramasamy R, Besada S, Lamb DJ. Fluorescent in situ hybridization of human sperm: diagnostics, indications, and therapeutic implications. *Fertil Steril* 2014; **102**(6): 1534–9. doi:10.1016/j.fertnstert.2014.09.013

20. Rubio C, Gil-Salom M, Simon C, Vidal F, Rodrigo L, Minguez Y, ... Pellicer A. Incidence of sperm chromosomal abnormalities in a risk population: relationship with sperm quality and ICSI outcome. *Hum Reprod* 2001; **16**(10): 2084–92. doi:10.1093/humrep/16.10.2084

21. World Health Organization. (1999) *WHO Laboratory Manual for the Examination of Human Semen and Sperm-Cervical Mucus Interaction*, 4th ed. Cambridge: Cambridge University Press.

22. Pang MG, Hoegerman SF, Cuticchia AJ, Moon SY, Doncel GF, Acosta AA, Kearns WG. Detection of aneuploidy for chromosomes 4, 6, 7, 8, 9, 10, 11, 12, 13, 17, 18, 21, X and Y by fluorescence in-situ hybridization in spermatozoa from nine patients with oligoasthenoteratozoospermia undergoing intracytoplasmic sperm injection. *Hum Reprod* 1999; **14**(5): 1266–73. doi:10.1093/humrep/14.5.1266

23. Caseiro AL, Regalo A, Pereira E, Esteves T, Fernandes F, Carvalho J. Implication of sperm chromosomal abnormalities in recurrent abortion and multiple implantation failure. *Reprod Biomed Online* 2015; **31**(4): 481–5. doi:10.1016/j.rbmo.2015.07.001

24. Bernardini L, Gianaroli L, Fortini D, Conte N, Magli C, Cavani S, ... Venturini PL. Frequency of hyper-, hypohaploidy and diploidy in ejaculate, epididymal and testicular germ cells of infertile patients. *Hum Reprod* 2000; **15**(10): 2165–72. doi:10.1093/humrep/15.10.2165

25. Burrello N, Calogero AE, De Palma A, Grazioso C, Torrisi C, Barone N, ... Vicari E. Chromosome analysis of epididymal and testicular spermatozoa in patients with azoospermia. *Eur J Hum Genet* 2002; **10**(6): 362–6. doi:10.1038/sj.ejhg.5200814

26. Mateizel I, Verheyen G, Van Assche E, Tournaye H, Liebaers I, Van Steirteghem A. FISH analysis of chromosome X, Y and 18 abnormalities in testicular sperm from azoospermic patients. *Hum Reprod* 2002; **17**(9): 2249–57. doi:10.1093/humrep/17.9.2249

27. Palermo GD, Colombero LT, Hariprashad JJ, Schlegel PN, Rosenwaks Z. Chromosome analysis of epididymal and testicular sperm in azoospermic patients undergoing ICSI. *Hum Reprod* 2002; **17**(3): 570–5. doi:10.1093/humrep/17.3.570

28. Rodrigo L, Rubio C, Mateu E, Simon C, Remohi J, Pellicer A, Gil-Salom M. Analysis of chromosomal abnormalities in testicular and epididymal spermatozoa from azoospermic ICSI patients by fluorescence in-situ hybridization. *Hum Reprod* 2004; **19**(1): 118–23. doi:10.1093/humrep/deh012

29. Gunes S, Hekim GN, Arslan MA, Asci R. Effects of aging on the male reproductive system. *J Assist Reprod Genet* 2016; **33**(4): 441–54. doi:10.1007/s10815-016-0663-y

30. Garcia-Ferreyra J, Hilario R, Luna D, Villegas L, Romero R, Zavala P, Duenas-Chacon J. In vivo culture system using the INVOcell device shows similar pregnancy and implantation rates to those obtained from in vivo culture system in ICSI procedures. *Clin Med Insights Reprod Health* 2015; **9**: 7–11. doi:10.4137/CMRH.S25494

31. Garcia-Ferreyra J, Luna D, Villegas L, Romero R, Zavala P, Hilario R, Duenas-Chacon J. High aneuploidy rates observed in embryos derived from donated oocytes are related to male aging and high percentages of sperm DNA fragmentation. *Clin Med Insights Reprod Health* 2015; **9**: 21–7. doi:10.4137/CMRH.S32769

32. Collodel G, Moretti E. Morphology and meiotic segregation in spermatozoa from men of proven fertility. *J Androl* 2008; **29**(1): 106–14. doi:10.2164/jandrol.107.002998

33. Mehdi M, Gmidene A, Brahem S, Guerin JF, Elghezal H, Saad A. Aneuploidy rate in spermatozoa of selected men with severe teratozoospermia. *Andrologia* 2012; **44**(Suppl. 1): 139–43. doi:10.1111/j.1439-0272.2010.01152.x

34. Calogero AE, De Palma A, Grazioso C, Barone N, Romeo R, Rappazzo G, D'Agata R. Aneuploidy rate in spermatozoa of selected men with abnormal semen parameters. *Hum Reprod* 2001; **16**(6): 1172–9. doi:10.1093/humrep/16.6.1172

35. Lewis-Jones I, Aziz N, Seshadri S, Douglas A, Howard P. Sperm chromosomal abnormalities are linked to sperm morphologic deformities. *Fertil Steril* 2003; **79**(1): 212–15. doi:10.1016/s0015-0282(02)04411-4

36. Tempest HG, Griffin DK. The relationship between male infertility and increased levels of sperm disomy. *Cytogenet Genome Res* 2004; **107**(1–2): 83–94. doi:10.1159/000079575

37. Keymolen K, Staessen C, Verpoest W, Liebaers I, Bonduelle M. Preimplantation genetic diagnosis in female and male carriers of reciprocal translocations: clinical outcome until delivery of 312 cycles. *Eur J Hum Genet* 2012; **20**(4): 376–80. doi:10.1038/ejhg.2011.208

38. Munne S, Sandalinas M, Escudero T, Fung J, Gianaroli L, Cohen J. Outcome of preimplantation genetic diagnosis of translocations. *Fertil Steril* 2000; **73**(6): 1209–18. doi:10.1016/s0015-0282(00)00495-7

39. Tempest HG. Meiotic recombination errors, the origin of sperm aneuploidy and clinical recommendations. *Syst Biol Reprod Med* 2011; **57**(1–2): 93–101. doi:10.3109/19396368.2010.504879

40. O'Flynn O'Brien KL, Varghese AC, Agarwal A. The genetic causes of male factor infertility: a review. *Fertil Steril* 2010; **93**(1): 1–12. doi:10.1016/j.fertnstert.2009.10.045

41. Chatziparasidou A, Christoforidis N, Samolada G, Nijs M. Sperm aneuploidy in infertile male patients: a systematic review of the literature. *Andrologia* 2015; **47**(8): 847–60. doi:10.1111/and.12362

42. Nicopoullos JD, Gilling-Smith C, Almeida PA, Homa S, Nice L, Tempest H, Ramsay JW. The role of sperm aneuploidy as a predictor of the success of intracytoplasmic sperm injection? *Hum Reprod* 2008; **23**(2): 240–50.

Chapter 24

Clinical Value of Sperm Function Tests

Ahmad Majzoub

24.1 Introduction

Infertility is a major public health concern affecting up to 25 percent of couples worldwide [1]. It is defined by the failure of a couple to achieve conception after one year of regular, unprotected intercourse. The male contributes to roughly 50 percent of the causes of infertility among couples highlighting the importance of research and development in this field of medicine [2]. Conventional semen analysis is the cornerstone test for evaluating the male factor [3]. While the test can provide a general understanding of the male fertility potential, it cannot be used as an accurate predictor of fecundity. About 10 percent of men with normal semen analysis are unable to conceive. On the contrary, an equal percentage of men with abnormal semen analysis have no issues with fertility [4]. Therefore, during the past few decades, the low predictive power of standard semen analysis has triggered researchers to look for more sensitive and specific tests of sperm function. This chapter aims to explore the clinical utility of various tests of sperm function that have been described in literature.

24.2 Sperm Function Tests in the Clinical Setting

24.2.1 Measures of Oxidative Stress

24.2.1.1 Background on the Implications of Oxidative Stress on Male Fertility

Oxidative stress (OS) is believed to be an important common mechanism, through which various etiologies of male factor infertility may cause sperm dysfunction. It results from the imbalance between oxidants and reductants in any given medium. Oxidants, also known as reactive oxygen species (ROS) are the products of aerobic metabolism that, under normal physiologic levels, play an important role in cell signaling [5]. However, several disease processes such as varicocele, genitourinary infection or trauma, malignancy and its treatment as well as various environmental exposures can cause an excessive production of ROS [6]. Antioxidants, on the other hand, are compounds that are capable of eliminating excessive ROS, thereby minimizing their unwanted effects. Nonetheless, when ROS production exceeds the antioxidant neutralizing capacity, OS occurs resulting in detrimental effects on sperm function. OS is believed to aggravate sperm lipid peroxidation, DNA fragmentation and abortive apoptosis thereby causing infertility [7, 8].

Due its small amount of cytoplasm with only little antioxidants available that can protect it from excessive ROS, the sperm cell is highly susceptible to OS [9, 10]. Furthermore, its plasma membrane contains large amounts of polyunsaturated fatty acids that are extraordinarily prone to peroxidation by ROS [11, 12]. High levels of ROS were detected in semen samples from up to 40 percent of men with infertility [5].

Studies have revealed a significant negative impact of OS on various semen parameters. Homa et al. [13] compared the ROS levels between three groups of patients; normal semen without leukocytospermia, abnormal semen without leukocytospermia and any semen with leukocytospermia. The authors reported the highest ROS levels in patients with leukocytospermia. More importantly, in patients without leukocytospermia, significantly higher levels of ROS were identified in men with abnormal semen than those with normal semen parameters. Similarly, Agarwal et al. [14] compared semen parameters and ROS levels between infertile patients and normal fertile controls. The authors confirmed the presence of higher ROS levels in semen samples of infertile patients in comparison to the fertile controls and reported significant positive associations between ROS levels and sperm concentration and total motility.

Excessive ROS can also impact sperm morphology. Venkatesh et al. [15] examined ROS between infertile patients and fertile men. The median ROS level was 124 times higher in infertile patients who had a significantly higher percentage of sperm with cytoplasmic droplets indicating that it might be secondary to OS. Recently, we have examined OS measures in semen samples obtained from 1168 infertile patients and 100 fertile men and detected a significantly negative correlation between OS measures and sperm normal morphology and a significantly positive correlation between OS measures and percentage of head defects [16].

Finally, several studies have confirmed the relationship between OS and sperm DNA fragmentation (SDF) [7, 17, 18, 19, 20]. SDF is an important cause of male factor infertility and will be discussed later in this chapter.

24.2.1.2 Tests Used for the Measurement of Oxidative Stress

Oxidative stress testing has gained much interest in recent years, especially after understanding its negative effects on male factor infertility. Various tests for OS measurement are available and can be roughly classified into direct and indirect methods. Direct methods assess the extent of oxidation within a spermatozoon, while indirect methods measure the detrimental consequences of OS such as lipid peroxidation or SDF. Table 24.1 lists the various methods for OS measurement. The technical aspects of the different OS measurement methods are discussed in Chapter 7, Sections 7.1 and 7.2.

Table 24.1 Types of Reactive Oxygen Species Measurement Assays

Direct assays	Indirect assays
Chemiluminescence	Total antioxidant capacity
Flow cytometry	Sperm DNA fragmentation
Nitroblue tetrazolium test	Chemokines
Thiobarbituric acid assay	Oxidation reduction potential
Cytochrome C reduction test	Myeloperoxidase/Endtz test
Electron spin resonance	

24.2.1.3 Indications and Clinical Value of Oxidative Stress Measurement

Although measuring OS in semen is not indicated during the routine evaluation of male fertility potential, it may provide valuable information in specific clinical scenarios. These include patients with clinical varicocele, lifestyle or environmental risk factors, genitourinary infections or leukocytospermia and couples going for assisted reproductive therapy.

Varicocele is the most common correctable cause of male infertility occurring in 40 percent and 80 percent of men with primary and secondary infertility, respectively [21]. Current evidence suggests that OS plays an integral role in the pathophysiology of sperm dysfunction in varicocele patients [22]. Several studies have confirmed the presence of elevated levels of OS markers in semen samples of men with varicocele compared to normal controls [22, 23, 24, 25]. Allamaneni et al. [26] reported a positive correlation between seminal ROS levels and varicocele grade, meaning that men with larger varicoceles had significantly higher seminal ROS levels than men with small varicoceles. Among healthy fertile men, varicocele appears to be associated with significantly higher levels of ROS in comparison to men without varicocele [27]. Specific free radicals such as NO [25, 28, 29, 30] and H_2O_2 [31, 32] were found to be significantly higher in semen samples from infertile men with varicocele in comparison to normal fertile controls.

Interestingly, surgical treatment of varicocele has been shown to reduce seminal oxidative stress in varicocele patients [33]. In one study, Sakamoto et al. [25] found that a time lag of approximately six months is required to achieve a marked improvement in seminal ROS markers after varicocele repair. Mostafa et al. [34] demonstrated a significant reduction of markers of seminal OS and an elevation of antioxidant levels three and six months after varicocele ligation. Finally, Hurtado de Catalfo et al. [35] reported normalization of seminal levels of antioxidant enzymes compared with age-matched fertile controls after varicocele ligation. These data indicate that OS measurement could play a vital role in evaluating surgical candidates for varicocele ligation and in following up the response to the treatment.

Oxidative stress measurement may also be indicated in patients with lifestyle/environmental exposures. Smoking is one factor that has been associated with significantly increased seminal ROS levels. Saleh et al. [36] compared infertile smokers and non-smokers with a group of healthy non-smoking fertile men. These authors observed 107 percent higher ROS levels among the smoking group in comparison to the infertile and fertile non-smoker groups. Another study has revealed that even among fertile men, smoking tends to be associated with significant elevations in seminal ROS levels [37]. Patients with certain occupational exposures may also benefit from OS measurement. Examples of such exposures include polyvinyl chloride (PVC) [38], heavy metals such as cadmium and lead [39], and polycyclic aromatic hydrocarbons (PAHs) [40], which have been associated with increased levels of seminal ROS and worse semen quality among exposed patients.

Finally, seminal OS measurement may also be considered in couples opting for ART especially in cases who had prior history of ART failure or recurrent miscarriages following ART. High seminal OS measures can aggravate SDF and alter the outcome of fertilization and embryogenesis [41]. Furthermore, many of the procedures performed during the course of in vitro fertilization or intra-cytoplasmic sperm injection may expose the sperm, oocyte and/or the embryo to exogenous sources of ROS. Examples of these procedures include the degree of illumination [42], culture media being used [43], the incubator temperature [44], centrifugation time [45] and the process of cryopreservation [46]. Therefore, prior identification and treatment of seminal OS in patients undergoing ART could help in ameliorating its negative effects on the ART outcome.

24.2.2 Sperm DNA Fragmentation Testing

24.2.2.1 Background on the Effects of High Sperm DNA Fragmentation on Male Fertility

The study of SDF has certainly gained a lot of attention over the past couple of decades. Sperm DNA integrity is believed to play an important role in fertilization, early embryo development and pregnancy [47, 48]. The human sperm is a unique cell as its DNA is in a highly compacted state aided by the replacement of its histones as nucleoproteins with protamines during spermiogenesis [49]. This compact state provides protection to the DNA as the sperm travels through the male and female reproductive tracts. However, a number of etiologies can trigger SDF such as errors in chromatin compaction during

spermiogenesis, elevated seminal ROS levels or aggravated apoptosis during the sperm transit through the epididymis [50, 51]. There is a large body of evidence suggesting a significant relationship between SDF and abnormal semen parameters and worse fertility outcomes both naturally and following ART [49, 52, 53, 54, 55, 56]. A meta-analysis of 28 studies involving 2883 infertile men and 1294 fertile men revealed significantly higher SDF levels among infertile patients in comparison to fertile controls [57].

24.2.2.2 Tests Used in the Measurement of Sperm DNA Fragmentation

There are two types of assays that have been developed to measure SDF: those that can directly measure the extent of DNA fragmentation through the use of probes and dyes and those that measure the susceptibility of DNA to denaturation, which occurs more commonly in fragmented DNA. The eight described methods to assess SDF are briefly presented below and summarized in Table 24.2. The most commonly used tests are terminal deoxynucleotidyl transferase dUTP nick end labeling (TUNEL), the sperm chromatin dispersion test (SCD), and the sperm chromatin structure assay (SCSA).

24.2.2.3 Indications and Clinical Value of Sperm DNA Fragmentation Testing

The significant impact SDF plays on fertility potential yielded the publication of society endorsed guidelines on the utility of SDF testing in clinical practice [58]. SDF testing is indicated in patients with unexplained infertility, recurrent miscarriages, varicocele, recurrent intrauterine insemination (IUI) and IVF failure, and recurrent miscarriages following ICSI [59].

Unexplained infertility is observed in about 10–30 percent of couples seeking fertility and is perhaps a true demonstration of the limitations of conventional semen analysis [60]. While the SDF value is inversely related to conventional semen parameters, high SDF levels may as well be detected in patients with normal semen analysis result [61]. Oleszczuk et al. confirmed the presence of significantly higher SDF levels in patients with unexplained infertility (18 percent) in comparison to fertile controls (10 percent) (p=0.005) [62]. Similarly, Saleh et al. observed a SDF index of 23 percent (assessed with SCSA) in men with unexplained infertility

Table 24.2 Principle, Advantages and Disadvantages of Various Sperm DNA Fragmentation Testing Methods

Test	Principle	Advantage	Disadvantage
(1) AO test	Metachromatic shift in fluorescence of acridine orange when bound to ss DNA. Uses fluorescent microscopy.	Rapid, simple and inexpensive.	Inter-laboratory variations and lack of reproducibility.
(2) AB staining	Increased affinity of AB dye to loose chromatin of sperm nucleus. Uses optical microscopy.	Rapid, simple and inexpensive.	Inter-laboratory variations and lack of reproducibility.
(3) CMA3 staining	CMA3 competitively binds to DNA indirectly visualizing protamine deficient DNA. Uses fluorescent microscopy.	Yields reliable results as it is strongly correlated with other assays.	Inter-observer variability.
(4) TB staining	Increased affinity of TB to sperm DNA phosphate residues. Uses optical microscopy.	Rapid, simple and inexpensive.	Inter-observer variability.
(5) TUNEL	Quantifies the enzymatic incorporation of dUTP into DNA breaks. Can be done using both optical microscopy or fluorescent microscopy. Uses optical microscopy, fluorescent microscopy and flow cytometry.	Sensitive, reliable with minimal inter-observer variability. Can be performed on few sperm.	Requires standardization between laboratories.
(6) SCSA	Measures the susceptibility of sperm DNA to denaturation. The cytometric version of the AO test. Uses flow cytometry.	Reliable estimate of the percentage of DNA-damaged sperm.	Requires the presence of expensive instrumentation (flow cytometer) and highly skilled technicians.
(7) SCD or Halo test	Assess dispersion of DNA fragments after denaturation. Uses optical or fluorescent microscopy.	Simple test.	Inter-observer variability.
(8) SCGE or Comet assay	Electrophoretic assessment of DNA fragments of lysed DNA. Uses fluorescent microscopy.	Can be done in very low sperm count. It is sensitive and reproducible.	Requires an experienced observer. Inter-observer variability.

(1) Acridine orange (AO) stains normal DNA fluoresces green, whereas denatured DNA fluoresces orange-red. (2) Aniline blue (AB) staining showing sperm with fragmented DNA and normal sperm. (3) Chromomycin A3 (CMA3) staining: protamine deficient spermatozoa appear bright yellow, spermatozoa with normal protamine appear yellowish green. (4) Toluidine blue (TB) staining: normal sperm appear light blue and sperm with DNA fragmentation appear violet. (5) Terminal deoxynucleotidyl transferase-mediated fluorescein-deoxyuridine triphosphate-nick end labeling (TUNEL).

which was significantly higher than the values measured in fertile controls (15 percent) [19].

A number of studies have linked the SDF level to recurrent early miscarriages, defined by three consecutive pregnancy losses before 20 weeks' gestation [55, 63, 64]. Khadem et al. measured SDF using the SCD assay in 30 patients with recurrent spontaneous abortions (RSA) and an equal number of fertile men [63]. The authors observed significantly higher SDF levels in patients with RSA (43.3 percent) compared with fertile controls (16.7 percent) (p=0.027). A recent systematic review and meta-analysis by Tan et al. conducted on 12 prospective and two retrospective studies involving 530 men with a history of RSA and 639 fertile controls revealed significantly higher SDF levels in patients with RSA compared with fertile men (mean difference 11.98, p<0.001) [65].

Varicocele is another condition in which SDF testing is indicated. A literature review by Zini and Dohle examined 16 case-control studies and reported that varicocele is associated with higher SDF levels regardless of the patients' fertility status [66]. A multicenter study by Esteves et al. examining SDF levels among patients with different etiologies of infertility observed the highest SDF levels in patients with varicocele (35.7±18.3 percent) [67]. Similarly, Smith et al. have echoed similar results and identified high SDF values in varicocele patients with normal or abnormal semen parameter results [68].

More importantly, varicocelectomy has been associated with a sound and significant reduction in SDF results [24, 69, 70]. A literature review by Zini and Dohle observed reductions in SDF levels in all the studies included in their study [71]. Another meta-analysis reported a significant reduction in SDF with a mean difference of −3.37 percent (95 percent CI, −4.09 to −2.65; p<0.00001) in patients undergoing varicocelectomy [72]. The reductions in SDF levels following varicocele treatment have been linked with improved pregnancy rates in a study by Smit et al [73]. The authors examined 49 patients who underwent varicocelectomy after a one-year history of infertility. A significant decrease in SDF from 35.2 percent to 30.2 percent (p=0.019) measured by SCSA was observed postoperatively. Natural pregnancy was observed in 37 percent of patients who had a significantly lower SDF than patients who did not conceive naturally or who conceived with assisted reproduction [73].

As for ARTs, a direct relationship has been observed between the SDF level and poor IUI, IVF and ICSI outcomes. Duran et al. evaluated the outcome of 154 IUI cycles and detected significantly higher SDF levels among patients with failed cycles [74]. Similarly, Bungum et al. reported lower pregnancy (3 percent versus 23.7 percent) and delivery (1 percent versus 19 percent) rates among patients with higher versus lower SDF levels [75]. With regards to IVF and ICSI, the current evidence features a significantly negative impact for SDF only on IVF pregnancy rates with reported odds ratios ranging between 1.27 (95 percent CI, 1.05–1.52; p=0.01) [76] and 1.57 (95 percent CI, 1.18–2.07; p<0.05) [77]. Nonetheless, higher SDF levels were associated with increased risk of pregnancy loss following both IVF and ICSI with a combined OR ranging between 2.16

(95 percent CI, 1.54–3.03, p<0.001) [78] and 2.48 (95 percent CI, 1.52–4.04; p<0.0001) [77].

24.2.3 Sperm Penetration Assay

24.2.3.1 Rational for Conducting the Sperm Penetration Assay

The SPA is one of the first tests utilized to assess sperm function. It is an in vitro test that combines sperm subjected to capacitating conditions with hamster eggs that are enzymatically devoid of their zona pellucida. The SPA assesses the sperm ability to perform capacitation and acrosome reaction and to fuse and penetrate through the oolemma and decondensate within the cytoplasm of hamster oocytes [79].

24.2.3.2 Indications and Clinical Value

The SPA has been thoroughly investigated in the pre-ICSI era [80, 81]. However, interest in this time-consuming and expensive test soon faded away principally because of its inconsistent results and the presence of significantly high false-positive and false-negative rates [82]. The reason behind these findings is believed to be related to dissimilarity the SPA has from the normal physiologic process in which the zona pellucida is absent.

A meta-analysis by Oehninger et al. performed to determine the predictive value of various sperm function tests on fertilization outcome with IVF reported a poor clinical value for the SPA [79]. The authors investigated a total of 2906 cycles, and found that although the SPA had a fairly good sensitivity, it suffered from very high false-positive rates averaging about 50 percent. Another meta-analysis by Bol et al. exploring 647 patients from 24 studies reported a SPA sensitivity of only 37 percent and highlighted the heterogenous nature of the reported results [83].

24.2.4 Sperm Zona Pellucida Binding Assays

24.2.4.1 Rational for Conducting the Sperm Zona Pellucida Binding Assay

The interaction between the sperm and the zona pellucida is an important step in the process of conception that can highlight fundamental sperm functional ability; namely capacitation and acrosome reaction. The most commonly used sperm-zona pellucida binding tests are the hemizona assay (HZA) and the competitive intact zona sperm binding test [84, 85]. Both tests are conducted to assess the tight binding of the sperm to the zona pellucida. The HZA uses matching halves of a human zona pellucida from stored or cadaveric oocytes to compare the binding ability of spermatozoa between infertile patients and fertile controls [84]. Studies have shown that sperm from fertile men have significantly higher binding capacity to the zona pellucida than sperm from infertile men [84, 86]. Results of the HZA are expressed as the hemizona index (HZI) which is calculated as follows: bound sperm from infertile male divided by bound sperm from fertile male × 100. The competitive intact zona sperm binding test, on the other hand, uses oocytes that failed to fertilize in vitro to compare control and test spermatozoa [87]. Both of these tests have been shown to demonstrate a high power in predicting fertilization in vitro [88, 89].

24.2.4.2 Indications and Clinical Value

Sperm zona pellucida binding assays are indicated in patients with recurrent fertilization failure during IVF or in the presence of moderate to severe derangement of semen parameters. A meta-analysis investigating 978 couples reported a significantly high predictive power for sperm zona pellucida binding assays for fertilization outcome with a positive predictive value >80 percent and a negative predictive value >70 percent [79]. Studies have reported a HZI cut-off of 35 percent to be a predictive value for IVF outcome [90–92]. Furthermore, a HZI <30 percent was associated with a significantly lower pregnancy rate following IUI in comparison to patients with a HZI >30 percent (11.1 percent versus 40.6 percent, respectively; p<0.05) [93]. Sperm from oligozoospermic men have significantly lower sperm – zona pellucida binding capacity consistent with their lower fertility potential both naturally and following ARTs [94]. Therefore, the result of these sperm function tests could help in counseling patients with moderate to severely abnormal semen parameters before deciding the most appropriate ART method for them. ICSI would be more reasonable for patients with abnormal sperm zona pellucida binding test results [95, 96].

24.2.5 Acrosome Reaction

24.2.5.1 Rational for Testing the Acrosome Reaction

Acrosome reaction occurs as a result of the release of hydrolyzing enzymes triggered by sperm binding to the zona pellucida. It is a crucial step for successful fertilization as only acrosome-reacted sperm are able to traverse the zona pellucida and fuse with the oolemma [97]. The acrosome of mammalian sperm contains large amounts of acrosin, an essential enzyme for gamete fusion [97]. About 25 percent of men with unexplained infertility were found to have a defective acrosome reaction [98]. Acrosome reaction can be assessed on spermatozoa removed from the surface of the zona pellucida or those exposed to zona pellucida disaggregated proteins using microscopy, flow cytometry, or fluorescently labeled lectins [97].

24.2.5.2 Indications and Clinical Value

Although acrosome reaction testing is more commonly utilized for research purposes, the test could provide some helpful information in couples opting for ART especially when there is prior history of recurrent fertilization failure. Studies have shown that acrosome reaction is a good predictor of fertilization, having a positive predictive value of >75 percent and a negative predictive value of >65 percent [79, 99].

24.2.6 Hyaluronic Binding Assay

24.2.6.1 Rational for Conducting the Hyaluronic Binding Assay

Hyaluronic acid (HA) is a substance that is naturally present around the oocyte acting as a biologic sperm selector [100]. Human sperm contain HA receptors and only mature sperm with normal morphology, minimal DNA fragmentation and chromosomal aneuploidy are able to bind with HA [100]. In other words, the test examines the function of sperm having a normal morphology and an intact acrosome which are more likely to traverse the extracellular matrix, bind to the zona pellucida and fertilize the ovum [101].

24.2.6.2 Indications and Clinical Value

Hyaluronic binding assay (HBA) is mainly utilized in the in vitro setting to aid in selecting sperm from candidates for IVF or ICSI. Despite that, evidence extracted from systematic reviews and meta-analyses did not reveal an improvement in fertilization and pregnancy rates with ICSI when HA binding sperm selection is used. Beck-Fruchter et al. investigated seven studies including 1437 cycles in which HBA was used for selecting sperm prior to ICSI [102]. The authors compared HA-selected sperm for ICSI to conventional ICSI and found no improvement in fertilization rate (relative risk 1.02, 95 percent CI 0.99–1.06) nor in pregnancy rate (relative risk 1.10,

95 percent CI 0.93–1.29). A Cochrane systematic review investigating the efficacy of advanced sperm selection techniques for ARTs also failed to find a significant improvement in clinical pregnancy, miscarriage rate or live birth rate in HA selected sperm ICSI versus conventional ICSI [103].

24.2.7 Hypo-Osmotic Swelling Test

24.2.7.1 Rational for Conducting Hypo-Osmotic Swelling Test

The hypo-osmotic swelling (HOS) test is based on the ability of live spermatozoa with an intact cytoplasmic membrane to endure hypo-osmotic stress. Water permeability is an essential physiologic property of all living cells making the HOS test a measure of sperm viability. Viable sperm swell to various degrees when exposed to hypotonic solution, while dead sperm which have lost their membrane permeability fail to do so [87, 104]. Sperm viability is a pre-requisite for fertilization and certainly a significant correlation has been observed in vitro between the percentage of viable sperm and the percentage of penetrated hamster oocytes (r=0.90) [104].

24.2.7.2 Indications and Clinical Value

The HOS test is most commonly used to assess sperm viability in patients with little or no motile sperm in their ejaculates and/or in selecting sperm for ICSI. Studies have shown that a high fertilization rate with ICSI can be achieved using sperm selected through the HOS test [105, 106]. Another utility for the HOS stems from its ability to indirectly assess the degree of SDF. Low sperm viability has been well correlated with high SDF levels [107].

24.3 Conclusion

Understanding the intricate functions of human spermatozoa during conception is fundamental for unraveling the ambiguities of human reproduction. The extensive research witnessed in the field of male infertility led to the discovery of various sperm function tests that helped in modifying various treatments and improving fertility outcome. Of all tests that have been investigated in literature, SDF testing and oxidative stress measurement are most commonly utilized in clinical practice.

References

1. Boivin J, Bunting L, Collins JA, Nygren KG. International estimates of infertility prevalence and treatment-seeking: potential need and demand for infertility medical care. *Hum Reprod* 2007; **22**: 1506–12.

2. Brugh VM, Lipshultz LI. Male factor infertility: evaluation and management. *Med Clin North Am* 2004; **88**: 367–85.

3. Cooper TG, Noonan E, von Eckardstein S, Auger J, Baker HW et al. World Health Organization reference values for human semen characteristics. *Hum Reprod Update* 2010; **16**: 231–45.

4. Sadeghi MR. The state of semen analysis over time. *J Reprod Infertil* 2014; **15**: 1.

5. Agarwal A, Gupta S, Sikka S. The role of free radicals and antioxidants in reproduction. *Curr Opin Obstet Gynecol* 2006; **18**: 325–32.

6. Agarwal A, Saleh RA, Bedaiwy MA. Role of reactive oxygen species in the pathophysiology of human reproduction. *Fertil Steril* 2003; **79**: 829–43.

7. Agarwal A, Said TM. Oxidative stress, DNA damage and apoptosis in male infertility: a clinical approach. *BJU International* 2005; **95**: 503–7.

8. Agarwal A, Virk G, Ong C, du Plessis SS. Effect of oxidative stress on male reproduction. *World J Mens Health* 2014; **32**: 1–17.

9. Aitken RJ, Jones KT, Robertson SA. Reactive oxygen species and sperm function–in sickness and in health. *J Androl* 2012; **33**: 1096–106.

10. Aitken RJ, Wingate JK, De Iuliis GN, McLaughlin EA. Analysis of lipid peroxidation in human spermatozoa using BODIPY C11. *Mol Hum Reprod* 2007; **13**: 203–11.

11. Bansal AK, Bilaspuri GS. Impacts of oxidative stress and antioxidants on semen functions. *Vet Med Int* 2010; 2010.

12 . Dandekar SP, Nadkarni GD, Kulkarni VS, Punekar S. Lipid peroxidation and antioxidant enzymes in male infertility. *J Postgrad Med* 2002; **48**: 186–9; discussion 9–90.

13. Homa ST, Vessey W, Perez-Miranda A, Riyait T, Agarwal A. Reactive Oxygen Species (ROS) in human semen: determination of a reference range. *J Assist Reprod Genet* 2015; **32**: 757–64.

14. Agarwal A, Sharma RK, Sharma R, Assidi M, Abuzenadah AM et al. Characterizing semen parameters and their association with reactive oxygen species in infertile men. *Reprod Biol Endocrinol* 2014; **12**: 33.

15. Venkatesh S, Singh G, Gupta NP, Kumar R, Deecaraman M et al. Correlation of sperm morphology

and oxidative stress in infertile men. *Iran J Reprod Med* 2009; **7**: 29–34.

16. Majzoub A, Arafa M, Mahdi M, Agarwal A, Al Said S et al. Oxidation-reduction potential and sperm DNA fragmentation, and their associations with sperm morphological anomalies amongst fertile and infertile men. *Arab J Urol* 2018; **16**: 87–95.

17. Aitken RJ, De Iuliis GN. On the possible origins of DNA damage in human spermatozoa. *Mol Hum Reprod* 2010; **16**: 3–13.

18. Aitken RJ, Krausz C. Oxidative stress, DNA damage and the Y chromosome. *Reproduction* 2001; **122**: 497–506.

19. Saleh RA, Agarwal A, Nada EA, El-Tonsy MH, Sharma RK et al. Negative effects of increased sperm DNA damage in relation to seminal oxidative stress in men with idiopathic and male factor infertility. *Fertil Steril* 2003; **79**(Suppl. 3): 1597–605.

20. Wright C, Milne S, Leeson H. Sperm DNA damage caused by oxidative stress: modifiable clinical, lifestyle and nutritional factors in male infertility. *Reprod Biomed Online* 2014; **28**: 684–703.

21. Agarwal A, Esteves SC. Varicocele and male infertility: current concepts and future perspectives. *Asian J Androl* 2016; **18**: 161–2.

22. Cho CL, Esteves SC, Agarwal A. Novel insights into the pathophysiology of varicocele and its association with reactive oxygen species and sperm DNA fragmentation. *Asian J Androl* 2016; **18**: 186–93.

23. Agarwal A, Prabakaran S, Allamaneni SS. Relationship between oxidative stress, varicocele and infertility: a meta-analysis. *Reprod Biomed Online* 2006; **12**: 630–3.

24. Majzoub A, Esteves SC, Gosalvez J, Agarwal A. Specialized sperm

function tests in varicocele and the future of andrology laboratory. *Asian J Androl* 2016; **18**: 205–12.

25. Sakamoto Y, Ishikawa T, Kondo Y, Yamaguchi K, Fujisawa M. The assessment of oxidative stress in infertile patients with varicocele. *BJU International* 2008; **101**: 1547–52.

26. Allamaneni SS, Naughton CK, Sharma RK, Thomas AJ, Jr., Agarwal A. Increased seminal reactive oxygen species levels in patients with varicoceles correlate with varicocele grade but not with testis size. *Fertil Steril* 2004; **82**: 1684–6.

27. Mostafa T, Anis T, Imam H, El-Nashar AR, Osman IA. Seminal reactive oxygen species-antioxidant relationship in fertile males with and without varicocele. *Andrologia* 2009; **41**: 125–9.

28. Mehraban D, Ansari M, Keyhan H, Sedighi Gilani M, Naderi G et al. Comparison of nitric oxide concentration in seminal fluid between infertile patients with and without varicocele and normal fertile men. *J Urol* 2005; **2**: 106–10.

29. Xu Y, Xu QY, Yang BH, Zhu XM, Peng YF. Relationship of nitric oxide and nitric oxide synthase with varicocele infertility. *Zhonghua nan ke xue* [National Journal of Andrology] 2008; **14**: 414–17.

30. Abd-Elmoaty MA, Saleh R, Sharma R, Agarwal A. Increased levels of oxidants and reduced antioxidants in semen of infertile men with varicocele. *Fertil Steril* 2010; **94**: 1531–4.

31. Mostafa T, Anis T, El Nashar A, Imam H, Osman I. Seminal plasma reactive oxygen species-antioxidants relationship with varicocele grade. *Andrologia* 2012; **44**: 66–9.

32. Mazzilli F, Rossi T, Marchesini M, Ronconi C, Dondero F. Superoxide anion in human semen related to seminal

parameters and clinical aspects. *Fertil Steril* 1994; **62**: 862–8.

33. Hamada A, Esteves SC, Agarwal A. Insight into oxidative stress in varicocele-associated male infertility: part 2. *Nat Rev Urol* 2013; **10**: 26–37.

34. Mostafa T, Anis TH, El-Nashar A, Imam H, Othman IA. Varicocelectomy reduces reactive oxygen species levels and increases antioxidant activity of seminal plasma from infertile men with varicocele. *Int J Androl* 2001; **24**: 261–5.

35. Hurtado de Catalfo GE, Ranieri-Casilla A, Marra FA, de Alaniz MJ, Marra CA. Oxidative stress biomarkers and hormonal profile in human patients undergoing varicocelectomy. *Int J Androl* 2007; **30**: 519–30.

36. Saleh RA, Agarwal A, Sharma RK, Nelson DR, Thomas AJ, Jr. Effect of cigarette smoking on levels of seminal oxidative stress in infertile men: a prospective study. *Fertil Steril* 2002; **78**: 491–9.

37. Taha EA, Ez-Aldin AM, Sayed SK, Ghandour NM, Mostafa T. Effect of smoking on sperm vitality, DNA integrity, seminal oxidative stress, zinc in fertile men. *Urology* 2012; **80**: 822–5.

38. Jurewicz J, Radwan M, Sobala W, Radwan P, Bochenek M et al. Effects of occupational exposure - is there a link between exposure based on an occupational questionnaire and semen quality? *Syst Biol Reprod Med* 2014; **60**: 227–33.

39. Taha EA, Sayed SK, Ghandour NM, Mahran AM, Saleh MA et al. Correlation between seminal lead and cadmium and seminal parameters in idiopathic oligoasthenozoospermic males. *Cent European J Urol* 2013; **66**: 84–92.

40. Jeng HAC, Lin WY, Chao MR, Lin WY, Pan CH. Semen quality and sperm DNA damage

associated with oxidative stress in relation to exposure to polycyclic aromatic hydrocarbons. *J Environ Sci Health A Tox Hazard Subst Environ Eng* 2018; **53**: 1221–8.

41. Ghaleno LR, Valojerdi MR, Hassani F, Chehrazi M, Janzamin E. High level of intracellular sperm oxidative stress negatively influences embryo pronuclear formation after intracytoplasmic sperm injection treatment. *Andrologia* 2014; **46**: 1118–27.

42. Takenaka M, Horiuchi T, Yanagimachi R. Effects of light on development of mammalian zygotes. *Proc Natl Acad Sci U S A* 2007; **104**: 14289–93.

43. Guerin P, El Mouatassim S, Menezo Y. Oxidative stress and protection against reactive oxygen species in the pre-implantation embryo and its surroundings. *Hum Reprod Update* 2001; **7**: 175–89.

44. Larkindale J, Knight MR. Protection against heat stress-induced oxidative damage in Arabidopsis involves calcium, abscisic acid, ethylene, and salicylic acid. *Plant Physiol* 2002; **128**: 682–95.

45. Shekarriz M, DeWire DM, Thomas AJ, Jr., Agarwal A. A method of human semen centrifugation to minimize the iatrogenic sperm injuries caused by reactive oxygen species. *Eur Urol* 1995; **28**: 31–5.

46. Alvarez JG, Storey BT. Evidence for increased lipid peroxidative damage and loss of superoxide dismutase activity as a mode of sublethal cryodamage to human sperm during cryopreservation. *J Androl* 1992; **13**: 232–41.

47. Alvarez JG. DNA fragmentation in human spermatozoa: significance in the diagnosis and treatment of infertility. *Minerva Ginecol* 2003; **55**: 233–9.

48. Irvine DS, Twigg JP, Gordon EL, Fulton N, Milne PA et al. DNA integrity in human spermatozoa: relationships with semen quality. *J Androl* 2000; **21**: 33–44.

49. Erenpreiss J, Spano M, Erenpreisa J, Bungum M, Giwercman A. Sperm chromatin structure and male fertility: biological and clinical aspects. *Asian J Androl* 2006; **8**: 11–29.

50. Sakkas D, Moffatt O, Manicardi GC, Mariethoz E, Tarozzi N et al. Nature of DNA damage in ejaculated human spermatozoa and the possible involvement of apoptosis. *Biol Reprod* 2002; **66**: 1061–7.

51. Moustafa MH, Sharma RK, Thornton J, Mascha E, Abdel-Hafez MA et al. Relationship between ROS production, apoptosis and DNA denaturation in spermatozoa from patients examined for infertility. *Hum Reprod* 2004; **19**: 129–38.

52. Agarwal A, Cho CL, Esteves SC. Should we evaluate and treat sperm DNA fragmentation? *Curr Opin Obstet Gynecol* 2016; **28**: 164–71.

53. Arafa M, AlMalki A, AlBadr M, Burjaq H, Majzoub A et al. ICSI outcome in patients with high DNA fragmentation: testicular versus ejaculated spermatozoa. *Andrologia* 2018; **50**(1). doi: 10.1111/and.12835.

54. Benchaib M, Lornage J, Mazoyer C, Lejeune H, Salle B et al. Sperm deoxyribonucleic acid fragmentation as a prognostic indicator of assisted reproductive technology outcome. *Fertil Steril* 2007; **87**: 93–100.

55. Kumar K, Deka D, Singh A, Mitra DK, Vanitha BR et al. Predictive value of DNA integrity analysis in idiopathic recurrent pregnancy loss following spontaneous conception. *J Assist Reprod Genet* 2012; **29**: 861–7.

56. Lopez G, Lafuente R, Checa MA, Carreras R, Brassesco M. Diagnostic value of sperm DNA fragmentation and sperm high-magnification for predicting outcome of assisted reproduction treatment. *Asian J Androl* 2013; **15**: 790–4.

57. Santi D, Spaggiari G, Simoni M. Sperm DNA fragmentation index as a promising predictive tool for male infertility diagnosis and treatment management – meta-analyses. *Reprod Biomed Online* 2018; **37**: 315–26.

58. Agarwal A, Cho CL, Majzoub A, Esteves SC. The Society for Translational Medicine: clinical practice guidelines for sperm DNA fragmentation testing in male infertility. *Transl Androl Urol* 2017; **6**: S720–S33.

59. Agarwal A, Majzoub A, Esteves SC, Ko E, Ramasamy R et al. Clinical utility of sperm DNA fragmentation testing: practice recommendations based on clinical scenarios. *Transl Androl Urol* 2016; **5**: 935–50.

60. Collins JA, Crosignani PG. Unexplained infertility: a review of diagnosis, prognosis, treatment efficacy and management. *Int J Gynaecol Obstet* 1992; **39**: 267–75.

61. Bareh GM, Jacoby E, Binkley P, Chang TC, Schenken RS et al. Sperm deoxyribonucleic acid fragmentation assessment in normozoospermic male partners of couples with unexplained recurrent pregnancy loss: a prospective study. *Fertil Steril* 2016; **105**: 329–36 e1.

62. Oleszczuk K, Augustinsson L, Bayat N, Giwercman A, Bungum M. Prevalence of high DNA fragmentation index in male partners of unexplained infertile couples. *Andrology* 2013; **1**: 357–60.

63. Khadem N, Poorhoseyni A, Jalali M, Akbary A, Heydari ST. Sperm DNA fragmentation in couples with unexplained recurrent spontaneous abortions. *Andrologia* 2014; **46**: 126–30.

64. Leach M, Aitken RJ, Sacks G. Sperm DNA fragmentation

abnormalities in men from couples with a history of recurrent miscarriage. *Aust N Z J Obstet Gynaecol* 2015; **55**: 379–83.

65. Tan J, Taskin O, Albert A, Bedaiwy MA. Association between sperm DNA fragmentation and idiopathic recurrent pregnancy loss: a systematic review and meta-analysis. *Reprod Biomed Online* 2019; **38**: 951–60.

66. Zini A. Are sperm chromatin and DNA defects relevant in the clinic? *Syst Biol Reprod Med* 2011; **57**: 78–85.

67. Esteves SC, Gosalvez J, Lopez-Fernandez C, Nunez-Calonge R, Caballero P et al. Diagnostic accuracy of sperm DNA degradation index (DDSi) as a potential noninvasive biomarker to identify men with varicocele-associated infertility. *Int Urol Nephrol* 2015; **47**: 1471–7.

68. Smith R, Kaune H, Parodi D, Madariaga M, Rios R et al. Increased sperm DNA damage in patients with varicocele: relationship with seminal oxidative stress. *Hum Reprod* 2006; **21**: 986–93.

69. Ni K, Steger K, Yang H, Wang H, Hu K et al. Sperm protamine mRNA ratio and DNA fragmentation index represent reliable clinical biomarkers for men with varicocele after microsurgical varicocele ligation. *J Urol* 2014; **192**: 170–6.

70. Roque M, Esteves SC. Effect of varicocele repair on sperm DNA fragmentation: a review. *Int Urol Nephrol* 2018; **50**: 583–603.

71. Zini A, Dohle G. Are varicoceles associated with increased deoxyribonucleic acid fragmentation? *Fertil Steril* 2011; **96**: 1283–7.

72. Wang YJ, Zhang RQ, Lin YJ, Zhang RG, Zhang WL. Relationship between varicocele and sperm DNA damage and the effect of varicocele repair: a meta-analysis. *Reprod Biomed Online* 2012; **25**: 307–14.

73. Smit M, Romijn JC, Wildhagen MF, Veldhoven JL, Weber RF et al. Decreased sperm DNA fragmentation after surgical varicocelectomy is associated with increased pregnancy rate. *J Urol* 2013; **189**: S146–50.

74. Duran EH, Morshedi M, Taylor S, Oehninger S. Sperm DNA quality predicts intrauterine insemination outcome: a prospective cohort study. *Hum Reprod* 2002; **17**: 3122–8.

75. Bungum M, Humaidan P, Axmon A, Spano M, Bungum L et al. Sperm DNA integrity assessment in prediction of assisted reproduction technology outcome. *Hum Reprod* 2007; **22**: 174–9.

76. Osman A, Alsomait H, Seshadri S, El-Toukhy T, Khalaf Y. The effect of sperm DNA fragmentation on live birth rate after IVF or ICSI: a systematic review and meta-analysis. *Reprod Biomed Online* 2015; **30**: 120–7.

77. Zini A, Sigman M. Are tests of sperm DNA damage clinically useful? Pros and cons. *J Androl* 2009; **30**: 219–29.

78. Robinson L, Gallos ID, Conner SJ, Rajkhowa M, Miller D et al. The effect of sperm DNA fragmentation on miscarriage rates: a systematic review and meta-analysis. *Hum Reprod* 2012; **27**: 2908–17.

79. Oehninger S, Franken DR, Sayed E, Barroso G, Kolm P. Sperm function assays and their predictive value for fertilization outcome in IVF therapy: a meta-analysis. *Hum Reprod Update* 2000; **6**: 160–8.

80. Ulstein M. In vitro sperm penetration of cervical mucus and male fertility. *Andrology* 1973; **5**: 189–91.

81. Barros C, Gonzalez J, Herrera E, Bustos-Obregon E. Human sperm penetration into zona-free hamster oocytes as a test to evaluate the sperm fertilizing ability. *Andrologia* 1979; **11**: 197–210.

82. Oehninger S, Franken DR, Ombelet W. Sperm functional tests. *Fertil Steril* 2014; **102**: 1528–33.

83. Mol BW, Meijer S, Yuppa S, Tan E, de Vries J et al. Sperm penetration assay in predicting successful in vitro fertilization. A meta-analysis. *J Reprod Med* 1998; **43**: 503–8.

84. Burkman LJ, Coddington CC, Franken DR, Krugen TF, Rosenwaks Z et al. The hemizona assay (HZA): development of a diagnostic test for the binding of human spermatozoa to the human hemizona pellucida to predict fertilization potential. *Fertil Steril* 1988; **49**: 688–97.

85. Liu DY, Lopata A, Johnston WI, Baker HW. A human sperm-zona pellucida binding test using oocytes that failed to fertilize in vitro. *Fertil Steril* 1988; **50**: 782–8.

86. Oehninger S, Morshedi M, Franken D. The hemizona assay for assessment of sperm function. *Methods Mol Biol* 2013; **927**: 91–102.

87. Kizilay F, Altay B. Sperm function tests in clinical practice. *Turk J Urol* 2017; **43**: 393–400.

88. Oehninger S. Clinical and laboratory management of male infertility: an opinion on its current status. *J Androl* 2000; **21**: 814–21.

89. Liu DY, Garrett C, Baker HW. Clinical application of sperm-oocyte interaction tests in in vitro fertilization – embryo transfer and intracytoplasmic sperm injection programs. *Fertil Steril* 2004; **82**: 1251–63.

90. Oehninger S, Coddington CC, Scott R, Franken DA, Burkman LJ et al. Hemizona assay: assessment of sperm dysfunction and

prediction of in vitro fertilization outcome. *Fertil Steril* 1989; **51**: 665–70.

91. Franken DR, Kruger TF, Oehninger S, Coddington CC, Lombard C et al. The ability of the hemizona assay to predict human fertilization in different and consecutive in-vitro fertilization cycles. *Hum Reprod* 1993; **8**: 1240–4.

92. Franken DR, Oehninger S. The clinical significance of sperm-zona pellucida binding: 17 years later. *Front Biosci* 2006; **11**: 1227–33.

93. Arslan M, Morshedi M, Arslan EO, Taylor S, Kanik A et al. Predictive value of the hemizona assay for pregnancy outcome in patients undergoing controlled ovarian hyperstimulation with intrauterine insemination. *Fertil Steril* 2006; **85**: 1697–707.

94. Liu DY, Baker HW. High frequency of defective sperm-zona pellucida interaction in oligozoospermic infertile men. *Hum Reprod* 2004; **19**: 228–33.

95. Oehninger S, Franken D, Kruger T. Approaching the next millennium: how should we manage andrology diagnosis in the intracytoplasmic sperm injection era? *Fertil Steril* 1997; **67**: 434–6.

96. Oehninger S, Mahony M, Ozgur K, Kolm P, Kruger T et al. Clinical significance of human sperm-zona pellucida binding. *Fertil Steril* 1997; **67**: 1121–7.

97. Brucker C, Lipford GB. The human sperm acrosome reaction: physiology and regulatory mechanisms. An update. *Hum Reprod Update* 1995; **1**: 51–62.

98. Liu DY, Clarke GN, Martic M, Garrett C, Baker HW. Frequency of disordered zona pellucida (ZP)-induced acrosome reaction in infertile men with normal semen analysis and normal spermatozoa-ZP binding. *Hum Reprod* 2001; **16**: 1185–90.

99. Sanchez R, Toepfer-Petersen E, Aitken RJ, Schill WB. A new method for evaluation of the acrosome reaction in viable human spermatozoa. *Andrologia* 1991; **23**: 197–203.

100. Parmegiani L, Cognigni GE, Ciampaglia W, Pocognoli P, Marchi F et al. Efficiency of hyaluronic acid (HA) sperm selection. *J Assist Reprod Genet* 2010; **27**: 13–16.

101. Myles DG, Primakoff P. Why did the sperm cross the cumulus? To get to the oocyte. Functions of the sperm surface proteins PH-20 and fertilin in arriving at, and fusing with, the egg. *Biol Reprod* 1997; **56**: 320–7.

102. Beck-Fruchter R, Shalev E, Weiss A. Clinical benefit using sperm hyaluronic acid binding technique in ICSI cycles: a systematic review and meta-analysis. *Reprod Biomed Online* 2016; **32**: 286–98.

103. Lepine S, McDowell S, Searle LM, Kroon B, Glujovsky D et al. Advanced sperm selection techniques for assisted reproduction. *Cochrane Database Syst Rev* 2019; **7**: CD010461.

104. Jeyendran RS, Van der Ven HH, Perez-Pelaez M, Crabo BG, Zaneveld LJ. Development of an assay to assess the functional integrity of the human sperm membrane and its relationship to other semen characteristics. *J Reprod Fertil* 1984; **70**: 219–28.

105. Liu J, Tsai YL, Katz E, Compton G, Garcia JE et al. High fertilization rate obtained after intracytoplasmic sperm injection with 100% nonmotile spermatozoa selected by using a simple modified hypo-osmotic swelling test. *Fertil Steril* 1997; **68**: 373–5.

106. Charehjooy N, Najafi MH, Tavalaee M, Deemeh MR, Azadi L et al. Selection of sperm based on hypo-osmotic swelling may improve ICSI outcome: a preliminary prospective clinical trial. *Int J Fertil Steril* 2014; **8**: 21–8.

107. Stanger JD, Vo L, Yovich JL, Almahbobi G. Hypo-osmotic swelling test identifies individual spermatozoa with minimal DNA fragmentation. *Reprod Biomed Online* 2010; **21**: 474–84.

Chapter 25

Future Developments: Sperm Proteomics

Manesh Panner, Selvam Kumar, Saradha Baskaran, Ashok Agarwal

25.1 Background

Spermatozoa are mature male gametes that are produced in the testes of a healthy man by spermatogenesis, with further maturation of sperm taking place during their transit through the epididymis. In the human, approximately 20 to 240 million sperm are produced per day [1]. Unlike other somatic cells present in the human body, spermatozoa contain a head, neck, mid-piece and tail region. The head region contains the genetic material which is transferred to the oocyte during the fertilization process. Apart from DNA, spermatozoa also deliver additional subcellular materials such as oocyte activating factors, RNA, microRNAs and exosomal proteins that are essential for the development of the oocyte into a zygote.

Disturbance in the molecular events related to testicular spermatogenesis or post-testicular maturation may result in infertility. In general, infertility evaluation in men is based on conventional semen analysis which is considered as the cornerstone in the assessment of male infertility. Typically, semen parameters such as sperm concentration, total motility, normal morphology and vitality are examined according to the fifth edition reference values established by the WHO laboratory manual [2]. In addition to basic semen analysis, specialized sperm function tests (SSFT) such as oxidation-reduction potential (ORP) [3] and terminal deoxynucleotidyl transferase-mediated dUTP nick-end labeling (TUNEL) or sperm chromatin structure assay (SCSA) are carried out to evaluate the seminal oxidative stress and sperm DNA fragmentation (SDF), respectively [3, 4]. High levels of oxidative stress and SDF are associated with fertilization failure and male infertility [4]. Both semen analysis and SSFT fail to identify molecular mechanisms and subcellular pathways that are dysfunctional in the spermatozoa of infertile men [5].

Recently, proteomic approaches are being used widely to understand the molecular factors that are associated with male infertility. Proteomic studies are of different types: structural proteomics, functional proteomics and expressional proteomics. In particular, global/expressional proteomic analysis of the ejaculated spermatozoa enables us to understand the patho-physiological state of spermatozoa. The mitochondrial proteome of sperm reflects the mitochondrial membrane integrity [6]. Similarly, the expression of energy metabolism-related proteins are directly associated with sperm motility. As spermatozoa are transcriptionally and translationally silent, their proteome reflects the outcome of spermatogenesis and maturation process. Furthermore, integration of proteomics with bioinformatics serves as a promising tool in the identification of potential diagnostic and therapeutic biomarkers for the management of male infertility. The availability of advanced proteomic tools such as matrix-assisted laser desorption/ionization time-of-flight (MALDI-TOF) and liquid chromatography-tandem mass spectrometry (LC-MS/MS) has increased the knowledge and understanding of the causes of male infertility. This chapter provides a brief overview of advanced proteomic techniques and highlights the general steps involved in processing of sperm cells for proteomics and bioinformatic analysis of the proteomic data. Furthermore, proteomic-based studies on sperm and seminal plasma are discussed in detail, along with the potential role of biomarkers in the prognosis and diagnosis of male infertility.

25.2 Proteomics of Sperm Cells

Proteomics is defined as the complete protein profiling of a tissue or cell. Sperm proteins are detected using both conventional and advanced proteomic techniques. Two-dimensional (2D) gel electrophoresis is the most commonly used technique to separate sperm proteins based on their isoelectric focusing point and molecular weight. Advanced proteomic techniques include analysis of sperm proteins using MALDI-TOF and LC-MS/MS. Semen contains cellular (spermatozoa) and non-cellular (seminal plasma) components. Other than spermatozoa, semen also contains round cells including leukocytes and immature germ cells. Round cells are of two types: spermatogenic and non-spermatogenic round cells. Hence, two types of samples are being used in sperm proteomic studies: 1) processed semen sample and 2) unprocessed or neat semen sample.

Processed semen samples contain pure fraction of spermatozoa. Density gradient technique is used to separate out the seminal plasma, round cells and leukocytes from spermatozoa. Few studies indicate that the use of sperm with round cells in the protein extraction process may contaminate the sperm proteome [7, 8, 9, 10, 11, 12]. The processing of neat semen samples for proteomic studies involves separation of spermatozoa from seminal fluid by centrifugation and subsequently, washing with phosphate buffer saline (PBS) to completely remove the seminal plasma. Recent studies explained the effect on biological pathways associated with sperm function due to the presence of round cell proteins in the proteome of sperm [13, 14]. The influence of non-spermatogenic round cell proteins was found to be very negligible or insignificant as they were masked by the sperm proteome [14]. Furthermore, the presence of these round cells and leukocyte proteins did not interfere in the molecular pathways associated with sperm function [13].

Initially, the sperm pellet is mixed with lysis buffer such as radioimmunoprecipitation assay (RIPA) and left overnight for complete lysis of spermatozoa [14]. Purity and concentration of the sperm proteins are checked prior to electrophoresis (either one-dimensional or 2D gel). Proteins separated by electrophoresis are subjected to in-gel digestion using trypsin. Further, the peptides are eluted and injected into the mass spectrometry (MS) system that detects the peptides and proteins using an unbiased approach by analyzing the mass shifts without any prior information about the structure [15]. The proteins are identified based on their mass/charge ratio (m/z) and with a very low false discovery rate. Next, the proteins and peptides detected by MS are scanned completely and compared with previously annotated and sequenced proteins available in a global database.

Lists of proteins are computed using softwares such as SEQUEST, Mascot and X!-Tandem that are operated using different algorithms [16]. The proteins are then categorized as differentially expressed proteins (DEPs) based on spectral counts and abundance of each protein. These DEPs are subjected to bioinformatic analysis to identify their role in different biological processes [17]. Gene ontology (GO) analysis is used to obtain the information related to localization and distribution of proteins. Furthermore, open access bioinformatics tools such as the Search Tool for the Retrieval of Interacting Genes/Proteins (STRING) are used to display the interaction between proteins [18]. Commercially available authenticated software such as Ingenuity Pathway Analysis (IPA) and Metacore™ are used to identify interactions between the functional pathways, biological processes, proteins and the transcriptional factors regulating their expression [18].

25.3 Review of Sperm Proteomic Studies

Characterization of sperm proteome and its implication in deciphering the molecular and cellular pathways in male infertility have gained increasing attention among reproductive researchers and andrologists. Although earlier proteomic studies mainly examined specific sperm surface proteins, the first comprehensive report on human sperm proteome was published in 2005 [19]. The study reported 1760 distinct proteins using 1D-SDS-PAGE coupled with LC-MS/MS analysis and indicated the presence of all 27 proteins constituting the 26S proteasome in the sperm. However, the study did not provide a complete list of proteins identified [19]. Later, Martinez-Heredia et al. characterized the sperm proteome and reported 98 distinct proteins using 2D-PAGE coupled with MALDI-TOF MS analysis [10]. Furthermore, the study revealed the functional distribution of these proteins to be energy production (23 percent), transcription, protein synthesis, transport, folding and turnover (23 percent), cell cycle, apoptosis and oxidative stress (10 percent), signal transduction (8 percent), cytoskeleton, flagella and cell movement (10 percent), cell recognition (7 percent) and metabolism (6 percent) [10]. The sperm proteomic study conducted by Baker et al. identified 1053 proteins, which included nicotinamide adenine dinucleotide phosphate oxidase (NOX), and its homolog, dual oxidase 2 (DUOX2), and various classes of receptors that are potential regulators of sperm function [20]. Gilany et al. retrieved the human sperm proteome from the literature and analyzed it by the Database for Annotation Visualization and Integrated Discovery (DAVID) software [21]. The analysis revealed a collection of 1300 proteins involved in various metabolic pathways that were primarily localized to cytoplasm [21].

Lately, in addition to whole sperm proteomics, subcellular proteomics has also gained significant attention as it provides in-depth information regarding the sperm protein content and their exact localization. Furthermore, it allows identification of less abundant proteins. Proteomic analysis of the head and flagellar regions of spermatozoa conducted by Baker et al. identified a total of 1429 proteins with 721 proteins exclusively localized in the tail and 521 proteins exclusively localized in the head fractions [22]. This was the first study that provided novel insight into the compartmentalization of proteins, particularly receptors [22]. Analysis of isolated tail fractions of spermatozoa resulted in the identification of 1049 proteins that were mainly involved in metabolism and energy production, and sperm tail structure and motility [7]. Interestingly, the analysis also revealed a high number of peroxisomal proteins in sperm, which are believed to be lacking peroxisomes [7].

Proteomic characterizations of membrane fractions of spermatozoa led to the elucidation of proteins involved in sperm-oocyte interaction [23]. de Mateo et al. isolated and analyzed human sperm nuclei by LC-MS/MS approach and reported 403 nuclear proteins [24]. The most abundant family of proteins were histones, followed by ribosome proteins, proteasome subunits, cytokeratins, tubulins, SPANX proteins, HSPs and Tektins. This was the first study to provide an in-sight on the nuclear proteins that are potentially related to sperm epigenetic functions, proper fertilization and embryo development [24]. Furthermore, de Mateo et al. were the first to report correlation between proteomics, DNA integrity and protamine content [25]. In 2014, Amaral et al. analyzed 30 different sperm proteomic studies and reported 6198 proteins, of which 30 percent are known to be expressed in the testis [8]. The proteins were cataloged based on their functional pathways including metabolism, cell cycle, apoptosis, membrane trafficking, RNA metabolism and post-translational protein modifications [8].

25.4 Sperm Proteome Profile and Male Infertility

25.4.1 Molecular Pathways and Proteins Affected in Varicocele

Varicocele is one of the most common and correctable causes of male infertility and is prevalent in 15 percent of normal men and 40 percent of infertile men of reproductive age groups [26]. Sperm proteome analysis in these subjects have facilitated in interpreting the cellular and molecular pathways implicated in the pathophysiology of varicocele. The first proteomic study that analyzed the differences in the sperm proteome of men with and without varicocele was published by Hosseinifar et al. [27]. The study revealed 15 DEPs that predominantly included heat shock proteins (HSPs), mitochondrial and cytoskeleton proteins. Sperm proteome characterization in infertile men with unilateral varicocele against healthy controls revealed 369 DEPs that were associated with major functional pathways such as metabolism, disease, immune system, gene expression, signal transduction and apoptosis [28]. Of the 369 DEPS, 29 proteins were identified to be involved in spermatogenesis and other fundamental reproductive processes such as sperm maturation, acquisition of sperm motility, hyperactivation, capacitation, acrosome reaction and fertilization. Furthermore, it was reported that unilateral varicocele mostly affected small molecule biochemistry and post-translational modification proteins [28].

Sperm proteome characterization in infertile men with bilateral varicocele against controls resulted in the identification of 73 DEPs. The majority of the DEPs were associated with metabolic processes, stress responses, oxidoreductase activity, enzyme regulation, and immune system processes [29]. Seven DEPs (Outer dense fiber protein 2 (ODF2); Tektin-3 (TEKT3); T-complex protein 11 homolog (TCP11); Protein-glutamine gamma-glutamyl transferase 4 (TGM4); Calmegin (CLGN); Mitochondrial import receptor subunit TOM22 homolog (TOM22); Apolipoprotein A-I (APOA1)) were involved in key sperm functions such as capacitation, motility and sperm-zona binding.

For the first time, Agarwal et al. compared the sperm proteome of unilateral and bilateral varicocele in men and reported the differences in expression of

247

proteins that were mostly involved in post-translational modification, protein folding, protein ubiquitination, free-radical scavenging, lipid and nucleic acid metabolism, small molecule biochemistry and mitochondrial dysfunction [30]. In fact, mitochondrial dysfunction is considered as one of the major mechanisms implicated in the pathophysiology of clinical varicocele and associated infertility [31, 32]. A recent study conducted by Samanta et al. examined the proteomic signatures of sperm mitochondria in varicocele subjects and reported 23 DEPs associated with mitochondrial structure (LETM1, EFHC, MIC60, PGAM5, ISOC2 and TOM22) and function (NDFSU1, UQCRC2 and COX5B), as well as core enzymes of carbohydrate and lipid metabolism [32]. Additionally, protein associated with sperm functions (ATPase1A4, HSPA2, SPA17 and APOA1) were reported to be under-expressed. Furthermore, mitochondrial electron transport chain (ETC) proteins along with testis-specific pyruvate dehydrogenase (PDH) have been suggested as biomarkers of sperm function in varicocele subjects [32].

25.4.2 Proteomic Signature of Sperm in Testicular Cancer

The incidence of testicular cancer (TC) has been increasing drastically for decades and most commonly reported in men of reproductive age group [33]. According to the American Cancer Society, the number of newly diagnosed cases of TC is estimated to be 9560 and about 410 related deaths in 2019 [33]. The most common form of TC is germ cell tumors (GCTs), which account for about 90–95 percent of all cases. The major types of GCTs are seminomas and non-seminomas. TC is associated with decline in semen quality and fertilizing potential of spermatozoa [34]. Proteomic studies have revealed that this reduction in semen quality is associated with alterations in the expression of sperm proteins [35, 36].

A few sperm proteomic studies have been conducted to identify the potential biomarkers and molecular mechanism(s) associated with the reduced fertilizing ability of TC subjects [35, 36, 37, 38, 39]. Dias et al. compared the sperm proteomic profile of men with testicular cancer seminoma against healthy fertile men [36]. Quantitative proteomic analysis revealed 393 DEPs between the groups that were associated with spermatogenic dysfunction, reduced sperm kinematics and motility, failure in capacitation

and fertilization. Comparative analysis of sperm proteome of men with non-seminoma testicular cancer and healthy fertile men revealed 189 DEPs with under expression of proteins crucial for mitochondrial function, sperm motility and fertilization [35]. About 198 proteins were identified as DEPs between normozoospermic (motility>40 percent) and asthenozoospermic (motility<40 percent) in TC patients who had cryopreserved semen samples before initiation of cancer therapy [39]. The study revealed under-expression of proteins associated with the binding to zona pellucida (CCT3), mitochondrial function (ATP5A1 and UQCRC2), sperm motility (ATP1A4) and exosomal pathway in asthenozoospermic TC patients. Another recent study reported under-expression of NDUFS1 associated with mitochondrial function and overexpression of CD63 involved in sperm maturation in both normozoospermic and asthenozoospermic TC patients when compared to normozoospermic infertile men without cancer [38].

25.4.3 Cellular Changes in Sperm of Unexplained Male Infertility

Infertility of unknown origin in men with normal semen parameters and without involvement of any female infertility factor is categorized as unexplained male infertility (UMI) [40]. Although semen analysis is the cornerstone for the evaluation of male infertility, 30 percent of normozoospermic men are diagnosed with UMI [40, 41]. This clearly indicates the limitations of conventional semen analysis in predicting the male fertility potential and reproductive outcome in couples. Sperm proteomic studies in these subjects may pave the way for identifying the etiologies as well as cellular and molecular changes associated with UMI. Frapsauce et al. analyzed the proteins in normal but non-fertilizing sperm using 2D fluorescence DIGE (difference gel electrophoresis) and reported 15 DEPs [42]. Furthermore, laminin receptor (LR67) and L-xylulose reductase (P34H) proteins involved in gamete interactions were proposed as potential targets for diagnosis and prognosis of fertilization failure in IVF [42]. Several sperm proteomic studies have been conducted in normozoospermic infertile men with IVF failure and mostly, the proteins associated with sexual reproduction, metabolic process, cell growth and/or maintenance, protein metabolism and protein transport, chromosome organization, capacitation, acrosome reaction and sperm-oocyte interaction were reported to be dysregulated [43, 44, 45, 46]. A recent study compared the sperm proteome of UMI subjects against normozoospermic fertile men using LC-MS/MS and reported 162 DEPs between the groups [47]. Analysis revealed under-expression of proteins associated with reproductive system development and function, and ubiquitination pathway in UMI subjects. Furthermore, serine protease inhibitor (SERPINA5), annexin A2 (ANXA2), and sperm surface protein Sp17 (SPA17) were suggested as biomarkers for screening the fertilization potential of spermatozoa in UMI subjects [47].

25.4.4 Sperm Proteome in Oligoasthenozoospermia

Oligoasthenozoospermia (OAT) is characterized by reduced sperm concentration and motility. Very few studies have been published on the seminal plasma proteomics, and none in the sperm proteomics of OAT subjects [47, 48, 49]. Herwig et al. identified the proteins involved in the etiology of OAT due to oxidative stress [48]. Seminal plasma proteins associated with multiple biological functions such as binding activity (lactotransferrin (LTF); prolactin-induced protein (PIP); extracellular matrix protein 1 (ECM1)), transporter activity (human epididymis-specific protein 1 (HE1); prostaglandin D2 synthase (PTGDS)), immune activity (CD177), and hydrolase activity (prostate-specific antigen (PSA)) were reported to be dysregulated in OAT subjects [49].

25.4.5 Sperm Proteome in Asthenozoospermia

Asthenozoospermia, or reduced progressive motility of spermatozoa, is the most common finding in infertile men. Several sperm proteomic studies have been conducted in these subjects that have shed light on the DEPs (Table 25.1) and related pathways implicated in the pathophysiology of asthenozoospermia [50, 51, 52, 53, 54, 55, 56]. The reduced motility has been attributed to several factors including dysregulation of energy metabolism, structural defects in sperm-tail protein components and differential expression of proteins involved in sperm motility [57]. Siva et al. compared the sperm proteome of asthenozoospermic and normozoospermic subjects using 2D-PAGE MALDI MS/MS approach. The DEPs were categorized into three functional groups, namely: "energy

and metabolism" (triose-phosphate isomerase (TPIS); testis-specific glycerol kinase 2 (GKP2); and succinyl-CoA:3-ketoacid co-enzyme A transferase 1 (OXCT1), mitochondrial precursor); "movement and organization" (tubulin beta 2C (TUBB2C) and tektin 1 (TEKT1)); and "protein turnover, folding and stress response" (proteasome alpha 3 subunit (PSMA3) and heat shock-related 70 kDa protein 2 (HSPA2)) [55]. Similar categorization of key DEPs was reported by other sperm proteomic studies conducted in asthenozoospermic subjects [50, 56].

Parte et al. compared the expression of phosphoproteins associated with sperm motility in asthenozoospermic and normozoospermic subjects [52]. Comparative sperm proteome analysis between normozoospermic and asthenozoospermic subjects resulted in the identification of pathways associated with altered expression of proteins (Table 25.1), which included axoneme activation and focal adhesion assembly, glycolysis, gluconeogenesis, cellular response to stress and nucleosome assembly [53]. The reported DEPs were HSPs, cytoskeletal proteins, proteins involved with fibrous sheath and energy metabolism. A recent proteomic study conducted by Nowicka-Bauer et al. using 2-DE and MALDI-TOF MS, correlated the DEPs identified with the sperm mitochondrial activity [51]. The findings of this study indicated the possible role of sperm mitochondrial dysfunction and oxidative stress in the etiology of asthenozoospermia [51]. Another recent study revealed decreased expression of proteins related to calcium ion entry (TEX40) and acrosomal acidification (ATP6V0A2) in asthenozoospermic men [54]. Lower expression of TEX40 and ATP6V0A2 leads to fewer entries of calcium ion into the spermatozoa and acrosomal de-acidification, which in turn results in diminution of sperm motility in asthenozoospermic men [54].

25.4.6 Sperm Proteome in Globozoospermia

Globozoospermia is a rare and severe form of teratozoospermia that is responsible for <0.1 percent of male infertility [61]. It is characterized by the presence of round-headed spermatozoa lacking an acrosome with deranged mid-piece and tail. Sperm proteomic studies have provided molecular insight into round-headed spermatogenesis and proteins implicated in the pathophysiology of globozoospermia. Liao et al. analyzed the difference in the

Table 25.1 Potential Sperm Protein Biomarkers Associated with Male Infertility

Clinical condition	Method	DEPs	Reference
Varicocele	2D PAGE MALDI-TOF/TOF-MS	HSPA5, ATP5D, SOD1, ACPP, CLU, PARK7, KLK3, PIP, SEMG2, SEMG2pre	Hosseinifar et al. 2013 [27]
	1D PAGE LC-MS/MS	CABYR, AKAP, APOPA1, SEMG1, ACR, SPA17, RSPH1, RSPH9 DNAH17, DLD, GSTM3, TGM4, NPC23, ODF2GPR64, PSMA8, HIST1H2BA, PARK7	Agarwal et al. 2015 [28]
	1D PAGE LC-MS/MS	GSTM3, SPANXB1, PARK7, PSMA8, DLD, SEMG1, SEMG2	Agarwal et al. 2015 [30]
	1D PAGE LC-MS/MS	ODF2, TEKT3, TCP11, TGM4, CLGN, TOM22, APOA1	Agarwal et al. 2016 [29]
	1D PAGE LC-MS/MS	PKAR1A, AK7, CCT6B, HSPA2, ODF2	Agarwal et al. 2016b [31]
	LC-MS/MS	LETM1, EFHC, MIC60, PGAM5, ISOC2, TOM22, NDFSU1, UQCRC2, COX5B, ATPase1A4, HSPA2, SPA17, APOA1	Samanta et al. 2018 [32]
	1D PAGE LC-MS/MS	HSPA2. HSP90B1, OXPHOS complex proteins	Swain et al. 2019 [58]
Testicular cancer	LC-MS/MS	PSA, PAcP, ZAG, SEMG 1 and 2, AKAP4, DNAH17	Agarwal et al. 2015 [37]
	1D PAGE LC-MS/MS	NDUFS1, UQCRC2, ATP1A4, ANXA2, ATP1A2, ACR	Dias et al. 2018 [35]
	1D PAGE LC-MS/MS	CCT3, ATP5A1, UQCRC2, ATP1A4, MMP9	Panner Selvam et al. 2019 [39]
	1D PAGE LC-MS/MS	NDUFS1, CD63	Panner Selvam et al. 2019 [38]
	1D PAGE LC-MS/MS	HSPA2, ATP1A4, UQCRC2, ACE	Dias et al. 2019 [36]
UMI	1D PAGE LC-MS/MS	SERPINA5, ANXA2, SPA17	Panner Selvam et al. 2019 [46]
	MALDI-TOF/TOF	PAEP, ODFP, SEGI, PSA, and GPx4pre	Xu et al. 2012 [45]
Normozoospermic men with IVF failure	2D-DIGE MS	P34H	Frapsauce et al. 2014 [42]
	iTRAQ LC-MS/MS	SEMG1, PIP, GAPDHS, PGK2	Légaré et al. 2014 [44]
	TMT LC-MS/MS	SRPK1	Azpiazu et al. 2014 [43]
Asthenozoospermia	2-DE MALDI-TOF MS	IDH-α, ODF, SEMG1, ARHGDIB, GOT1, PGAM2, TPI1, CA2, GS10, MSS1	Zhao et al. 2007 [56]
	2D PAGE MS	ACTB, ANXA5, COX6B, H2A, PIP, PIPpre, S100A9, CLUpre, DLDpre, FHpre, HSPA2, IMPA1, MPST/ECH1pre, PSMB3, SEMG1pre, TEX12	Martinez-Heredia et al. 2008 [50]
	2D PAGE MALDI MS/MS	TPIS, PSMA3, GKP2, HSPA2, OXCT1, TUBB2C, TEKT1	Siva et al. 2010 [55]
	Nano UPLC–MS^E tandem mass spectrometry	GRP78, GAPDHS, HSP70-2, TUBA4A, TUBA3C, TUBA8, ODF1, AKAP3, AKAP4, ROPN1B, SPANXB, CLU, PIP, ATP5B, ALDOA, ARGDIA	Parte et al. 2012 [52]
	2-DE MALDI-TOF/TOF MS	UBB2B, ODF2, AKAP4, KRT1, CLU, COX6B, GAPDS, PHGPx, HSPA2, HSPA9, VDAC2, GSTMu3, ASRGL1, SPANXB	Hashemitabar et al 2015 [59]

Table 25.1 (*cont.*)

Clinical condition	Method	DEPs	Reference
	UPLC-MS	PLXNB2, POTEKP, NIN, PHF3, DYNLL1, PROCA1, FASCIN-3; LRRC37B, PLC	Saraswat et al 2017 [53]
	2-DE MALDI-TOF MS	LFT, ATP5B, DJ-1, PARK7, ODF, TEKT1, AKAP4, ELSPBP1, PDHB, NDUS1, SUCLA2, SDHA	Nowicka-Bauer et al. 2018 [51]
	2D-DIGE MALDI -TOF-MS	TEX40, ATP6V0A2, SERPINB9, PSA	Sinha et al. 2019 [54]
Globozoospermia	2D DIGE MALDI-TOF/ TOF MS/MS	SAMP1, ODF2, SPANXa/d, TUBA2, TPI1, PIP	Liao et al. 2009 [60]

Nano UPLC–MS^E: nanoflow ultra-performance chromatography tandem mass spectrometry.

proteome of normal and round-headed spermatozoa using 2-D fluorescence difference gel electrophoresis (DIGE) coupled with MS/MS [60]. About 35 protein spots were noted to be differentially expressed in round-headed spermatozoa when compared to normal spermatozoa. These DEPs (Table 25.1) were recognized to play an important role in spermatogenesis, cell skeleton, metabolism and motility [60].

25.4.7 Sperm Protein Biomarkers of Male Infertility

Recent advancement and development in proteomics may help in the identification of biomarkers associated with several male infertility conditions. In general, sperm protein biomarkers can be used to understand the molecular mechanisms involved in the patho-physiology related to sperm function. For accurate prediction and classification of infertile men, the biomarker must be highly sensitive, specific and non-invasive [62]. Proteomic analysis of spermatozoa has resulted in the identification of DEPs associated with various male infertility conditions. These key proteins could serve as potential biomarkers in the diagnosis of male infertility (Table 25.1).

25.4.8 Integrating Sperm Proteomics and Sperm Function Tests

Currently, andrology laboratories use several sperm function tests to assess the functional quality of the spermatozoa used in ART. These tests were developed to overcome the limitations of conventional semen analysis. Additional sperm function tests include hypo-osmotic swelling test, anti-sperm antibody test, reactive oxygen species (ROS) tests, and sperm chromatin integrity tests [63]. Sperm proteomics can be used as a tool to understand and identify the biomarkers that reflect the molecular changes occurring in dysfunctional spermatozoa. To date, the majority of the proteomic studies on spermatozoa have been able to identify the DEPs associated with acrosome reaction, oxidative stress, SDF, and mitochondrial dysfunction (Table 25.2). Use of these protein biomarkers along with the available sperm function tests will improve the efficiency and accuracy of diagnosis.

25.4.9 The Future of Sperm Proteomics

Currently, research on sperm proteomics has identified several biomarkers associated with a number of male infertility conditions. Advancement in the field of sperm proteomics has significantly helped our understanding of the molecular pathology involved in various male infertility conditions. However, one of the main challenges at present is to translate these findings into the clinical setting as the translational research is moving very slowly, especially in the field of male infertility [70]. Further development in the technology and introduction of large scale proteomic experiments at affordable cost may help accelerate translating the findings from bench to bed side. Another key challenge is to identify a unique biomarker specific to each infertility condition. This can be addressed by using protein biomarker panels for the prognosis and diagnosis of male infertility [71]. In fact, a combination of biomarkers has the potential to deliver a higher predictive power than a single biomarker [72, 73]. Such panels can be developed by selecting the key proteins involved in various biological processes associated with the pathophysiology of a particular male infertility condition. The final challenge would be the clinical validation of the sperm

Table 25.2 Potential Protein Biomarkers Associated with Sperm Dysfunction

Sperm dysfunction	DEPs	Reference
Oxidative stress	HIST1H2BA, MDH2, TGM4, GPX4, GLUL, HSP90B1, HSPA5, ACE, HSPA2, RPS27A, MAP3K3 and APP, PRDX1, AKAP4	Hamada et al. 2013 [64]; Sharma et al. 2013 [65]; Ayaz et al. 2018 [66]
Mitochondrial dysfunction	PKAR1A, AK7, CCT6B, HSPA2, ODF2, DLD, ATP5D, NDUFS1, UQCRC2, COX5B, PDH, PHGPx, VDAC, COX6B, AKAP4	Hosseinifar et al. 2014 [67]; Hashemitabar et al. 2015 [59]; Agarwal et al. 2016 [68]; Samanta et al. 2018 [32]
Sperm DNA damage	CRISPLD2, CRISPLD2, RARRES1	Intasqui et al. 2016 [69]

protein biomarker panels for individual infertility conditions. This can be achieved by developing strategies to conduct clinical trials to validate the biomarkers in infertile men.

25.2 Conclusion

Sperm proteomic studies have significantly improved our understanding about the molecular events associated with the spermatozoa. The use of sophisticated and expensive proteomic instruments, and requirement of skilled and well trained bioinformaticians to interpret the proteomic data has limited its availability in clinical set-up. Furthermore, the results from clinical trials might validate the biomarkers, which in turn will help the physicians to offer better treatment and care for their patients.

References

1. Plant TM, Zeleznik AJ. (2014). *Knobil and Neill's Physiology of Reproduction*. Amsterdam: Elsevier Academic Press.

2. World Health Organization. (2010). *WHO Laboratory Manual for the Examination and Processing of Human Semen*. Geneva: The WHO Press.

3. Agarwal A, Gupta S, Sharma R. (2016). Oxidation–reduction potential measurement in ejaculated semen samples. In Agarwal A, Gupta S and Sharma R, eds., *Andrological Evaluation of Male Infertility: A Laboratory Guide*. London: Springer International Publishing, pp. 165–70.

4. Agarwal A, Sharma R, Roychoudhury S, Du Plessis S, Sabanegh E. MiOXSYS: a novel method of measuring oxidation reduction potential in semen and seminal plasma. *Fertil Steril* 2016; **106**: 566–73.e510.

5. Bracke A, Peeters K, Punjabi U, Hoogewijs D, Dewilde S. A search for molecular mechanisms underlying male idiopathic infertility. *Reprod BioMed Online* 2018; **36**: 327–39.

6. Amaral A, Lourenço B, Marques M, Ramalho-Santos J. Mitochondria functionality and sperm quality. *Reproduction* 2013; **146**: R163–R174.

7. Amaral A, Castillo J, Estanyol JM, Ballesca JL, Ramalho-Santos J, Oliva R. Human sperm tail proteome suggests new endogenous metabolic pathways. *Mol Cell Proteom* 2013; **12**: 330–42.

8. Amaral A, Paiva C, Attardo Parrinello C, Estanyol JM, Ballescà JLS, Ramalho-Santos JO, Oliva R. Identification of proteins involved in human sperm motility using high-throughput differential proteomics. *J Proteome Res* 2014; **13**: 5670–84.

9. Intasqui P, Camargo M, Del Giudice PT, Spaine DM, Carvalho VM, Cardozo KHM, Cedenho AP, Bertolla RP. Unraveling the sperm proteome and post-genomic pathways associated with sperm nuclear DNA fragmentation. *J Assist Reprod Genet* 2013; **30**: 1187–202.

10. Martínez-Heredia J, Estanyol JM, Ballescà JL, Oliva R. Proteomic identification of human sperm proteins. *Proteomics* 2006; **6**: 4356–69.

11. Wang S, Wang W, Xu Y, Tang M, Fang J, Sun H, Sun Y, Gu M, Liu Z, Zhang Z. Proteomic characteristics of human sperm cryopreservation. *Proteomics* 2014; **14**: 298–310.

12. Wang XM, Xiang Z, Fu Y, Wu HL, Zhu WB, Fan LQ. Comparative proteomics reveal the association between SPANX proteins and clinical outcomes of artificial insemination with donor sperm. *Scientific Reports* 2018; **8**: 6850.

13. Panner Selvam MK, Agarwal A, Dias TR, Martins AD, Baskaran S,

Samanta L. Molecular pathways associated with sperm biofunction are not affected by the presence of round cell and leukocyte proteins in human sperm proteome. *J Proteome Res* 2018; **18**: 1191−7.

14. Panner Selvam MK, Agarwal A, Dias TR, Martins AD, Samanta L. Presence of round cells proteins do not interfere with identification of human sperm proteins from frozen semen samples by LC-MS/MS. *Int J Mol Sci* 2019; **20**: 314.

15. Glish GL, Vachet RW. The basics of mass spectrometry in the twenty-first century. *Nat Rev Drug Discov* 2003; **2**: 140.

16. Zhou T, Zhou Z-M, Guo X-J. Bioinformatics for spermatogenesis: annotation of male reproduction based on proteomics. *Asian J Androl* 2013; **15**: 594.

17. Lan N, Montelione GT, Gerstein M. Ontologies for proteomics: towards a systematic definition of structure and function that scales to the genome level. *Curr Opin Chem Biol* 2003; **7**: 44–54.

18. Agarwal A, Durairajanayagam D, Halabi J, Peng J, Vazquez-Levin M. Proteomics, oxidative stress and male infertility. *Reprod BioMed Online* 2014; **29**: 32–58.

19. Johnston DS, Wooters J, Kopf GS, Qiu Y, Roberts KP. Analysis of the human sperm proteome. *Ann NY Acad Sci* 2005; **1061**: 190–202.

20. Baker MA, Reeves G, Hetherington L, Müller J, Baur I, Aitken RJ. Identification of gene products present in Triton X-100 soluble and insoluble fractions of human spermatozoa lysates using LC-MS/MS analysis. *Proteom Clin Appl* 2007; **1**: 524–32.

21. Gilany K, Lakpour N, Vafakhah M, Sadeghi MR. The profile of human sperm proteome: a mini-review. *J Reprod Infertil* 2011; **12**: 193–9.

22. Baker MA, Naumovski N, Hetherington L, Weinberg A, Velkov T, Aitken RJ. Head and flagella subcompartmental proteomic analysis of human spermatozoa. *Proteomics* 2013;**13**: 61–74.

23. Nixon B, Mitchell LA, Anderson AL, Mclaughlin EA, O'Bryan MK, Aitken RJ. Proteomic and functional analysis of human sperm detergent resistant membranes. *J Cell Physiol* 2011; **226**: 2651–65.

24. de Mateo S, Castillo J, Estanyol JM, Ballescà JL, Oliva R. Proteomic characterization of the human sperm nucleus. *Proteomics* 2011; **11**: 2714–26.

25. de Mateo S, Martínez-Heredia J, Estanyol JM, Domíguez-Fandos D, Vidal-Taboada JM, Ballescà JL, Oliva R. Marked correlations in protein expression identified by proteomic analysis of human spermatozoa. *Proteomics* 2007; **7**: 4264–77.

26. Kupis Ł, Dobroński PA, Radziszewski P. Varicocele as a source of male infertility – current treatment techniques. *Cent European J Urol* 2015; **68**: 365–70.

27. Hosseinifar H, Gourabi H, Salekdeh GH, Alikhani M, Mirshahvaladi S, Sabbaghian M, Modarresi T, Gilani MAS. Study of sperm protein profile in men with and without varicocele using two-dimensional gel electrophoresis. *Urology* 2013; **81**: 293–300.

28. Agarwal A, Sharma R, Durairajanayagam D, Ayaz A, Cui Z, Willard B, Gopalan B, Sabanegh E. Major protein alterations in spermatozoa from infertile men with unilateral varicocele. *Reprod Biol Endocrinol* 2015; **13**: 8.

29. Agarwal A, Sharma R, Durairajanayagam D, Cui Z, Ayaz A, Gupta S, Willard B, Gopalan B, Sabanegh E. Spermatozoa protein alterations in infertile men with

bilateral varicocele. *Asian J Androl* 2016; **18**: 43–53.

30. Agarwal A, Sharma R, Durairajanayagam D, Cui Z, Ayaz A, Gupta S, Willard B, Gopalan B, Sabanegh E. Differential proteomic profiling of spermatozoal proteins of infertile men with unilateral or bilateral varicocele. *Urology* 2015; **85**: 580–8.

31. Agarwal A, Sharma R, Samanta L, Durairajanayagam D, Sabanegh E. Proteomic signatures of infertile men with clinical varicocele and their validation studies reveal mitochondrial dysfunction leading to infertility. *Asian J Androl* 2016; **18**: 282–91.

32. Samanta L, Agarwal A, Swain N, Sharma R, Gopalan B, Esteves SC, Durairajanayagam D, Sabanegh E. Proteomic signatures of sperm mitochondria in varicocele: clinical use as biomarkers of varicocele associated infertility. *J Urol* 2018; **200**: 414–22.

33. Siegel RL, Miller KD, Jemal A. Cancer statistics. *CA Cancer J Clin* 2019; **69**: 7–34.

34. Rives N, Perdrix A, Hennebicq S, Saïas-Magnan J, Melin MC, Berthaut I, Barthélémy C, Daudin M, Szerman E, Bresson JL. The semen quality of 1158 men with testicular cancer at the time of cryopreservation: results of the French National CECOS Network. *J Androl* 2012; **33**: 1394–401.

35. Dias TR, Agarwal A, Pushparaj PN, Ahmad G, Sharma R. New insights on the mechanisms affecting fertility in men with non-seminoma testicular cancer before cancer therapy. *World J Mens Health* 2018; **38**: 198–207.

36. Dias TR, Agarwal A, Pushparaj PN, Ahmad G, Sharma R. Reduced semen quality in patients with testicular cancer seminoma is associated with alterations in the expression of sperm proteins. *Asian J Androl* 2020; **22**: 88–93.

37. Agarwal A, Tvrda E, Sharma R, Gupta S, Ahmad G, Sabanegh ES. Spermatozoa protein profiles in cryobanked semen samples from testicular cancer patients before treatment. *Fertil Steril* 2015; **104**: e260.

38. Panner Selvam MK, Agarwal A, Pushparaj PN. Altered molecular pathways in the proteome of cryopreserved sperm in testicular cancer patients before treatment. *Int J Mol Sci* 2019; **20**: 677.

39. Panner Selvam MK, Agarwal A, Pushparaj PN. A quantitative global proteomics approach to understanding the functional pathways dysregulated in the spermatozoa of asthenozoospermic testicular cancer patients. *Andrology* 2019; **7**: 454–62.

40. Hamada A, Esteves SC, Agarwal A. Unexplained male infertility: potential causes and management. *Hum Androl* 2011; **1**: 2–16.

41. Wallach EE, Moghissi KS, Wallach EE. Unexplained infertility. *Fertil Steril* 1983; **39**: 5–21.

42. Frapsauce C, Pionneau C, Bouley J, Delarouziere V, Berthaut I, Ravel C, Antoine J-M, Soubrier F, Mandelbaum J. Proteomic identification of target proteins in normal but nonfertilizing sperm. *Fertil Steril* 2014; **102**: 372–80.

43. Azpiazu R, Amaral A, Castillo J, Estanyol JM, Guimerà M, Ballescà JL, Balasch J, Oliva R. High-throughput sperm differential proteomics suggests that epigenetic alterations contribute to failed assisted reproduction. *Hum Reprod* 2014; **29**: 1225–37.

44. Légaré C, Droit A, Fournier F, Bourassa S, Force A, Cloutier F, Tremblay R, Sullivan R. Investigation of male infertility using quantitative comparative proteomics. *J Proteom Res* 2014; **13**: 5403–14.

45. Xu W, Hu H, Wang Z, Chen X, Yang F, Zhu Z, Fang P, Dai J, Wang L, Shi H et al. Proteomic characteristics of spermatozoa in normozoospermic patients with infertility. *J Proteom* 2012; **75**: 5426–36.

46. Panner Selvam MK, Agarwal A, Pushparaj PN, Baskaran S, Bendou H. Sperm proteome analysis and identification of fertility-associated biomarkers in unexplained male infertility. *Genes* 2019; **10**: 522.

47. Giacomini E, Ura B, Giolo E, Luppi S, Martinelli M, Garcia RC, Ricci G. Comparative analysis of the seminal plasma proteomes of oligoasthenozoospermic and normozoospermic men. *Reprod Biomed Online* 2015; **30**: 522–31.

48. Herwig R, Knoll C, Planyavsky M, Pourbiabany A, Greilberger J, Bennett KL. Proteomic analysis of seminal plasma from infertile patients with oligoasthenoteratozoospermia due to oxidative stress and comparison with fertile volunteers. *Fertil Steril* 2013; **100**: 355–66.e352.

49. Liu X, Wang W, Zhu P, Wang J, Wang Y, Wang X, Liu J, Li N, Lin C, Liu F. In-depth quantitative proteome analysis of seminal plasma from men with oligoasthenozoospermia and normozoospermia. *Reprod Biomed Online* 2018; **37**: 467–79.

50. Martínez-Heredia J, de Mateo S, Vidal-Taboada JM, Ballescà JL, Oliva R. Identification of proteomic differences in asthenozoospermic sperm samples. *Hum Reprod* 2008; **23**: 783–91.

51. Nowicka-Bauer K, Lepczynski A, Ozgo M, Kamieniczna M, Fraczek M, Stanski L, Olszewska M, Malcher A, Skrzypczak W, Kurpisz M. Sperm mitochondrial dysfunction and oxidative stress as possible reasons for isolated asthenozoospermia. *J Physiol Pharmacol* 2018; **69**(3). doi: 10.26402/jpp.2018.3.05

52. Parte PP, Rao P, Redij S, Lobo V, D'Souza SJ, Gajbhiye R, Kulkarni V. Sperm phosphoproteome profiling by ultra performance liquid chromatography followed by data independent analysis (LC–MSE) reveals altered proteomic signatures in asthenozoospermia. *J Proteom* 2012; **75**: 5861–71.

53. Saraswat M, Joenväärä S, Jain T, Tomar AK, Sinha A, Singh S, Yadav S, Renkonen R. Human spermatozoa quantitative proteomic signature classifies normo- and asthenozoospermia. *Mol Cell Proteom* 2017; **16**: 57–72.

54. Sinha A, Singh V, Singh S, Yadav S. Proteomic analyses reveal lower expression of TEX40 and ATP6V0A2 proteins related to calcium ion entry and acrosomal acidification in asthenozoospermic males. *Life Sciences* 2019; **218**: 81–8.

55. Siva AB, Kameshwari DB, Singh V, Pavani K, Sundaram CS, Rangaraj N, Deenadayal M, Shivaji S. Proteomics-based study on asthenozoospermia: differential expression of proteasome alpha complex. *Mol Hum Reprod* 2010; **16**(7): 452–62. doi: 10.1093/molehr/gaq009

56. Zhao C, Huo R, Wang F-Q, Lin M, Zhou Z-M, Sha J-H. Identification of several proteins involved in regulation of sperm motility by proteomic analysis. *Fertil Steril* 2007; **87**: 436–8.

57. Cao X, Cui Y, Zhang X, Lou J, Zhou J, Bei H, Wei R. Proteomic profile of human spermatozoa in healthy and asthenozoospermic individuals. *Reprod Biol Endocrinol* 2018;**16**: 16.

58. Swain N, Samanta L, Agarwal A, Kumar S, Dixit A, Gopalan B, Durairajanayagam D, Sharma R, Puspharaj PN, Baskaran S. Aberrant upregulation of compensatory redox molecular machines may contribute to sperm dysfunction in infertile men with unilateral varicocele: a

proteomic insight. *Antioxid Redox Signal* 2019; **32**: 504–21.

59. Hashemitabar M, Sabbagh S, Orazizadeh M, Ghadiri A, Bahmanzadeh M. A proteomic analysis on human sperm tail: comparison between normozoospermia and asthenozoospermia. *J Assist Reprod Genet* 2015; **32**: 853–63.

60. Liao TT, Xiang Z, Zhu WB, Fan LQ. Proteome analysis of round-headed and normal spermatozoa by 2-D fluorescence difference gel electrophoresis and mass spectrometry. *Asian J Androl* 2009; **11**: 683–93.

61. Dam AHDM, Feenstra I, Westphal JR, Ramos L, van Golde RJT, Kremer JAM. Globozoospermia revisited. *Hum Reprod Update* 2006; **13**: 63–75.

62. Kovac JR, Lipshultz LI. The significance of insulin-like factor 3 as a marker of intratesticular testosterone. *Fertil Steril* 2013; **99**: 66–7.

63. Oehninger S, Franken DR, Ombelet W. Sperm functional tests. *Fertil Steril* 2014; **102**: 1528–33.

64. Hamada A, Sharma R, du Plessis SS, Willard B, Yadav SP, Sabanegh E, Agarwal A. Two-dimensional differential in-gel electrophoresis-based proteomics of male gametes in relation to oxidative stress. *Fertil Steril* 2013; **99**: 1216–26. e1212.

65. Sharma R, Agarwal A, Mohanty G, Hamada AJ, Gopalan B, Willard B, Yadav S, du Plessis S. Proteomic analysis of human spermatozoa proteins with oxidative stress. *Reprod Biol Endocrinol* 2013; **11**: 48.

66. Ayaz A, Agarwal A, Sharma R, Kothandaraman N, Cakar Z, Sikka S. Proteomic analysis of sperm proteins in infertile men with high levels of reactive oxygen species. *Andrologia* 2018; **50**: e13015.

67. Hosseinifar H, Sabbaghian M, Nasrabadi D, Modarresi T, Dizaj AV, Gourabi H, Gilani MA. Study of the effect of varicocelectomy on sperm proteins expression in patients with varicocele and poor sperm quality by using two-dimensional gel electrophoresis. *J Assist Reprod Genet* 2014; **31**: 725–9.

68. Agarwal A, Sharma R, Samanta L, Durairajanayagam D, Sabanegh E. Proteomic signatures of infertile men with clinical varicocele and their validation studies reveal mitochondrial dysfunction leading to infertility. *Asian J Androl* 2016; **18**: 282–91.

69. Intasqui P, Camargo M, Antoniassi MP, Cedenho AP, Carvalho VM, Cardozo KHM, Zylbersztejn DS, Bertolla RP. Association between the seminal plasma proteome and sperm functional traits. *Fertil Steril* 2016; **105**: 617–28.

70. Schiza CG, Jarv K, Diamandis EP, Drabovich AP. An emerging role of TEX101 protein as a male infertility biomarker. *EJIFCC* 2014; **25**: 9–26.

71. Bieniek JM, Drabovich AP, Lo KC. Seminal biomarkers for the evaluation of male infertility. *Asian J Androl* 2016; **18**: 426–33.

72. Huang Z, Lin L, Gao Y, Chen Y, Yan X, Xing J, Hang W. Bladder cancer determination via two urinary metabolites: a biomarker pattern approach. *Mol Cell Proteom* 2011; **10**: M111.007922.

73. Zhang J, Mu X, Xia Y, Martin FL, Hang W, Liu L, Tian M, Huang Q, Shen H. Metabolomic analysis reveals a unique urinary pattern in normozoospermic infertile men. *J Proteom Res* 2014; **13**: 3088–99.

Conclusion

Ahmad Majzoub, Ralf Henkel, Ashok Agarwal

The second half of the twentieth century witnessed major advancements in the study of infertility. Perhaps the most prominent breakthrough was the birth of Louise Brown on July 25, 1978, the result of the first successful in vitro fertilization in humans. This marked a new era where the molecular interplay between spermatozoa and oocytes became the primary topic of interest. Since 1980, the World Health Organization (WHO) has published five editions of their *Laboratory Manual for the Examination and Processing of Human Semen*, which formed the basis for the evaluation of male fertility potential [1, 2, 3, 4, 5].

Conventional semen analysis is regarded as the cornerstone for male fertility evaluation. Its results can provide vital information about the functions of the male reproductive organs and can thereby offer clues regarding the choice of subsequent management modalities. Despite that, about 30–45 percent of infertile men are still diagnosed with unexplained or idiopathic infertility based on their semen analysis results and the presence of a female infertility factor [6, 7, 8]. This limitation of conventional semen analysis testing, in addition to the continued refinement in sperm selection techniques prior to assisted reproductive procedures, were the main driving force for the search for advanced tests of sperm function.

Oxidative stress was recognized as an important common etiology for a variety of clinical conditions resulting in infertility [9]. It is the end result of the imbalance between reactive oxygen species (oxidants) and antioxidant capacity in any given medium in favor of the oxidants. Studies have shown that oxidative stress does not only lead to lipid peroxidation of sperm membrane lipids [10], but also impairs protein synthesis, disrupts sperm DNA integrity and trigger and promotes apoptosis of developing sperm [11]. Agarwal et al. have recently described the term male oxidative stress infertility (MOSI) after denoting its

prevalence in 40 percent of patients with idiopathic infertility and 50 percent of patients with unexplained infertility [8]. Oxidative stress can be measured through a number of tests including chemiluminescence for ROS, total antioxidant capacity for antioxidants, the malondialdehyde assay for lipid peroxidation and oxidation reduction potential [12].

Sperm DNA fragmentation testing is another assay that has been extensively investigated in recent years. The sperm DNA is uniquely structured and compacted within the very confined space of the sperm head. Histones that envelope the DNA in somatic cells are replaced by protamines, basic proteins that form disulfide bridges and are therefore able to highly condense and compact the sperm chromatin, thus providing it with protection during its transport through male and female reproductive tracts [13, 14]. However, sperm DNA damage can still occur secondary to errors in chromatin compaction or when exposed to excessive amounts of reactive oxygen species in the male genital tract or the seminal fluid. Considerable evidence has linked sperm DNA fragmentation with male infertility due to decreased fertilization and embryogenesis and increased incidence of early pregnancy loss and miscarriage [14, 15].

Several tests for sperm DNA fragmentation have been described in the literature and are increasingly being utilized in the evaluation of infertile men. A recent cross-sectional survey performed on 65 reproductive specialists revealed that sperm DNA fragmentation testing was utilized by 79.6 percent of responders and that terminal deoxynucleotidyl transferase nick end labeling (TUNEL) and sperm chromatin structure assay (SCSA) were the most commonly utilized methods (30.6 percent for both), followed by sperm chromatin dispersion (SCD) (20.4 percent), single cell gel electrophoresis (Comet) (6.1 percent) and other methods (12.2 percent) (16). Recent clinical practice guidelines endorsed by the society of translational medicine recommended the utility of sperm DNA fragmentation testing in patients with unexplained infertility, clinical varicocele, and recurrent spontaneous abortion, prior to assisted reproductive therapies and in those with lifestyle risk factors [17].

A number of sperm function tests have been developed to specifically assess the sperm fertilizing ability aiming to better understand the sperm contribution to assisted reproductive procedures. Acrosome reaction is one example, which is a process triggered by either progesterone [18] or the zona pellucida protein 3 [19]. As a result, hydrolyzing enzymes aiding in the penetration of the cumulus and the zona pellucida are released. Acrosome reaction is a crucial step for successful fertilization as only acrosome-reacted sperm are able to traverse the zona pellucida and fuse with the oolemma [20]. About 25 percent of men with unexplained infertility were found to have a defective acrosome reaction [21]. Acrosome reaction can be assessed in spermatozoa removed from the surface of the zona pellucida or those exposed to zona pellucida disaggregated proteins using microscopy, flow cytometry, or fluorescently labeled lectins.

Zona pellucida binding tests are another example of assays that can assess the interaction between the sperm and the zona pellucida, which is a crucial step in the process of conception. The most commonly used sperm-zona pellucida binding tests are the hemizona assay (HZA) [22, 23] and the competitive intact zona sperm binding test [24]. Studies have shown that sperm from fertile men have significantly higher binding capacity to the zona pellucida than sperm from infertile men [24, 25, 26].

Finally, the sperm penetration assay is another test, which assesses the ability of male germ cells to perform capacitation and acrosome reaction, penetrate through the oolemma and decondensate within the cytoplasm of hamster oocytes [27]. It is an in vitro test that combines sperm subjected to capacitating conditions with hamster eggs that are enzymatically devoid of their zona pellucida. While these tests may be indicated for couples with recurrent assisted reproductive failure, their laborious requirements and expensive nature make them more commonly performed in research activities rather than clinical practice.

Sperm vitality testing is another important test of sperm function that is commonly performed in clinical practice especially in patients with severe alteration in sperm motility [28]. In such patients, sperm vitality testing could help differentiate dead from alive sperm, which are selected for use in intra-cytoplasmic sperm injection (ICSI). Two methods for sperm vitality testing have been described; the hypo-osmotic swelling test and the dye exclusion test. While both tests are principally based on testing the sperm membrane permeability status, the former is more commonly utilized as it does not jeopardize sperm quality allowing live sperm selection for ICSI.

Sperm proteomics has gained a lot of attention in recent years, including the field of male infertility. Proteomic studies have revealed the role of key proteins in normal physiological functions of spermatozoa [29, 30]. As spermatozoa are transcriptionally and translationally inactive, their proteome reflects the outcome of spermatogenesis and the maturation process. Furthermore, integration of proteomics with bioinformatics serves as a promising tool in the identification of potential diagnostic and therapeutic biomarkers for the management of male infertility.

While our understanding of the functional properties of the sperm cell has increased significantly with the implementation of the abovementioned laboratory testing techniques, further research is required to develop the best diagnostic modality that can decode unexplained etiologies of male infertility.

References

1. World Health Organization. (1980) WHO Laboratory Manual for the Examination of Human Semen and Sperm-Cervical Mucus Interaction, 1st ed. Cambridge: Cambridge University Press.

2. World Health Organization. (1987) WHO Laboratory Manual for the Examination of Human Semen and Sperm-Cervical Mucus Interaction, 2nd ed. Cambridge: Cambridge University Press.

3. World Health Organization. (1992) WHO Laboratory Manual for the Examination of Human Semen and Sperm-Cervical Mucus Interaction, 3rd ed. Cambridge: Cambridge University Press.

4. World Health Organization. (1999) WHO Laboratory Manual for the Examination of Human Semen and Sperm-Cervical Mucus Interaction, 4th ed. Cambridge: Cambridge University Press.

5. World Health Organization. (2010) WHO Laboratory Manual for the Examination and Processing of Human Semen, 5th ed. Geneva: The WHO Press.

6. Isaksson R, Tiitinen A. Present concept of unexplained infertility.

Gynecol Endocrinol 2004; **18**: 278–90.

7. Jungwirth A, Giwercman A, Tournaye H, Diemer T, Kopa Z, Dohle G, Krausz C. European Association of Urology Working Group on Male Infertility. European Association of Urology guidelines on Male Infertility: the 2012 update. *Eur Urol* 2012; **62**: 324–32.

8. Agarwal A, Parekh N, Panner Selvam MK, Henkel R, Shah R et al. Male oxidative stress infertility (MOSI): proposed terminology and clinical practice guidelines for management of idiopathic male infertility. *World J Mens Health* 2019; **37**(3): 296–312.

9. Dutta S, Majzoub A, Agarwal A. Oxidative stress and sperm function: a systematic review on evaluation and management. *Arab J Urol* 2019; **17**(2): 87–97.

10. Twigg J, Fulton N, Gomez E, Irvine DS, Aitken RJ. Analysis of the impact of intracellular reactive oxygen species generation on the structural and functional integrity of human spermatozoa: lipid peroxidation, DNA fragmentation and effectiveness of antioxidants. *Hum Reprod* 1998; **13**: 1429–36.

11. Agarwal A, Virk G, Ong C, et al. Effect of oxidative stress on male reproduction. *World J Mens Health* 2014; **32**: 1–17.

12. Agarwal A, Majzoub A. Laboratory tests for oxidative stress. *Indian J Urol* 2017; **33**(3): 199–206.

13. Ward WS, Coffey DS. DNA packaging and organization in mammalian spermatozoa: comparison with somatic cells. *Biol Reprod* 1991; **44**: 569–74.

14. Agarwal A, Majzoub A, Esteves SC, Ko E, Ramasamy R, Zini A. Clinical utility of sperm DNA fragmentation testing: practice recommendations based on clinical scenarios. *Transl Androl Urol* 2016; **5**(6): 935–50.

15. Opuwari CS, Henkel RR, Agarwal A. (2019). Sperm DNA fragmentation index. In Arora M, Mukhopadhaya N, eds., *Recurrent Pregnancy Loss*, 3rd ed. New Delhi: Jaypee Brothers Publishers, pp. 45–53.

16. Majzoub A, Agarwal A, Cho CL, Esteves SC. Sperm DNA fragmentation testing: a cross sectional survey on current practices of fertility specialists. *Transl Androl Urol* 2017; **6**(Suppl. 4): S710–S719.

17. Agarwal A, Cho CL, Majzoub A, Esteves SC. The Society for Translational Medicine: clinical practice guidelines for sperm DNA fragmentation testing in male infertility. *Transl Androl Urol* 2017; **6**(Suppl. 4): S720–S733.

18. Sabeur K, Edwards DP, Meizel S. Human sperm plasma membrane progesterone receptor(s) and the acrosome reaction. *Biol Reprod* 1996; **54**: 993–1001.

19. Cross NL, Morales P, Overstreet JW, Hanson FW. Induction of acrosome reactions by the human zona pellucida. *Biol Reprod* 1988; **38**: 235–44.

20. Hirohashi N, Yanagimachi R. Sperm acrosome reaction: its site and role in fertilization. *Biol Reprod* 2018; **99**(1): 127–33.

21. Peedicayil J, Deendayal M, Sadasivan G, Shivaji S. Assessment of hyperactivation, acrosome reaction and motility characteristics of spermatozoa from semen of men of proven fertility and unexplained infertility. *Andrologia* 1997; **29**(4): 209–18.

22. Burkman LJ, Coddington CC, Franken DR, Kruger TF, Rosenwaks Z, Hodgen GD. The hemizona assay (HZA): development of a diagnostic test for the binding of human spermatozoa to the human hemizona pellucida to predict fertilization potential. *Fertil Steril* 1988; **49**: 688–97.

23. Franken DR, Coddington CC, Burkman LJ, Oosthuizen WT, Oehninger SC, Kruger TF, Hodgen GD. Defining the valid hemizona assay: accounting for binding variability within zonae pellucidae and within semen samples from fertile males. *Fertil Steril* 1991; **56**: 1156–60.

24. Liu DY, Baker HW. High frequency of defective sperm-zona pellucida interaction in oligozoospermic infertile men. *Hum Reprod* 2004; **19**: 228–33.

25. Oehninger S, Franken D, Kruger T. Approaching the next millennium: how should we manage andrology diagnosis in the intracytoplasmic sperm injection era? *Fertil Steril* 1997a; **67**: 434–6.

26. Oehninger S, Mahony M, Ozgur K, Kolm P, Kruger T et al. Clinical significance of human sperm-zona pellucida binding. *Fertil Steril* 1997b; **67**: 1121–7.

27. Liu DY, Garrett C, Baker HW. Clinical application of sperm-oocyte interaction tests in in vitro fertilization – embryo transfer and intracytoplasmic sperm injection programs. *Fertil Steril* 2004; **82**: 1251–63.

28. Lepine S, McDowell S, Searle LM, Kroon B, Glujovsky D et al. Advanced sperm selection techniques for assisted reproduction. *Cochrane Database Syst Rev* 2019; **7**: CD010461.

29. Panner Selvam MK, Agarwal A, Pushparaj PN, Baskaran S, Bendou H. *Sperm proteome analysis and identification of fertility-associated biomarkers in unexplained male infertility. Genes* 2019; **11**: 10.

30. Samanta L, Sharma R, Cui Z, Agarwal A. Proteomic analysis reveals dysregulated cell signaling in ejaculated spermatozoa from infertile men. *Asian J Androl* 2019; **21**(2): 121–30.

Index

259